Internet of Things in Bioelectronics

Scrivener Publishing
100 Cummings Center, Suite 541J
Beverly, MA 01915-6106

Publishers at Scrivener
Martin Scrivener (martin@scrivenerpublishing.com)
Phillip Carmical (pcarmical@scrivenerpublishing.com)

Internet of Things in Bioelectronics

Emerging Technologies and Applications

Edited by

Hari Murthy

Dept. of Electronics and Communication Engineering, School of Engineering and Technology, CHRIST (Deemed to be University), Bangalore, India

Marta Zurek-Mortka

Dept. of Control Systems, Institute for Sustainable Technologies, Radom, Poland

Vinay Jha Pillai

Dept. of Electronics and Communication Engineering, School of Engineering and Technology, CHRIST (Deemed to be University), Bangalore, India

and

Kukatlapalli Pradeep Kumar

Dept. of Electronics and Communication Engineering, School of Engineering and Technology, CHRIST (Deemed to be University), Bangalore, India

Scrivener Publishing

WILEY

This edition first published 2024 by John Wiley & Sons, Inc., 111 River Street, Hoboken, NJ 07030, USA and Scrivener Publishing LLC, 100 Cummings Center, Suite 541J, Beverly, MA 01915, USA

For more information about Scrivener publications please visit www.scrivenerpublishing.com.

Wiley Global Headquarters
111 River Street, Hoboken, NJ 07030, USA

For details of our global editorial offices, customer services, and more information about Wiley products visit us at www.wiley.com.

Library of Congress Cataloging-in-Publication Data

ISBN 978-1-394-24187-3

Front cover image provided by Wikimedia Commons
Cover design by Russell Richardson

Set in size of 11pt and Minion Pro by Manila Typesetting Company, Makati, Philippines

Printed in the USA

10 9 8 7 6 5 4 3 2 1

Contents

Preface

The rapid convergence of technology and biology heralds a new era of evolution in the Internet of Things (IoT), a transformative force enabling interconnected devices to communicate and operate with unparalleled synergy. This is particularly true in the groundbreaking field of bioelectronics, where the fusion of biological systems with electronic devices and IoT is reshaping the landscape of bioelectronics, promising to open up new frontiers in healthcare, diagnostics, and personalized medicine.

This book aims to provide a comprehensive exploration of this exciting intersection. It delves into the principles, applications, and future directions of IoT in the realm of bioelectronics, and it is designed to serve as both an introduction for those new to the field and as a detailed reference for experienced professionals seeking to deepen their knowledge.

This timely resource explores the numerous ways in which IoT-enabled bioelectronic devices are used to monitor and enhance human health, from wearable sensors that track vital signs to implantable devices that can communicate with healthcare providers in real-time. One central theme of this book is the transformative impact of IoT on healthcare. By enabling continuous, remote monitoring of patients, IoT technologies are not only improving the accuracy of diagnostics but also making healthcare more accessible and personalized. The book also addresses the critical issues of securing health records on the internet, which are of paramount importance as we increasingly rely on interconnected devices to collect and transmit sensitive health information. Additional attention is paid to the future directions of IoT in bioelectronics and the integration of innovative areas, such as artificial intelligence, machine learning, and big data analytics, in driving the development of ever more sophisticated and capable bioelectronic systems.

We extend our heartfelt thanks to all those who have contributed to this book, including our collaborators, reviewers, and the many experts whose work has informed our understanding of this field. We also thank our readers, whose curiosity and passion for innovation drive the ongoing exploration and development of these transformative technologies. Finally, I am most grateful to Martin Scrivener of Scrivener Publishing for his help and for making this book possible.

The Editors

Acknowledgement

The editors would like to thank the management at CHRIST University for providing the necessary resources and the motivation to complete the proposed title. Rev. Dr. Fr. Jose CC, Vice Chancellor, CHRIST University and Dr. Anil Pinto, Registrar, CHRIST University for their unwavering support. Rev. Dr. Fr. Sony J Chundattu, Director, School of Engineering and Technology, CHRIST University and Dr. Iven Jose, Dean, School of Engineering and Technology, CHRIST University for ensuring that the resources required for the book are available at all times. Dr. Inbanila K, Head of Department, Department of Electronics and Communication Engineering, School of Engineering and Technology, CHRIST University and Dr. Mary Anita, Associate Dean, Head of Department, Department of Computer Science and Engineering, School of Engineering and Technology, CHRIST University for encouraging us to go ahead with the interdisciplinary topic and providing all the support to ensure that the book comes out in due time. Last and not the least, we would like to thank our family who has been the greatest source of inspiration and who have put up with our antics.

1

IoT-Based Implant Devices in Humans/Animals for Therapeutic Reasons

Chetankumar Kalaskar

Department of CSE, Poojya Doddappa Appa College of Engineering Kalaburgi, Karnataka, India

Abstract

IoT-based implant devices have revolutionized therapeutic applications in both humans and animals. These cutting-edge implants enable real-time remote monitoring and personalized treatment adjustments, reducing the need for frequent physical visits to healthcare providers. With the power of continuous data streams and real-time analysis, these implants enhance patient engagement and adherence to treatment plans. The ability to detect anomalies and device malfunctions early through data-driven insights ensures timely interventions, improving patient outcomes. Despite their transformative potential, challenges related to power management, data security, and regulatory compliance must be addressed for seamless integration. Overall, IoT-based implants hold the promise to reshape healthcare delivery and elevate patient care to new levels.

Keywords: Implantable medical devices, IoT healthcare, remote patient monitoring, continuous health monitoring

1.1 Introduction

The Internet of Things (IoT) is a term used to describe the concept of connecting physical objects to the internet and enabling them to communicate with other devices and systems [1]. It refers to the network of devices, vehicles, appliances, and other items embedded with electronics, software,

Email: chetankalaskar@pdaengg.com

Hari Murthy, Marta Zurek-Mortka, Vinay Jha Pillai and Kukatlapalli Pradeep Kumar (eds.) Internet of Things in Bioelectronics: Emerging Technologies and Applications, (1–16) © 2024 Scrivener Publishing LLC

sensors, and connectivity which enables them to connect and exchange data with other devices over the internet. The ultimate goal of IoT is to make everyday objects smarter and more connected, improving the way we live and work.

IoT technology has revolutionized the way we interact with our surroundings and has enabled us to collect and process data in ways that were previously impossible. With the help of IoT, devices can communicate with each other, share data, and take action based on that data. This technology has far-reaching implications across various industries such as healthcare, transportation, agriculture, and manufacturing. It has the potential to improve the efficiency and effectiveness of various systems and processes, leading to increased productivity and reduced costs [2].

IoT-based implant devices are a rapidly growing field in healthcare, with the potential to revolutionize the way medical treatment is delivered. These devices, which are implanted inside the body, use IoT technology to collect and transmit data on a patient's vital signs and other health-related information. This information can then be used by healthcare providers to monitor the patient's health, detect potential issues, and provide timely interventions. The use of IoT-based implant devices in animals and humans for therapeutic reasons has the potential to greatly improve patient outcomes, reduce costs, and increase access to healthcare services. These devices can be used for a variety of purposes, such as monitoring vital signs, delivering medication, and providing electrical stimulation for conditions such as Parkinson's disease.

Another benefit of IoT-based implant devices is their ability to deliver medication directly to the site of the problem. For example, an implantable device could be used to deliver insulin to a patient with diabetes, or to deliver medication to a patient with a chronic pain condition. This can greatly improve the effectiveness of the medication and reduce the need for frequent injections or oral medications. While IoT-based implant devices have the potential to greatly improve patient outcomes, there are also several challenges that need to be addressed.

The Technology behind IoT-based implants rely on a combination of hardware and software technologies. The hardware components include small sensors, microprocessors, wireless communication devices, and power sources such as batteries. These components are carefully designed to fit within the constraints of the implantable device and to withstand the harsh environment inside the body.

The software components include the algorithms that process the data collected by the sensors, and the communication protocols that enable the device to transmit data to external devices. These algorithms must be

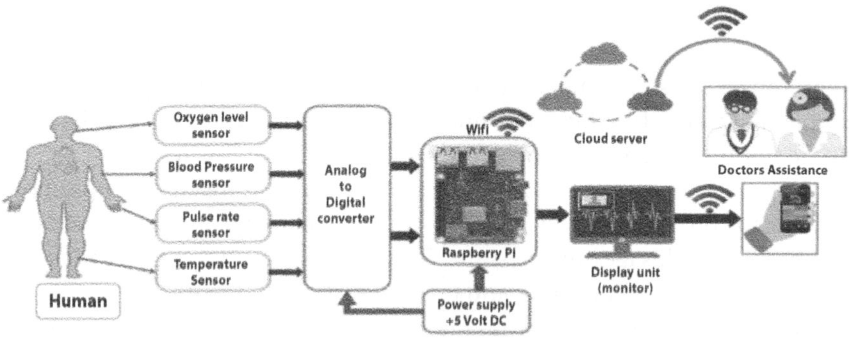

Figure 1.1 Technical framework of IoT-based implant devices in humans for therapeutic reasons.

optimized for low power consumption and high efficiency, as the devices are often powered by small batteries that must last for years. In addition, the software must be highly secure to prevent unauthorized access to the device and the sensitive data it collects shows the evidence of Technical framework of IoT-based implant devices in humans for therapeutic reasons.

Advances in microelectronics, wireless communication, and biomedical engineering have made it possible to develop increasingly sophisticated IoT-based implantable devices. These devices have the potential to revolutionize healthcare by enabling real-time monitoring of vital signs, drug delivery, and other critical parameters. The technology behind IoT-based implants is constantly evolving, driven by the need for smaller, more powerful, and more reliable devices that can provide accurate and timely information to healthcare professionals.

Some of IoT-based implant devices that are currently being developed or used for therapeutic purposes in humans.

This chapter outlines the significance of IoT-based implant devices for therapeutic purposes in both humans and animals. It covers various aspects related to these devices, including current developments, potential improvements, and future directions.

1.2 Application of IoT in Implantable Insulin Pumps

An insulin pump is a medical device that is used to deliver insulin to individuals with diabetes. This device replaces the need for multiple daily injections of insulin by delivering a continuous flow of insulin into the body. In recent years, implantable insulin pumps have gained popularity due to their ability to provide insulin therapy without the need for external tubing or devices. IoT technology is revolutionizing the field of healthcare, particularly in devices like implantable insulin pumps. These pumps, surgically implanted under the skin, continuously deliver insulin to manage diabetes IoT components enhance their functionality in the following ways:

Remote Monitoring and Adjustment: IoT-enabled insulin pumps allow healthcare professionals to remotely monitor patients' glucose levels and adjust insulin dosages in real-time. This remote connectivity reduces the need for frequent clinic visits and enables timely interventions.

Wireless Connectivity: The integration of wireless communication modules like Bluetooth or cellular connectivity facilitates seamless data transmission from the pump to external devices or cloud platforms. This connectivity ensures that patients and healthcare providers have access to critical health data.

Data Analytics and Insights: IoT-enabled pumps collect a wealth of data, including insulin delivery rates and glucose levels. Advanced analytics algorithms process this data to generate insights, enabling healthcare providers to make informed decisions about treatment adjustments.

1.3 Application of IoT in Implantable Heart Monitors

As shown in Figure 1.2, an implantable heart monitor device that is inserted beneath the skin of a patient's chest. The device is small and compact, roughly the size of a pacemaker, and is connected to leads that are implanted into the heart. The leads monitor the electrical activity of the

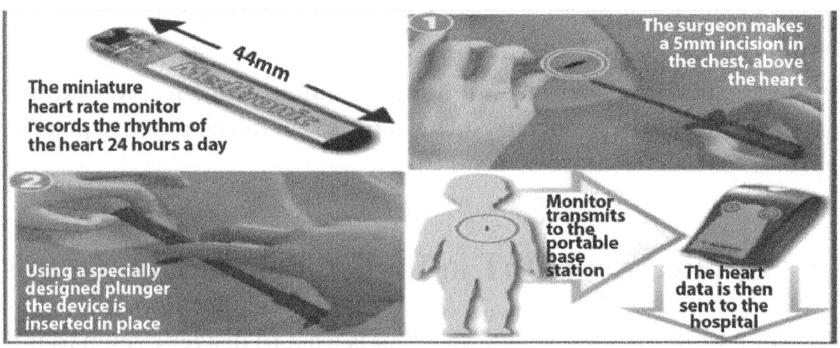

Figure 1.2 Implantable heart monitors.

heart and send this information to the device. An implantable heart monitor is a small device that is placed inside a patient's chest to continuously monitor their heart rhythm and detect any abnormalities. These devices are typically used in patients who have a history of heart disease or other cardiovascular issues, as they provide continuous monitoring of the heart's electrical activity and can help detect potential issues early on. Implantable heart monitors, also known as cardiac implants or pacemakers, are lifesaving devices used to monitor and regulate heart rhythms [4].

The application of IoT in these devices brings several benefits:

Remote Monitoring and Alerts: IoT-enabled heart monitors can transmit real-time heart rhythm data to healthcare providers. This remote monitoring allows for early detection of irregularities, enabling prompt medical intervention.

Alerts and Notifications: When abnormal heart rhythms are detected, IoT-enabled monitors can automatically send alerts to both patients and healthcare providers. This rapid communication ensures timely responses to critical situations.

Data-driven Insights: IoT components collect data on heart rhythm patterns over time. Analyzing this data helps healthcare professionals identify trends, triggers, and potential risk factors, leading to more personalized treatment plans.

1.4 Application of IoT in Implantable Nerve Stimulators

Implantable nerve stimulators are devices that use electrical impulses to stimulate the nerves in the body. These devices are typically used to treat chronic pain or other conditions that are resistant to traditional treatments. IoT integration offers the following advantages:

Remote Control and Adjustment: IoT-enabled nerve stimulators allow patients to adjust stimulation settings within prescribed limits. This remote control enhances patient comfort and minimizes the need for in-person adjustments.

Data-driven Optimization: The continuous collection of stimulation data enables healthcare providers to optimize therapy settings for individual patients. This data-driven approach enhances treatment outcomes and patient satisfaction.

1.5 Application of IoT in Implantable Drug Delivery Systems

Implantable drug delivery systems are a type of medical device that are designed to deliver medication directly into the body over an extended period of time. These devices have revolutionized the way we treat many chronic conditions, providing a more targeted and consistent drug delivery than traditional methods such as pills or injections. Implantable drug delivery systems have a wide range of applications, from treating chronic pain to managing diabetes, cancer, and other diseases. Incorporating IoT components enhances their effectiveness:

Dosing Personalization: IoT-enabled drug delivery systems can adapt dosing regimens based on real-time physiological data. This personalized approach ensures optimal drug delivery and therapeutic outcomes.

Adherence Monitoring: IoT technology allows healthcare providers to monitor patients' medication adherence. This ensures that patients receive the prescribed medications on time, leading to improved treatment effectiveness.

1.6 Application of IoT in Implantable Brain-Computer Interfaces

Implantable Brain-Computer Interfaces (BCIs) are devices that enable direct communication between the human brain and a computer. They are designed to help people who have lost motor function due to neurological injuries or disorders, such as injuries in spinal cord, stroke, or amyotrophic lateral sclerosis (ALS).

Implantable brain-computer interfaces establish direct communication pathways between the brain and external devices. The incorporation of IoT technology expands their capabilities:

Real-time Feedback: IoT-enabled brain-computer interfaces can provide real-time feedback to users based on brain activity. This feedback can be used to control external devices, enhancing user interaction and quality of life.

1.7 Application of IoT in Implantable Biosensors

Implantable Micro-Electro-Mechanical Systems (MEMS) are small devices that combine mechanical, electrical, and computational components to enable a wide range of biomedical applications. MEMS devices are typically smaller than a few millimeters and are implanted into the body to monitor or modulate various physiological processes. They are made up of microfabricated components that can sense, measure, and respond to physical and chemical stimuli.

Implantable biosensors are used to continuously monitor various physiological parameters within the body. Integrating IoT components enhances their functionality:

Continuous Monitoring: IoT-enabled biosensors can transmit real-time data on parameters like glucose levels, oxygen saturation, or pH. This continuous monitoring provides healthcare professionals with timely insights for treatment adjustments [6].

In conclusion, IoT technology is revolutionizing the healthcare landscape by enhancing the capabilities of implantable medical devices. From remote monitoring and personalized treatment to real-time insights and improved patient outcomes, the application of IoT is transforming the way these devices function and contribute to patient care.

1.8 IoT Revolutionizing Healthcare Devices: A Comparative Analysis of IoT-Based Implants vs. Conventional Medical Devices

The advent of IoT technology has introduced a new dimension to medical implants, revolutionizing the way we perceive healthcare devices. A compelling comparison between IoT-based implanted devices and conventional non-IoT devices highlights the transformative impact of IoT on medical implants [7].

Connectivity and Remote Monitoring:
IoT-Implanted Devices: IoT-based implants enable seamless wireless connectivity, allowing real-time data transmission to remote platforms. This enables healthcare providers to monitor patients' conditions and device functionality from a distance.

Conventional Devices: Non-IoT medical implants lack remote monitoring capabilities. Monitoring often requires in-person visits to healthcare facilities, limiting timely intervention and patient convenience.

Data Analysis and Insights:
IoT-Implanted Devices: Data collected by IoT implants can be analyzed for trends, patterns, and anomalies. These insights aid in personalized treatment plans and proactive healthcare management.
Conventional Devices: Conventional implants lack the ability to provide data-driven insights, often resulting in delayed reactions to medical conditions.

Real-time Alerts and Notifications:
IoT-Implanted Devices: IoT implants can generate real-time alerts and notifications to both patients and healthcare providers in case of critical events, ensuring timely medical attention.
Conventional Devices: Without IoT connectivity, conventional implants cannot provide immediate alerts, potentially leading to missed opportunities for urgent medical care.

Personalized Treatment:
IoT-Implanted Devices: IoT-enabled implants allow for personalized adjustments in treatment plans based on real-time data, optimizing patient outcomes.
Conventional Devices: Conventional implants rely on fixed settings, lacking the flexibility to adapt to changing patient needs.

User Engagement and Empowerment:
IoT-Implanted Devices: IoT devices engage patients by offering them access to their health data through mobile apps, fostering better understanding and active participation in their treatment journey.
Conventional Devices: Non-IoT implants may not provide patients with insights into their health data, limiting their involvement in healthcare decisions.

Predictive Maintenance:
IoT-Implanted Devices: IoT technology facilitates predictive maintenance of implants, identifying potential malfunctions and minimizing device failure risks.
Conventional Devices: Conventional implants may fail without warning, leading to unexpected complications for patients.

Timely Healthcare Interventions:
IoT-Implanted Devices: IoT implants enable early detection of anomalies, allowing healthcare providers to intervene promptly and prevent worsening conditions.
Conventional Devices: Conventional implants may not provide early indicators of problems, resulting in delayed medical interventions.

Long-term Monitoring and Historical Data:
IoT-Implanted Devices: IoT technology enables long-term data storage and analysis, offering a comprehensive view of patients' health history and trends.
Conventional Devices: Non-IoT implants lack the ability to provide a holistic view of patient health over time.

While IoT-based implanted devices offer unprecedented benefits, challenges such as power consumption, data security, and regulatory compliance must be carefully addressed. The comparison underscores the transformative potential of IoT in reshaping healthcare through continuous monitoring, real-time data analysis, and improved patient engagement. IoT components used in implantable devices for humans, along with examples and their working principles [8]:

Wireless Communication Module:
Example: Bluetooth Low Energy (BLE), Cellular Modem
Working: The wireless communication module enables the implantable device to establish a connection with external devices or networks. It can transmit data to remote servers, healthcare providers, or the patient's smartphone. This real-time communication allows for continuous monitoring and remote adjustments.

Sensors:
Example: Accelerometers, Temperature Sensors
Working: Sensors embedded in the implantable device collect various physiological data. For instance, accelerometers can measure movement or activity levels, while temperature sensors can monitor body temperature. These sensors convert physical data into digital information that can be processed and transmitted for analysis.

Microcontroller or Processor:
Example: ARM Cortex-M series microcontroller
Working: The microcontroller acts as the brain of the implantable device. It processes data from sensors, manages power usage, and controls data

transmission. It can execute algorithms for signal processing, data compression, or encryption, depending on the device's purpose.

Memory:
Example: Flash memory
Working: Memory storage is crucial for storing collected data, device settings, and firmware updates. It ensures that data is retained even if there is a temporary loss of communication. Healthcare providers can retrieve historical data for analysis.

Power Management System:
Example: Lithium-ion battery, Energy Harvesting
Working: The power management system is responsible for providing a stable and long-lasting power source. Implantable devices may use rechargeable batteries or energy harvesting techniques to harness energy from the body's movements or other sources, extending the device's lifespan.

Encryption and Security Features:
Example: Advanced Encryption Standard (AES), Secure Boot
Working: Security features are crucial to protect patient data and the device itself. Encryption methods like AES secure data during transmission, while secure boot processes ensure that only trusted software runs on the device, preventing unauthorized access.

External Communication Interface:
Example: USB, Proprietary Docking Station
Working: In some cases, external communication interfaces facilitate interactions between the implantable device and external devices or healthcare providers during check-ups or for device configuration, data retrieval, or firmware updates.

Biocompatible Materials:
Example: Titanium, Medical-grade Polymers
Working: Implantable devices are constructed using biocompatible materials to minimize the risk of tissue rejection or adverse reactions. These materials ensure the device can function safely within the human body.

Together, these IoT components enable implantable devices to collect, process, and transmit vital health data, allowing for remote monitoring, timely interventions, and improved patient care. They are pivotal in advancing the field of medical technology and enhancing the quality of life for individuals with various medical conditions.

1.9 Challenges in Therapeutic Implant Devices for Humans and Animals

Let us explore the typical challenges present in implant devices in animals/humans for therapeutic.

IoT-based implant devices in animals/humans for therapeutic reasons present unique security challenges, as they are designed to be implanted in the body and can potentially be accessed remotely by unauthorized individuals. Here are some of the main security challenges associated with these devices [3]:

Device hacking: IoT-based implant devices are vulnerable to hacking, which could lead to unauthorized access to patient data, manipulation of device settings, or even physical harm to the patient. Hackers could exploit vulnerabilities in the device's firmware or software to gain access to the device.

Data privacy: IoT-based implant devices collect and transmit sensitive patient data, such as medical history, biometric data, and other personal information. If this data falls into the wrong hands, it could be used for identity theft, fraud, or other malicious purposes.

Physical security: Implantable devices are physically attached to the body and can be difficult to access or replace if they are compromised. Patients must be vigilant about protecting their devices from theft or tampering.

Regulatory compliance: IoT-based implant devices must comply with various regulations and standards, such as HIPAA and FDA regulations. Failure to comply with these regulations could result in legal and financial penalties.

To address these security challenges, device manufacturers, healthcare providers, and regulatory bodies must work together to implement appropriate security measures. These measures may include:

- Strong authentication and encryption mechanisms to secure device communications and prevent unauthorized access.
- Regular software updates and security patches to address vulnerabilities and improve device security.
- Physical security measures, such as tamper-evident seals and anti-theft mechanisms, to protect the device from physical tampering.

- Patient education and training to raise awareness of device security risks and best practices for device management.
- Compliance with relevant regulations and standards to ensure that devices meet minimum security requirements.

Ensuring data security and cryptography for implanted materials is a rapidly evolving area, with several recent trends emerging to address the unique security challenges of these devices [5].

Here are some of the key trends:
Block chain technology: Block chain technology provides a secure and decentralized way to store and manage patient data. By using a block chain-based system, data can be securely stored, verified, and accessed by authorized parties without the need for a central authority.
Advanced cryptography: Advanced encryption techniques such as homomorphic encryption, zero-knowledge proofs, and multi-party computation are being developed and applied to implanted materials. These techniques allow for secure computation and data sharing without compromising patient privacy.
Cybersecurity regulations: Governments and regulatory bodies are increasingly implementing regulations and standards to ensure the cybersecurity of implanted materials. For example, the U.S. FDA has issued guidelines for medical device manufacturers to help ensure the security of medical devices, including implanted materials.
Machine learning and AI: Machine learning and AI can be used to detect and prevent cyber-attacks on implanted materials. By analyzing huge amounts of dataset, these technologies ML and AI can identify patterns which are irregular and unnatural that may indicate a security breach.
Physical security measures: In addition to digital security measures, physical security measures are also being developed to protect implanted materials. For example, researchers are developing nanoscale structures that can be embedded in materials to provide physical security and prevent tampering.

Overall, ensuring data security and cryptography for implanted materials is a complex and rapidly evolving field, with many promising technologies and strategies being developed to address the unique security challenges of these devices. By staying up-to-date with the latest trends and developments, researchers and practitioners can help ensure the safety and security of these devices for patients.

IoT-based implant devices in animals/humans for therapeutic reasons pose unique security challenges that must be addressed through a combination of technical, organizational, and regulatory measures. By implementing appropriate security measures, we can ensure that these devices are safe and effective for patients.

IoT-based implant devices in animals are increasingly being used for a variety of applications, including healthcare, research, and monitoring. These devices typically consist of small, implantable sensors or microchips that can communicate wirelessly with external devices or networks. Here are some examples of IoT-based implant devices in animals:

Implantable health monitors: Implantable health monitors can be used to monitor the health of animals in real-time. These devices can track vital signs such as heart rate, respiration, and temperature, as well as detect abnormalities or changes in behavior.

GPS tracking implants: GPS tracking implants can be used to monitor the location and movements of animals. These devices are commonly used in wildlife conservation efforts to track animal migrations and populations.

Smart collars: Smart collars are another type of IoT-based implant device that can be used to monitor the health and behavior of animals. These collars can track activity levels, monitor sleep patterns, and even detect changes in vocalizations or body language.

Implantable microchips: Implantable microchips are commonly used in pets for identification purposes. These devices can store information such as the owner's contact information and the pet's medical history.

Smart feeders: Smart feeders are IoT-based implant devices that can be used to regulate the feeding of animals. These devices can dispense food in controlled portions and can be programmed to provide meals at specific times.

IoT-based implant devices in animals offer a range of benefits for both animals and their owners, including improved healthcare, monitoring, and tracking capabilities. As these technologies continue to grow, it is likely that we will see even increase in innovative applications of IoT-based implant devices in animals in the future.

One of the key highlights of IoT-based implants for therapeutic reasons include:

Real-time monitoring: IoT-based implant devices can provide real-time monitoring of a patient's condition, allowing for early detection of potential problems or complications.

Improved accuracy: These devices can provide highly accurate measurements and data, improving the precision and effectiveness of medical treatment.
Personalized treatment: IoT-based implants can be customized to meet the unique needs of each patient, providing more targeted and personalized treatment options.
Enhanced patient comfort: Many IoT-based implant devices are designed to be minimally invasive and highly comfortable for the patient, reducing discomfort and improving overall satisfaction with medical treatment.
Reduced healthcare costs: By providing more targeted and effective treatment options, IoT-based implant devices can help to reduce healthcare costs over the long-term.
Improved patient outcomes: By providing early detection and targeted treatment options, IoT-based implant devices can help to improve outcomes of the patient and increase overall quality of life.

IoT-based implants for therapeutic reasons hold immense promise for the field of healthcare, providing clinicians and patients with highly targeted and personalized treatment options that can improve patient outcomes and reduce healthcare costs. The development of IoT-based implant devices has been driven by advances in technology such as miniaturization, wireless connectivity, and data analytics, enabling highly accurate and real-time monitoring of a patient's condition [9].

By leveraging IoT technology, implant devices can collect vast amounts of patient data and transmit it to healthcare providers in real-time, allowing for early stage detection of potential problems and complications. This can help to improve outcomes of the patient, reduce the need for hospitalization, and ultimately, reduce healthcare costs.

Moreover, IoT-based implants can be customized to meet the unique needs of each patient, providing more targeted and personalized treatment options. This can be especially valuable for patients with complex or chronic medical conditions, where a one-size-fits-all approach may not be effective.

Overall, the relevance of IoT-based implants for therapeutic reasons lies in their potential to transform the way we approach healthcare, providing clinicians with highly accurate and personalized treatment options that can improve patient outcomes and reduce healthcare costs. As these technologies continue to advance, it is likely that we will see even more innovative and impactful applications of IoT-based implants in the future.

1.10 Future Prospects

The future prospects for IoT-based implant devices in healthcare are vast and exciting. Advancements in miniaturization, sensor technology, wireless communication, and data analytics will further enhance the capabilities and functionalities of these devices. Future developments may include the integration of artificial intelligence and machine learning algorithms to enable real-time data analysis and predictive analytics for personalized treatment plans. Moreover, advancements in power management and energy harvesting technologies will lead to longer-lasting and more sustainable implantable devices [10].

Additionally, the focus on security and privacy will continue to be crucial to ensure the protection of patient data and the prevention of unauthorized access to implantable devices. Collaborative efforts among healthcare professionals, engineers, researchers, and policymakers will be essential in addressing these challenges and fostering the adoption of IoT-based implant devices on a larger scale.

Overall, IoT-based implant devices have opened up new possibilities in healthcare, revolutionizing patient care, remote monitoring, and treatment options. With ongoing advancements and research, the future holds great promise for the continued innovation and widespread adoption of these devices, ultimately leading to improved healthcare outcomes and enhanced quality of life for patients.

However, some statistics on the use of medical implants in general:

According to a report by Grand View Research, the global medical implant market size was valued at USD 85.6 billion in 2020 and is expected to grow at a compound annual growth rate (CAGR) of 5.8% from 2021 to 2028.

The report also notes that the cardiovascular segment is the largest revenue-generating segment, accounting for over 30% of the total market share.

Another report by Research and Markets estimates that the global implantable medical devices market will reach USD 54.1 billion by 2026, growing at a CAGR of 5.6% from 2021 to 2026.

In terms of specific implantable devices, the global market for implantable neurostimulation devices was valued at USD 4.2 billion in 2020 and is projected to reach USD 8.4 billion by 2027, growing at a CAGR of 9.4% from 2021 to 2027 (source: Data Bridge Market Research).

References

1. Al-Fuqaha, A., Guizani, M., Mohammadi, M., Aledhari, M., Ayyash, M., Internet of Things: A survey on enabling technologies, protocols, and applications. *IEEE Commun. Surv. Tutor.*, 17, 4, 2347–2376, 2015.
2. Bonomi, F., Milito, R., Zhu, J., Addepalli, S., Fog computing and its role in the internet of things, in: *Proceedings of the first edition of the MCC workshop on mobile cloud computing*, pp. 13–16, 2012.
3. Hou, Y.T. and Wu, L.Y., A review on the security of implantable medical devices. *J. Med. Syst.*, 43, 8, 1–11, 2019.
4. Huang, L., Li, X., Wang, X., An IoT-based wearable ECG monitoring system for smart healthcare. *J. Med. Syst.*, 40, 12, 286, 2016.
5. Kim, D., Lee, S., Kim, J., Security and privacy in the Internet of Things for Smart Healthcare: Challenges and solutions. *J. Med. Syst.*, 41, 3, 1–7, 2017.
6. Mokhtari, G., Gandomi, A.H., Kiani, M., Health monitoring systems: A review of recent advances in wearable sensors. *Sensors*, 15, 9, 23929–23972, 2015.
7. Shnayder, V., Chen, B.R., Lorincz, K., Fulford-Jones, T.R., Welsh, M., Sensor networks for medical care, in: *Proceedings of the 2005 ACM SIGCOMM workshop on experimental approaches to wireless network design and analysis*, pp. 1–6, 2005.
8. Wang, K. and Lu, R., Secure and privacy-preserving data sharing and collaboration in mobile healthcare social networks. *IEEE Trans. Inf. Forensics Secur.*, 12, 4, 865–877, 2017.
9. Yuce, M.R. and Nguyen, H.T., Wearable and implantable medical devices: Applications, challenges, and opportunities. *J. Med. Devices*, 12, 2, 020801, 2018.
10. Zhang, Y., Li, Y., Li, X., Zhang, Y., Privacy-preserving and secure data sharing framework for mobile healthcare social networks. *Future Gener. Comput. Syst.*, 83, 382–390, 2018.

2

IoT and Nano-Bioelectronics for Target Drug Delivery

Ambikesh Soni[1], Pratiksha Singh[2], Gagan Kant Tripathi[2*] and Priyanka Dixit[3]

[1]Regenerative Medicine and Stem Cell Laboratory (RMS), Department of Biomedical Engineering, Indian Institute of Technology Hyderabad, Telangana, India
[2]School of Nanotechnology, Rajiv Gandhi Proudyogiki Vishwavidyalaya (RGPV), Bhopal, Madhya Pradesh, India
[3]Computer Science and Engineering, University Institute of Technology, RGPV, Bhopal, Madhya Pradesh, India

Abstract
With the global expansion of several cancerous variants nowadays new drugs and treatments are desperately needed. The Internet of Things (IoT) has played a significant role in recent advancements in healthcare technologies. The research objectives in the field of nano-biotechnologies for drug delivery encompass several key goals. These include enhancing the precision and efficiency of drug targeting and delivery, minimizing toxicity levels while retaining therapeutic efficacy, ensuring optimal safety and biocompatibility, and accelerating the development process of new and secure medications. The healthcare field has undergone progressive change due to ubiquitous computing. By deploying such IoT-based devices, health professionals can better serve society. The study will introduce a model of a "Smart Portable Intensive Care Unit" based on the Internet of Things for remote drug distribution and real-time patient monitoring. The suggested paradigm allows medical staff and the patient's family to remotely monitor the patient's physiological data.

Keywords: Targeted drug delivery, IoT, nano-bioelectronics, nanofabrication, nano printing, gene therapy, nanoprobes, health care

**Corresponding author*: gagankanttripathi@gmail.com

Hari Murthy, Marta Zurek-Mortka, Vinay Jha Pillai and Kukatlapalli Pradeep Kumar (eds.) Internet of Things in Bioelectronics: Emerging Technologies and Applications, (17–40) © 2024 Scrivener Publishing LLC

2.1 Introduction

Drug delivery (DD) encompasses a range of approaches, formulations, technologies, and procedures employed to transport pharmaceutical substances within the body with the aim of achieving the desired therapeutic outcome. Its scope extends to the administration of medicinal compounds in both humans and animals, ultimately striving to attain optimal therapeutic effectiveness [1]. In recent times, significant advancements have been made in the field of drug delivery systems (DDSs), with a notable emphasis on smart drug delivery. This approach aims to administer drugs with utmost precision in terms of timing, dosage, and targeted location, ensuring optimal safety and efficacy. Targeted drug delivery systems (TDDSs) play a key role in this endeavor, enabling the delivery of drugs to specific locations within the body rather than distributing them throughout the entire organ or system. The advancement of targeted drug delivery systems (TDDSs) is the result of combining insights from a range of scientific fields. These include pharmacology, polymer science, molecular biology, and bioconjugate chemistry. The successful integration of these disciplines plays a crucial role in attaining enhanced outcomes in drug delivery [2]. The objective of targeted drug delivery (TDD) is to effectively manage and regulate various aspects of therapeutic agents, including pharmacokinetics, pharmacodynamics, specific toxicity, immunogenicity, and biorecognition. By doing so, the ultimate aim is to enhance the effectiveness of treatments while minimizing undesirable side effects. What sets targeted drug delivery systems (TDDSs) apart from conventional DDSs is their ability to achieve site-specific drug release from a particular dosage form, as opposed to relying on drug absorption through biological membranes as seen in the latter [3]. The chapter discusses about the core concepts of internet of things, nano bioelectronics, targeted drug delivery, its principles including relevance of work, and methodology.

2.2 Literature Study

2.2.1 Internet of Things

The advent of Internet of Things (IoT) technology has revolutionized communication between various objects within a network. IoT facilitates seamless connectivity and communication between objects as well as between objects and computers. In the context of targeted drug delivery, IoT plays a significant role by enabling the precise delivery of drugs to

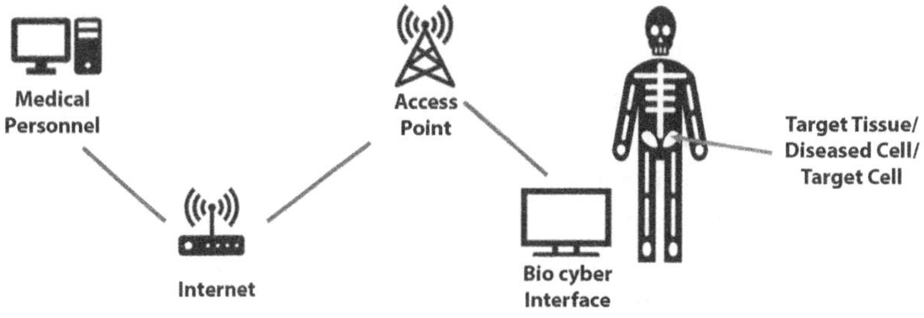

Figure 2.1 Illustration of IoT model for target drug delivery.

specific diseased sites within the human body. Figure 2.1 provides a visual representation of how IoT is involved in this process. Through IoT, sensors, devices, and objects present in the network can autonomously communicate and interact with one another, ensuring efficient and accurate drug delivery to the intended targets [3]. The combination of the body sensor area network (BSN) and Internet of Things (IoT) technology enables the real-time transmission of a patient's physiological data [4]. This allows doctors or the patient's relatives to monitor the patient's condition from any location and at any time. In this chapter, we delve into the investigation of an IoT-based model called the "Smart Portable Intensive Care Unit (SPICU)," which serves as a remote diagnostic unit. SPICU assists medical personnel in accessing and reviewing the patient's vital parameters, thereby aiding in making informed diagnostic decisions. This innovative model enhances patient care by providing convenient and timely access to critical health information [5]. A wirelessly reconfigurable micro pumping device based on Internet of Things (IoT) technology is being developed, specifically designed for personalized cancer therapy. This innovative device is aimed at being implanted directly into tumor tissue and features miniature size for optimal compatibility. The device incorporates refillable reservoirs that store anticancer drugs. By utilizing a wireless system, the device allows for real-time data analysis, enabling precise control and reconfiguration of the drug administration regimen.

2.2.2 Nanobioelectronics

Nanofabrication refers to the process of crafting functional structures with customized patterns, typically featuring dimensions smaller than 100 nm in at least two directions. Recent literature reviews showcase the latest advancements in this field. Creating nanostructured bioelectronic devices comes with its own set of challenges. Recent studies have highlighted the importance of developing synthetic biomaterials that possess a similar softness to the surrounding tissue when seamlessly integrated [6]. Moreover, there is a growing interest in fabricating nanostructures that closely mimic the characteristics of the extracellular matrix. Additionally, these devices can be engineered to incorporate systems capable of controlled release of anti-inflammatory agents or growth factors. In the future, it will be vital to integrate chemo-attractants into these devices to promote targeted interactions with specific types of cells [7]. The fabrication process of such devices involves creating structures at different scales, ranging from macro to micro to nano. It's unlikely that a single fabrication approach can meet all these requirements simultaneously. In this discussion, we specifically focus on fabricating nano-scale components. For more than thirty years, microelectrode arrays measuring 100 mm in diameter have been employed to monitor neuronal cell activity in laboratory settings. Nevertheless, the primary objective is to establish a direct interface between the electrodes and individual cells, with cell bodies measuring less than 30 mm in diameter, or even individual axons with a cross-section below 500 nm. Achieving such a high degree of miniaturization brings about new challenges in different aspects. To begin with, when choosing materials, one must consider how relevant properties transform with the reduction in electrode size. For instance, in the scaling down of gold or platinum electrodes, the constrained charge injection capacity of these noble metals starts to act as a restricting element [8].

2.2.2.1 Scanning Beam Lithography

Scanning beam lithography (SBL) is an advanced direct-write technique that employs a tightly focused beam to create intricate patterns through selective removal of materials or deposition of species. Although SBL operates at a slower pace, requiring approximately 24 hours per square centimeter for achieving 20 nm scale features, its exceptional resolution and unwavering pattern fidelity render it an indispensable technology in manufacturing photolithography masks. Moreover, SBL has found valuable applications in specialized research fields such as bioelectronics, where it serves unique purposes [9].

2.2.2.2 Jet Printing

Inkjet Printing is a micro-scale fabrication method primarily characterized by its ability to work with droplets as small as pico-liters, enabling

Table 2.1 Literature review table describing the IoT and nano bioelectronics related title, authors, journal, year, summary, and references.

Title	Authors	Journal	Year	Summary	References
"A digital nervous system aiming toward personalized IoT healthcare"	Armgarth, A. *et al.*	Scientific Reports	2021	The system envisions a transformative impact on healthcare by seamlessly merging digital technologies, offering unique and precise health monitoring and management tailored to each individual's needs.	[26]
"CRISPR/Cas Systems-Inspired Nano/Biosensors for Detecting Infectious Viruses and Pathogenic Bacteria"	Zhang, X. *et al.*	Small Methods	2022	Explores the role of CRISPR/Cas-based nano/biosensor technology, underscoring their promising applications in real-world scenarios.	[25]
"A self-powered triboelectric MXene-based 3D-printed wearable physiological biosignal sensing system for on-demand, wireless, and real-time health monitoring"	Yi, Q. *et al.*	Nano Energy	2022	The paper presents a self-powered wearable biosignal sensing system utilizing 3D-printed MXene, enabling real-time health monitoring through on-demand wireless capabilities.	[27]

(*Continued*)

Table 2.1 Literature review table describing the IoT and nano bioelectronics related title, authors, journal, year, summary, and references. (*Continued*)

Title	Authors	Journal	Year	Summary	References
"The Internet of Things (IoT) in healthcare: Taking stock and moving forward"	Rejeb, A. *et al.*	Internet of Things	2023	The current status and future directions of the Internet of Things (IoT) in healthcare offer insights into the progress made so far while outlining the potential pathways for further advancements in this dynamic field.	[28]
"Utilization of AI and IoT-based smart nanosystems for the control and management of COVID-19 pandemic"	Tripathi, G.K. *et al.*	Academic Press	2023	Smart nanosystems, integrated with AI and IoT, offer a promising avenue for pandemic control. These systems can provide real-time data collection, analysis, and monitoring of critical parameters, such as body temperature and respiratory patterns.	[13]

resolutions in the range of approximately 10 micrometers. Information provided in Table 2.1 Literature review table describing the IoT and nano bioelectronics related title, authors, journal, year, summary, and references. A closely related technique called electrohydrodynamic jet printing (e-JP) has been recently developed, allowing for even smaller droplets in the femto-liter and atto-liter range, with diameters around 200 nanometers. The resolution achievable through e-JP depends on factors such as liquid properties, substrate wettability, and the size of the jet nozzle. While e-JP shows promise, it does have a limitation in that it requires the use of a conductive substrate [10].

2.2.2.3 AFM Nano Printing

Several DPN (dip-pen nanolithography) techniques focus on creating patterns using metal nanoparticles, particularly functionalized gold (Au) nanoparticles, for applications such as sensing or bio-recognition. While these approaches offer diverse methods for ink transfer, such as ink-substrate hydrophobicity and nanografting, the insulating nature of capping agents used with the nanoparticles limits their ability to generate conductive lines [11]. One approach that focuses on nanoparticles involves incorporating silver nanoparticles into an ink formula thickened with glycerol, enabling the deposition of conductive traces. By annealing the mixture at a temperature of 150°C, a relatively high conductivity of 3×10^4 S cm^{-1} was achieved [10]. The another method known as the "surface-activated *in situ* redox approach" uses specific surface chemistry to decrease the metal precursor ink as it gets laid down. Dip-pen nanolithography (DPN) has been extensively researched for creating conductive metal patterns, and one widely employed method involves using thiol-resist nanopatterning to shield a metal coating from wet etching. This particular approach provides high resolution at micro- or nanoscale levels (less than 50 nm) and has the ability to scale up to millions of features across large areas using polymer pen lithography. A crucial point to note is that this technique preserves the electrical characteristics. This means that the pattern keeps the same conductivity as the metal thin film that's deposited through thermal evaporation [11].

2.3 Principles of Targeted Drug Delivery

The basic idea of drug targeting revolves around delivering a focused dose of medication to the desired location while minimizing its presence in non-targeted areas. This approach aims to enhance the therapeutic benefits of the drug while reducing side effects caused by interactions with unintended targets, higher dosages, and unintended concentrations in non-targeted regions. Targeting strategies also enhance the drug's interaction with the body's bioenvironmental factors, which can influence its accessibility to the intended sites. In Figure 2.2, drug targeting is depicted as a synchronized process involving the drug's behavior, a designated targeting site, and a pharmaceutical carrier. The targeting site refers to the particular organ, cell, or group of cells affected by chronic or acute conditions that necessitate treatment and will engage with the drug [11].

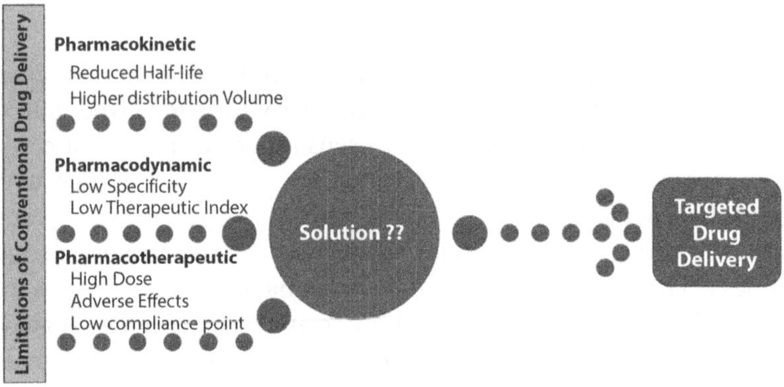

Figure 2.2 Illustrates the need for targeted drug delivery over conventional drug delivery.

2.3.1 Targeted Drug Delivery

The combination of targeted delivery and controlled drug release plays a crucial role in the future of personalized medicine. Targeted drug delivery (TDD) involves the direct administration of drugs to specific areas within the body, including organs, cells, and even subcellular levels [13]. This approach offers numerous advantages compared to conventional drug delivery systems. TDD has applications in pain management, cancer treatment, addressing chronic diseases, targeted gene therapy, and managing neurological disorders. By delivering drugs directly to the affected area, TDD aims to minimize the side effects associated with conventional drug delivery methods and enhance patient outcomes [14].

Unlike the usual method of drug delivery, where the drug is absorbed through a biological membrane, targeted release systems provide the drug in a precise and specific form of dosage. The advantages of targeted drug delivery (TDD) over conventional systems can be categorized into four aspects: addressing shortcomings in drug performance related to pharmacodynamics, pharmacokinetics, pharmaceutical properties, and pharmacotherapeutic features. Targeting drugs to specific areas using optimized drug delivery methods is an essential aspect of achieving targeted delivery, which requires overcoming certain challenges [15].

TDD can be used to provide adequate pain relief by eliminating systemic opioids. The Control Workflow for TDD is an approach that can be used for this purpose [16]. TDD can also be used to target cancer cells specifically, thereby reducing the side effects of chemotherapy. This is accomplished by delivering the medication straight to the tumor location. This raises the drug's concentration in the affected area compared to other parts of the body.

Targeted drug delivery (TDD) finds application in the treatment of chronic diseases like Alzheimer's disease, diabetes, and Parkinson's disease. By directly delivering drugs to the affected area, TDD offers the advantage of minimizing side effects associated with conventional drug delivery methods [9]. Additionally, TDD holds promise for targeted gene therapy, involving the delivery of therapeutic genes to specific cells or tissues in the body. This approach has the potential to address genetic disorders and diseases resulting from genetic mutations. Furthermore, targeted drug delivery (TDD) has the potential to address neurological disorders like chronic pain, spasticity, and dystonia. Through targeted drug delivery to the specific region in need, TDD can contribute to reducing the negative effects often linked with traditional drug delivery methods [16].

The development of targeting strategies for precise drug delivery to specific sites shows great potential in reducing off-target effects and improving the therapeutic effectiveness of drugs. Extensive research spanning the

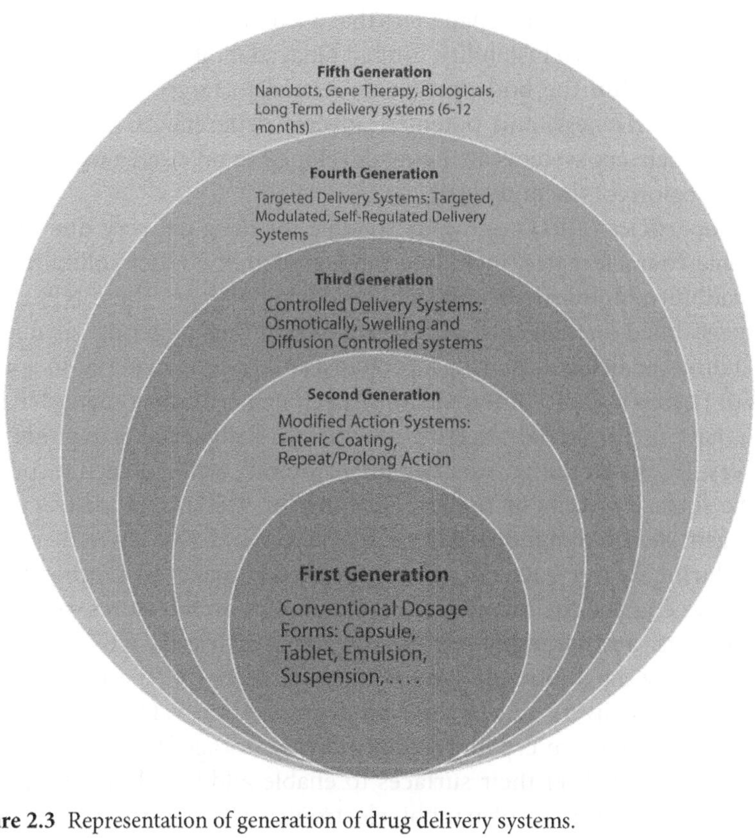

Figure 2.3 Representation of generation of drug delivery systems.

past thirty years has been dedicated to understanding the biological barriers that impede tissue-specific drug delivery and devising strategies to overcome them. In Figure 2.3, the progression of drug delivery systems is depicted, encompassing up to the 5th generation, which encompasses targeted drug delivery and extends to gene therapy. These efforts have resulted in the development of various targeting strategies that manipulate drug delivery in both preclinical and clinical settings. These strategies include approaches utilizing small molecules, nucleic acids, peptides, antibodies, and cell-based methods [17].

Nano-bioelectronics and the Internet of Things (IoT) play a crucial role in advancing targeted drug delivery by focusing on the development of more precise drug targeting and delivery systems. The main goals involve decreasing toxicity while preserving treatment effectiveness, improving safety and compatibility with the body, and making it easier to quickly create new medicines that are safe. Nanotechnology offers numerous advantages in treating chronic human diseases by enabling site-specific and target-oriented delivery of precise drug amounts to the affected area. However, there are several challenges that need to be addressed. These challenges include *in vivo* instability, limited bioavailability and solubility, poor absorption within the body, problems related to target-specific delivery, variable effectiveness, and potential adverse drug effects. Consequently, new drug delivery systems are being developed to precisely target drugs to specific regions of the body [18].

Nanoparticles (NPs) are highly suitable for drug delivery due to their desirable characteristics, including biodegradability, water solubility, biocompatibility, biomimicry, and stability during storage. These NPs can be easily modified on their surfaces to enable additional targeting capabilities, facilitating the delivery of drugs, proteins, and genetic material to specific cells or tissues [16]. To minimize non-specific distribution, many NP platforms have incorporated targeting moieties on their surfaces to guide their delivery. These targeting moieties often interact with molecules present on the surface of cells or tissues, allowing for site-specific delivery [17]. Intelligent design of nanoparticles can overcome various barriers encountered during delivery. Recent advancements in controlled synthesis strategies have enabled the incorporation of complex architectures, responsive components, and targeting agents into nanoparticle designs, enhancing their delivery capabilities. Polymeric nanoparticles (NPs) are highly suitable for drug delivery due to their biodegradability, water solubility, biocompatibility, biomimicry, and stability during storage [19]. These NPs can be easily modified on their surfaces to enable additional targeting capabilities. The integration of nanobioelectronics and IoT has the potential to bring significant advancements to drug delivery by developing more precise drug targeting and delivery systems that minimize toxicity while maintaining therapeutic efficacy. The overarching objective is to create safe and effective drug delivery systems that can be utilized for the treatment of various chronic human diseases [20].

2.3.2 Carriers for the Targeted Drug Delivery

Various drug carriers, including nanoparticles (NPs), colloidal systems, monoclonal antibodies (Abs), polymers, and cells, are available for drug delivery purposes. The selection of the carrier relies on factors like the drug's characteristics, the intended location in the body, and the state of the disease. Targeting moieties, such as proteins, antibodies, lipoproteins, polysaccharides, charged molecules, and hormones, can be incorporated with carriers to enhance their targeting capabilities [20]. Targeted drug delivery (TDD) is a method of delivering drugs directly to particular body areas, like organs, cells, or even smaller structures within cells. TDD has numerous benefits over regular drug delivery systems (DSs). These advantages encompass better accuracy in delivering drugs to their targets, reducing harm while keeping the treatment benefits, improved safety and compatibility with the body, and quicker creation of new, safe medicines [21]. However, several challenges associated with TDD need to be addressed. An important hurdle in drug delivery is ensuring that the drug reaches the intended location in the body, while minimizing potential side effects on healthy organs. To address this, scientists have devised different carrier systems for drug delivery, aiming to overcome these challenges. Nanoparticles (NPs) are one such carrier system that has been successfully employed recently. Nanoparticles (NPs) provide numerous advantages in the treatment of chronic human diseases by delivering therapeutic agents or natural-based active compounds to specific locations in a targeted and precise manner. This approach aims to effectively address various ailments [22].

Polymeric nanoparticles (NPs) are highly suitable for drug delivery due to their desirable characteristics. They are biodegradable, soluble in water, biocompatible, biomimetic, and exhibit stability during storage. Moreover, polymeric nanoparticles (NPs) can have their surfaces easily modified to facilitating the delivery of drugs, and improve targeting abilities, and genetic material to specific cells. In order to minimize unintended distribution, many NP platforms incorporate targeting components on their surfaces to ensure precise delivery [23]. Many targeting components engage with molecules found in both unhealthy and healthy cells. The quest for appropriate carriers as drug delivery systems comes with a range of main obstacles. These obstacles consist of instability within the body, restricted bioavailability and solubility, insufficient absorption within the body, challenges in accomplishing precise target delivery, inadequate therapeutic effectiveness, and the potential negative impacts of drugs. Addressing these issues is crucial to developing effective and efficient drug delivery systems [19].

2.4 Methodology

The approach for targeted drug delivery, start by crafting specialized bioelectronic devices encompassing nanoscale sensors and actuators, designed to control drug administration. Design bioelectronic devices incorporating nanoscale sensors and actuators for drug delivery control [17]. Utilize biocompatible materials to ensure compatibility with biological systems. Develop microfabrication techniques to create miniaturized devices for implantation or wearable integration. These devices are fashioned using biocompatible materials, ensuring compatibility with the human body [19]. Integrate nano sensors capable of detecting specific biomarkers or physiological changes indicative of drug efficacy. Implement IoT connectivity to establish a real-time data transmission link between the device and external monitoring systems. Incorporate feedback loops to continuously assess the patient's response to the delivered drug [20]. An intricate network of nano sensors to detect specific biomarkers, and through the power of IoT, establishes a real-time link for data transmission between the device and external monitoring systems. Employing machine learning, we analyze the data, making informed decisions based on patients' responses to the drugs [23]. Researchers design drug reservoirs and incorporate mechanisms for controlled drug release, often influenced by real-time monitoring and IoT-driven commands. Incorporate targeting ligands or biomolecules on the device's surface to enhance its interaction with specific cells or tissues [25]. Utilize diagnostic data to determine the optimal timing and location for drug delivery, ensuring targeted treatment. These mechanisms might include controlled diffusion, electrophoresis, or temperature-responsive systems. To enhance precision, researchers incorporate targeting ligands and biomolecules, optimizing interactions with desired cells or tissues [27]. Throughout the process, researchers maintain strict ethical and regulatory adherence, conducting *in vitro* and animal studies before venturing into human clinical trials. By following this comprehensive methodology, the integration of IoT and bioelectronics in targeted drug delivery can lead to

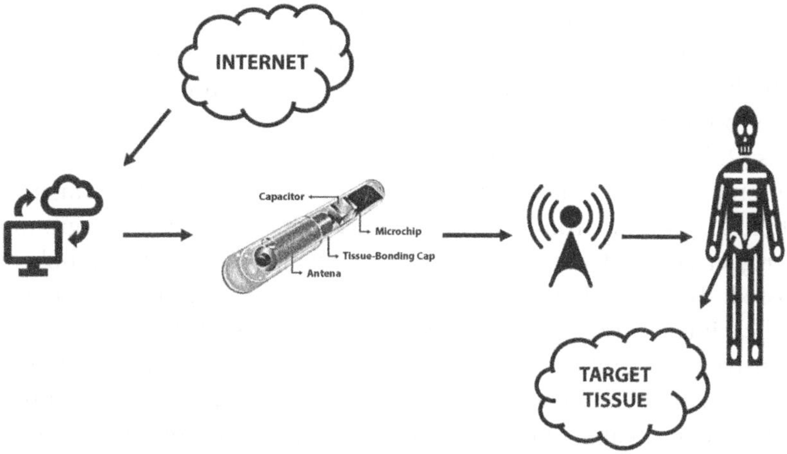

Figure 2.4 Integration of internet, device integration, sensing, data acquisition, and drug release mechanism in the target tissue for clinical trials.

more precise, effective, and personalized therapeutic interventions while ensuring patient safety and regulatory compliance as shown in Figure 2.4.

2.5 Smart Portable Intensive Care Unit

The Smart Portable Intensive Care Unit represents a groundbreaking advancement in healthcare, leveraging the synergy of IoT and nano bioelectronics. This concept envisions a compact, yet highly intelligent, medical solution designed to address the challenges of modern patient care [25]. By seamlessly integrating real-time monitoring, diagnostics, and treatment, this innovative approach has the potential to transform critical care scenarios. At the core of this concept lies the Internet of Things (IoT), a network of interconnected devices that can exchange data and information seamlessly. In healthcare, IoT offers the capability to create a dynamic and interconnected ecosystem where medical devices, sensors, and even wearable technologies can communicate and collaborate in real-time [26]. This connectivity enhances the ability to monitor patients remotely and gather a continuous stream of vital data, enabling healthcare providers to make informed decisions promptly. The Smart Portable Intensive Care Unit's design encompasses a compact and user-friendly device that can be easily transported and set up. It can continuously monitor the patient's vital signs, such as heart rate, blood pressure, oxygen levels, and temperature, while also tracking more specific indicators like glucose levels or specific biomarkers indicative of infections or other medical conditions. The real-time data generated by the device is transmitted securely through IoT connectivity to healthcare professionals, enabling them to remotely assess the patient's condition and make informed decisions [27]. The integration of IoT and nano bioelectronics in this portable unit empowers healthcare providers to detect any alarming changes in a patient's condition promptly. Furthermore, the device can be programmed to trigger automated responses or alerts when predefined thresholds are crossed. This functionality could potentially save lives by ensuring that medical interventions are administered swiftly. Overall, the Smart Portable Intensive Care Unit showcases the transformative potential of combining IoT and nano bioelectronics in healthcare. It offers a glimpse into a future where medical care is not only data-driven but also portable and proactive. By enabling continuous monitoring, timely interventions, and remote connectivity, this innovative approach has the capacity to redefine critical care, ultimately improving patient outcomes and the efficiency of healthcare delivery [28].

2.6 Applications of Targeted Drug Delivery

Targeted drug delivery (TDD) involves delivering medications straight to specific body regions, including organs, cells, and even the tiniest parts within cells. TDD has several applications in the field of medicine [16, 18]. Here are some of the applications of TDD:

a. TDD can provide effective pain relief by eliminating systemic opioids. The Control Workflow for TDD is an approach that can be used for this purpose.
b. TDD can target cancer cells specifically, thereby reducing the side effects of chemotherapy. This is accomplished by transporting the medicine directly to the tumor location, leading to higher medication concentrations in the affected area compared to other body regions.
c. Targeted drug delivery (TDD) has applications in treating chronic diseases like diabetes, Parkinson's disease, and Alzheimer's disease. Through direct delivery of drugs to the affected area, TDD has the potential to mitigate the side effects commonly associated with conventional drug delivery methods.

d. TDD can also be used for targeted gene therapy which involves delivering therapeutic genes to specific cells or tissues in the body. This approach has the potential to treat genetic disorders and other diseases that are caused by genetic mutations.
e. Targeted drug delivery (TDD) has applications in the treatment of neurological disorders like chronic pain, spasticity, and dystonia. By directly delivering drugs to the affected region, TDD can minimize the side effects commonly associated with conventional drug delivery methods.

Exploring targeting techniques to facilitate drug delivery to specific sites shows potential in reducing off-target effects, minimizing undesired toxicities, and improving the therapeutic effectiveness of drugs [6, 13]. Extensive research conducted over the past thirty years has been dedicated to comprehending the biological obstacles that impede tissue-specific drug delivery and devising strategies to overcome these challenges. The primary objective of nano-biotechnologies in drug delivery research is to achieve more precise targeting and delivery of drugs, while simultaneously reducing toxicity and maintaining therapeutic efficacy. The focus is on enhancing safety, biocompatibility, and the development process of new medications. The major challenges in finding suitable carrier systems as drug delivery platforms involve addressing concerns related to instability within the body, limited bioavailability and solubility, inefficient absorption, difficulties in achieving target-specific delivery, optimal therapeutic effectiveness, and potential adverse effects of drugs [7].

2.7 Applications of IoT and Nanobioelectronics

Targeted drug delivery (TDD) is a method that involves delivering medications directly to specific areas of the body, including organs, cells, or even at the subcellular level. TDD finds utility in various medical fields, such as pain management, cancer treatment, addressing chronic diseases, targeted gene therapy, and managing neurological disorders [11]. By delivering drugs directly to the affected area, TDD can help reduce the side effects of conventional drug delivery systems and improve patient outcomes. Over the past few years, advancements in nano-bioelectronics and the Internet of Things (IoT) have transformed drug delivery. These advancements have led to the creation of more precise drug targeting and delivery systems, which lower toxicity while upholding the desired treatment outcomes [12].

Applications of IoT and nano-bioelectronics for the field of targeted drug delivery include:

a. IoT technology can be used to develop smart drug delivery systems that can monitor patient health in real-time and adjust drug dosages accordingly. Once the patient receives the prescription and provides feedback, IoT technology can save the information and analyze the precise dosage needed for that particular patient. This can help reduce the risk of overdose or underdose and improve patient outcomes.
b. Controlled drug release devices are a type of TDD system that can release drugs at a specific rate over a period of time. These devices can be designed to respond to specific stimuli such as temperature, pH, or light. IoT technology can be used to monitor these stimuli in real-time and adjust drug release rates accordingly.
c. DNA nanoprobes are a type of nanoparticle that can be used for targeted drug delivery. These nanoprobes are designed to bind specifically to target cells or tissues and deliver drugs directly. IoT technology can be used to monitor the binding of these nanoprobes in real-time and adjust drug dosages accordingly.
d. A dual-channel iontophoretic drug delivery system is a type of TDD system that uses an electric current to deliver drugs directly to the affected area. IoT technology can be used to monitor the electric current in real-time and adjust drug dosages accordingly. This system has been specifically designed for elderly patients with difficulty managing their medication.
e. Nanoparticles (NPs) have been investigated as potential solutions for cancer therapy due to their ability to target cancer cells specifically while minimizing damage to healthy cells. Recent research has focused on improving NP-based studies by investigating new nanotechnology approaches that enhance drug delivery. Artificial intelligence (AI) has also been integrated into this field to optimize drug delivery platforms.

The fields of IoT and nano-bioelectronics have brought about a revolution in drug delivery. They have pioneered the creation of drug targeting and delivery systems that are highly specific, decreasing toxicity while still upholding the desired treatment effects [14]. The applications of these technologies in TDD include smart drug delivery systems, controlled drug release devices, DNA nanoprobes, dual-channel iontophoretic drug delivery systems, and nanoparticles for cancer therapy. These technologies can improve patient outcomes by reducing side effects and improving treatment efficacy [21, 23].

2.8 Use of IoT to Improve Drug Delivery System

IoT technology can improve drug delivery systems in several ways:

a. IoT technology can help connect patients to doctors through remote monitoring and virtual visits. This can help doctors monitor patients' health in real-time and adjust drug dosages accordingly. Once the patient receives the prescribed medication and provides feedback, IoT technology can store and analyze the data to determine the precise dosage needed for the individual. This approach reduces the chances of overdosing or underdosing, leading to enhanced patient outcomes [20].
b. IoT technology can create customized medicines for each patient. Utilization of 3D food printing technology, combined with drug delivery systems (DDSs), enables the incorporation of accurate drug doses into food compositions. This enables the production of medication-infused food in various shapes quickly, offering an accurate means of delivering drugs to patients even from remote locations [18].
c. IoT technology can be used to issue reminders for medication refills and dosage schedules. For example, AdhereTech smart pill bottles are used just like normal bottles but issue reminders for medication refills [16].
d. IoT technology can enable preventative care by tracking and transmitting patients' health data to providers in real-time. Medical apps paired with IoMT technology enable patients to track and transmit their health data to providers in real-time, allowing doctors to monitor patients' health and adjust drug dosages accordingly [13].

e. IoT technology can enable critical care response by providing real-time patient health status data. For example, IoT-enabled devices can monitor patients' vital signs and alert healthcare providers if any changes require immediate attention [9].

2.8.1 Examples of IoT-Based Drug Delivery Systems

In the healthcare sector, drug delivery systems empowered by IoT are gaining growing popularity. Here are some examples of IoT-enabled drug delivery systems:

a. Iontophoretic drug delivery device uses a low-level electric current to deliver drugs through the skin. It is connected to a smartphone app that allows doctors to monitor patients' medication adherence and adjust dosages as needed [7].
b. Prescription adverse drug event (prescADE) system improves patient safety by alerting healthcare providers of potential adverse drug events. It uses IoT technology to monitor patients' medication use and sends alerts to healthcare providers if there are any issues [5].
c. Enteral Feeding IoT platform allows doctors to preprogram devices, emergency staff to administer infusions on the go, and patients to self-infuse in the comfort of their own homes using a smartphone app [2].
d. AdhereTech smart pill bottle is used for medication refills. It issues reminders for patients to take their medication and sends alerts to healthcare providers if patients miss doses [12].

The potential of IoT technology to transform the medical field is immense, as it enhances the effectiveness of drugs while minimizing potential side effects. These IoT-enabled drug delivery systems are just some examples of how these technologies can be used in targeted drug delivery [11].

2.8.2 Role of IoT and Nanobioelectronics in Targeted Drug Delivery

The utilization of nanoparticles for drug delivery shows great promise in enhancing the effectiveness of drugs while reducing their potential side effects. Nanoparticles serve as an advantageous drug delivery system due to several key benefits over traditional drugs. These advantages include improved stability and biocompatibility, targeted delivery to specific sites, and controlled release of the drug. Scientists have achieved the development of suitable and biocompatible drug delivery vehicles through the use of various carriers such as liposomes, hydrogels, micelles, dendrimers, and mesoporous particles [24]. Furthermore, integrating IoT technology into drug delivery systems offers several advantages. As an illustration, a drug delivery system with dual-channel iontophoresis, integrated with IoT capabilities, has been created to support the medication management of elderly patients. This system uses a wearable device that delivers drugs through the skin using a low-level electric current. The device is connected to a smartphone app that allows doctors to monitor patients' medication adherence and adjust dosages as needed [22]. Moreover, 3D printing technology can be used to create patient-specific drug delivery systems. Through the incorporation of IoT technology, patients now have the convenience of receiving diagnoses and prescriptions from their doctors without needing to leave their homes [23]. Through the combination of 3D food printing and IoT, it becomes possible to incorporate precise drug dosages into food compositions, allowing for personalized medication production in various shapes and forms within a short period. This automation of food and drug delivery systems shows great potential for providing remote healthcare solutions. Nanotechnology plays a crucial role in the development of targeted drug delivery systems and the advancement of human therapeutics. Ongoing research focuses on exploring and enhancing nanotechnology in the field of medicine, with particular emphasis on NP-based studies. Novel approaches in nanotechnology continue to be investigated in order to improve drug delivery methods [19].

2.9 Challenges

The use of IoT and nano-bioelectronics technology in drug delivery systems can raise potential privacy and security concerns. Some of these concerns are:

a. Hackers can gain access to private patient data, which can lead to the theft of information or intentional or unintentional alteration of data [17].
b. Insecure communications and data storage can lead to data security concerns in IoT applications. Data encryption can

be used to protect data in motion and at rest, but it is only sometimes implemented. Insecure communications and data storage can lead to data security concerns in IoT applications, which are often used with nano-bioelectronics [15].

c. Hackers can develop malware to infect IoT devices, and phishing techniques can be used to provoke individuals to share sensitive data [3].
d. The widespread use of smart devices and the sharing and integration of data pose potential risks to privacy and data security, which can disrupt workflow. Similarly, the incorporation of nano-bioelectronics in drug delivery systems raises privacy concerns. Cybersecurity professionals express concerns about the potential for nanotechnology to introduce new cybersecurity threats. The extensive adoption of smart devices with data sharing and integration can also give rise to privacy and data breach risks [9].
e. Securing information is a critical aspect of IoT authentication, as the multitude of data collection in the IoT environment poses inherent risks. The widespread presence of applications in this context increases the vulnerability of information security [13].
f. Cybersecurity threats context of nanodevices, which are typically controlled by a program on a conventional electronic device, there are concerns among digital security experts regarding the potential vulnerability of a single nanoparticle with its own processor to hacking. Theoretically, if a patient has multiple nanoparticles within their body, a hacker could manipulate them to form a network within the body, utilizing the body's systems for communication and control. This technology presents a potential risk if weaponized, highlighting the importance of strict regulation and thorough penetration testing to mitigate the risk of hacking in nanotechnology applications [24].

2.10 Conclusion

The development of nanotechnology-based drug delivery systems has shown great promise in achieving site-specific drug delivery, reduced side effects, and better treatment outcomes. Nanoparticle-mediated drug delivery offers distinct benefits, including enhanced stability and compatibility with biological systems, improved functionality, and more precise targeting and delivery of drugs. Various types of drug carriers, such as liposomes, nanoparticles, hydrogels, micelles, dendrimers, and mesoporous particles, have demonstrated successful development as effective and biocompatible vehicles for drug delivery. Integrating nano-bioelectronics techniques and the Internet of Things (IoT) has also shown great potential in the targeted drug delivery system. The suggested paradigm of a "Smart Portable Intensive Care Unit" based on IoT makes it possible for medical staff and the patient's family to remotely monitor the patient's physiological data. Overall, nanotechnology-based drug delivery systems have brought new hope for targeted and efficient drug delivery in cancer treatment. The integration of IoT technology in healthcare has also shown great potential in improving patient care and outcomes.

Relevance of Work

The field of targeted drug delivery systems (TDDSs) using nanobioelectronics and the Internet of Things (IoT) is rapidly advancing, offering great potential in the field of advanced medicine and drug formulations. Nanobioelectronics provides numerous advantages in the treatment of chronic diseases by enabling precise and targeted delivery of medications. Nanotechnology-based drug delivery systems (DDSs) have the ability to improve the therapeutic efficacy of drugs through targeted and controlled release, addressing challenges such as instability, poor bioavailability, and suboptimal pharmacokinetic and pharmacodynamic features associated with conventional delivery methods.

The requirement for TDDSs instead of traditional DDSs stems from the constraints seen in how drugs perform in aspects like their pharmacokinetic, pharmacodynamic, pharmacotherapeutic, and pharmaceutical attributes when administered through conventional methods. The development of successful nanoparticulate systems relies on optimized DDS methods to target drugs to specific areas. Utilizing nanoparticle-based DDSs allows for controlled drug release, ensuring adequate time for drug action while minimizing toxicity. The choice of an optimal nano-drug delivery system depends on the specific biophysical and biochemical characteristics of the drugs used for treatment. Nanomedicines are increasingly being recognized for their ability to provide targeted and effective drug delivery, overcoming the limitations of conventional therapies. Both preclinical and clinical investigations have shown the potential of these nanomedicines in achieving site-specific drug delivery, minimizing side effects, and reducing toxicity to healthy cells. In the field of cancer therapy, nanoparticle-based drug delivery systems bring forth numerous advantages. These include enhanced stability and biocompatibility, utilization of the enhanced permeability and retention effect, and the ability to achieve precise targeting. Furthermore, the development of hybrid nanoparticles, which combine the unique properties of different types of nanoparticles, has propelled the advancement of drug-carrier systems to new heights.

The integration of Internet of Things (IoT) technology into Targeted Drug Delivery Systems (TDDSs) allows for real-time monitoring and feedback, enabling personalized and precise drug delivery. This integration not only improves patient compliance but also reduces the risk of adverse effects. The utilization of nanotechnology and IoT in the development of TDDSs plays a crucial role in enhancing the therapeutic effectiveness of drugs, minimizing toxicity, and addressing the limitations of conventional therapy.

References

1. Chen, Y., Kosmas, P., Anwar, P.S., Huang, L., A touch-communication framework for drug delivery based on a transient microbot system. *IEEE Trans. Nanobiosci.*, 14, 4, 397–408, 2015.
2. Wang, Z., Ju, Y., Ali, Z., Yin, H., Sheng, F., Lin, J., Wang, B., Hou, Y., Near-infrared light and tumor microenvironment dual responsive size-switchable nanocapsules for multimodal tumor theranostics. *Nat. Commun.*, 10, 1, 4418, 2019, doi: 10.1038/s41467-019-12142-4.
3. El-Fatyany, A., Wang, H., Abd El-atty, S.M., Efficient framework analysis for targeted drug delivery based on internet of bio-nanothings. *Arabian J. Sci. Eng.*, 46, 10, 9965–9980, 2021, doi: 10.1007/s13369-021-05651-2.
4. Rinaldi, A., Caraffi, R., Grazioli, M.V., Oddone, N., Giardino, L., Tosi, G., Vandelli, M.A., Calzà, L., Ruozi, B., Duskey, J.T., Applications of the ROS-responsive thioketal linker for the production of smart nanomedicines. *Polymers*, 14, 4, 687, 2022, doi: 10.3390/polym14040687.
5. Power, M., Seneci, C.A., Thompson, A.J., Yang, G.Z., *Modelling and characterization of a compliant tethered microgripper for microsurgical applications*, pp. 1–7, IEEE, 2017.
6. Soni, A., Bhandari, M.P., Tripathi, G.K., Bundela, P., Khiriya, P.K., Khare, P.S., Kashyap, M.K., Dey, A., Vellingiri, B., Sundaramurthy, S., Suresh, A., Nano-biotechnology in tumour and cancerous disease: A perspective review. *J. Cell. Mol. Med.*, 27, 6, 737–762, 2023.
7. Ilkhani, H., Zhong, C.J., Hepel, M., Magneto-plasmonic nanoparticle grid biosensor with enhanced raman scattering and electrochemical transduction for the development of nanocarriers for targeted delivery of

protected anticancer drugs. *Nanomaterials*, 11, 5, 1326, 2021, doi: 10.3390/nano11051326.

8. Soni, A., Tripathi, G.K., Bundela, P., Khiriya, P.K., Khare, P.S., Synthesis and characterization of assorted pH CdSe quantum dots by solvo-thermal method to determine its dye-degradation application. *Opt. Quantum Electron.*, 55, 3, 277, 2023, doi: 10.1007/s11082-022-04536-4.
9. Hossen, S., Hossain, M.K., Basher, M.K., Mia, M.N.H., Rahman, M.T., Uddin, M.J., Smart nanocarrier-based drug delivery systems for cancer therapy and toxicity studies: A review. *J. Adv. Res.*, 15, 1–18, 2019, doi: 10.1016/j.jare.2018.06.005.
10. Rahman, B.A., Viphavakit, C., Chitaree, R., Ghosh, S., Pathak, A.K., Verma, S., Sakda, N., Optical fiber, nanomaterial, and thz-metasurface-mediated nano-biosensors: A Review. *Biosensors*, 12, 1, 42, 2022, doi: 10.3390/bios12010042.
11. Tewabe, A., Abate, A., Tamrie, M., Seyfu, A., Abdela Siraj, E., Targeted drug delivery—from magic bullet to nanomedicine: principles, challenges, and future perspectives. *J. Multidiscip. Healthc.*, 14, 1711–1724, 2021, doi: 10.2147/JMDH.S313968.
12. Cicha, I., Priefer, R., Severino, P., Souto, E.B., Jain, S., Biosensor-Integrated Drug Delivery Systems as New Materials for Biomedical Applications. *Biomolecules*, 12, 9, 1198, 2022, doi: 10.3390/biom12091198.
13. Tripathi, G.K., Bundela, P., Soni, A., Dixit, P., Utilization of AI and IoT-based smart nanosystems for the control and management of COVID-19 pandemic, in: *Smart Nanomaterials to Combat the Spread of Viral Infections*, pp. 345–364, Academic Press, 2023, doi: 10.1016/b978-0-323-99148-3.00014-5.
14. Tregubov, A.A., Nikitin, P.I., Nikitin, M.P., Advanced smart nanomaterials with integrated logic-gating and biocomputing: dawn of theranostic nanorobots. *Chem. Rev.*, 118, 20, 10294–10348, 2018, doi: 10.1021/acs.chemrev.8b00198.
15. Zafar, S., Nazir, M., Bakhshi, T., Khattak, H.A., Khan, S., Bilal, M., Choo, K.K.R., Kwak, K.S., Sabah, A., A systematic review of bio-cyber interface technologies and security issues for internet of bio-nano things. *IEEE Access*, 9, 93529–93566, 2021, doi: 10.1109/ACCESS.2021.3093442.
16. Wang, J., Tao, W., Chen, X., Farokhzad, O.C., Liu, G., Emerging advances in nanotheranostics with intelligent bioresponsive systems. *Theranostics*, 7, 16, 3915, 2017, doi: 10.7150/thno.21317.
17. Jariwala, T., Ico, G., Tai, Y., Park, H., Myung, N.V., Nam, J., Mechano-responsive piezoelectric nanofiber as an on-demand drug delivery vehicle. *ACS Appl. Bio Mater.*, 4, 4, 3706–3715, 2021, doi: 10.1021/acsabm.1c00232.
18. Lam, C., van Velthoven, M.H., Meinert, E., Application of internet of things in cell-based therapy delivery: Protocol for a systematic review. *JMIR Res. Protoc.*, 9, 3, 16935, 2020, doi: 10.2196/16935.
19. Karimi, M., Eslami, M., Sahandi-Zangabad, P., Mirab, F., Farajisafiloo, N., Shafaei, Z., Ghosh, D., Bozorgomid, M., Dashkhaneh, F., Hamblin, M.R.,

pH-Sensitive stimulus-responsive nanocarriers for targeted delivery of therapeutic agents. *Wiley Interdiscip. Rev. Nanomed. Nanobiotechnol.*, 8, 5, 696–716, 2016, doi: 10.1002/wnan.

20. Genchi, G.G., Marino, A., Tapeinos, C., Ciofani, G., Smart materials meet multifunctional biomedical devices: Current and prospective implications for nanomedicine. *Front. Bioeng. Biotechnol.*, 5, 80, 2017, doi: 10.3389/fbioe.2017.00080.
21. Hoop, M., Mushtaq, F., Hurter, C., Chen, X.Z., Nelson, B.J., Pané, S., A smart multifunctional drug delivery nanoplatform for targeting cancer cells. *Nanoscale*, 8, 25, 12723–12728, 2016, doi: 10.3929/ethz-b-000118280.
22. Jha, A., Rama, A., Ladani, B., Verma, N., Kannan, S., Naha, A., Temperature and pH-responsive nanogels as intelligent drug delivery systems: A comprehensive review. *J. Appl. Pharm. Sci.*, 11, 12, 001–016, 2021, doi: 10.7324/JAPS.2021.1101201.
23. Aqra, M.W. and Ramanathan, A.A., Review of the recent advances in nano-biosensors and technologies for healthcare applications. *Chem. Proc.*, 5, 1, 76, 2022, doi: 10.3390/csac2021-10473.
24. Cleeton, C., Keirouz, A., Chen, X., Radacsi, N., Electrospun nanofibers for drug delivery and biosensing. *ACS Biomater. Sci. Eng.*, 5, 9, 4183–4205, 2019, doi: 10.1021/acsbiomaterials.9b00853.
25. Zhang, X., Shi, Y., Chen, G., Wu, D., Wu, Y., Li, G., CRISPR/Cas Systems-Inspired Nano/Biosensors for Detecting Infectious Viruses and Pathogenic Bacteria. *Small Methods*, 6, 10, 2200794, 2022.
26. Armgarth, A., Pantzare, S., Arven, P., Lassnig, R., Jinno, H., Gabrielsson, E.O., Kifle, Y., Cherian, D., Arbring Sjöström, T., Berthou, G., Dowling, J., A digital nervous system aiming toward personalized IoT healthcare. *Sci. Rep.*, 11, 1, 7757, 2021.
27. Yi, Q., Pei, X., Das, P., Qin, H., Lee, S.W., Esfandyarpour, R., A self-powered triboelectric MXene-based 3D-printed wearable physiological biosignal sensing system for on-demand, wireless, and real-time health monitoring. *Nano Energy*, 101, 107511, 2022.
28. Rejeb, A., Rejeb, K., Treiblmaier, H., Appolloni, A., Alghamdi, S., Alhasawi, Y., Iranmanesh, M., The Internet of Things (IoT) in healthcare: Taking stock and moving forward. *Internet Things*, 22, 100721, 2023.

3

Healthcare and Hygiene Monitoring Using Internet of Things (IoT) Enabled Technology

J. Sandhya* **and Lakshmi Sundeep**

Department of Biotechnology, Hindustan Institute of Technology and Science, Padur, Tamil Nadu, India

Abstract

The current work gives a comprehensive description on the role and scope of Internet of Things (IoT) for the benefit of healthcare and hygiene applications. This study offers important insights into the implementation of IoT in healthcare and its recent advancements for faster diagnosis, quality treatment and improved healthcare services. Although, numerous research is being done on IoT based medical systems, it is necessary to thoroughly understand the architecture of IoT in healthcare, from a viewpoint of the technology's potential in integrating IoT devices, various sensors and the healthcare professionals rendering an efficient patient-doctor interaction. This helps in establishing an improved treatment process with higher accuracy and reliability. The chapter has extensively covered the impact of IoT based applications on the aspects of health and hygiene, giving greater attention to the need for improving security constraints and authentication systems in medical data transfer and storage. Thus, it would ensure privacy and confidentiality in the patient's personal medical records. The presented information also points out the significance of the technology in remote monitoring of health conditions with increased accuracy, comfort and better patient experience. Emphasis on the coexistence of healthcare services along with hygiene care in the medical system has also been provided. It further explains the architecture of hygiene and healthcare system focusing on the need for implementing and adhering to these practices in maintaining the healthcare service quality. This chapter focusses on the benefits of IoT technology in ensuring strict implementation and

**Corresponding author*: jsandhya@hindustanuniv.ac.in

Hari Murthy, Marta Zurek-Mortka, Vinay Jha Pillai and Kukatlapalli Pradeep Kumar (eds.) Internet of Things in Bioelectronics: Emerging Technologies and Applications, (41–68) © 2024 Scrivener Publishing LLC

hygiene habits both at a personal level and at community level for efficient and reliable medical service and treatment results.

Through this chapter, an attempt has been made to create a greater emphasis on the fact that a technology driven application should operate concomitantly with increase in patient safety, accessibility to services together with reduced healthcare expenditure. Additionally, various challenges in terms of enabling technology and services, data security and perspectives on resolving them for a powerful domain in medical field have been explored. Overall, this section covers diverse information on the IoT enabled healthcare applications and IoT framework, guiding researchers and future academicians in gaining knowledge and exploring more in the field of IoT for healthcare system.

Keywords: Data, wireless, surveillance, healthcare, security, hygiene

3.1 Introduction

Internet of Things (IoT) is thriving to be the new paradigm that is a very promising and is influencing several domains at a rapid pace. Applications ranging from wearables, smart devices, fast and easy interconnectivity, robotic controlled facilities, distant monitoring, surveillance and several other IoT enabled advancements in healthcare have greatly revolutionized the medical industry. The impact of IoT has been tremendous in the healthcare and related services and this has directly influenced the quality of human lives. Internet of Things (IoT) has exhibited tremendous potential in interconnecting medical devices, real time functioning, sensor-based application, data storage and its access with the healthcare professionals to deliver an effective, faster and quality health services even in remote locations [1].

Healthcare is an essential component of any community. Through IoT, the prospects for enhancing healthcare related services and their operations are wider and can be operated more effectively. IoT in healthcare has gained immense attention as it advances in its features of ease in operating, enhanced precision and accuracy in functioning, reduced cost of operation, deploying lesser staff, credibility on predicting and forecasting consequences and events in future. Some of the important advantages of IoT in healthcare are shown in Figure 3.1. Technological developments in terms of software, applications, wireless technologies, broadband network connectivity, devices for storing, sharing, accessing and monitoring data and information all leading to a digital economy form the essential components in facilitating such IoT enabled facilities. Healthcare IoT (HIoT)

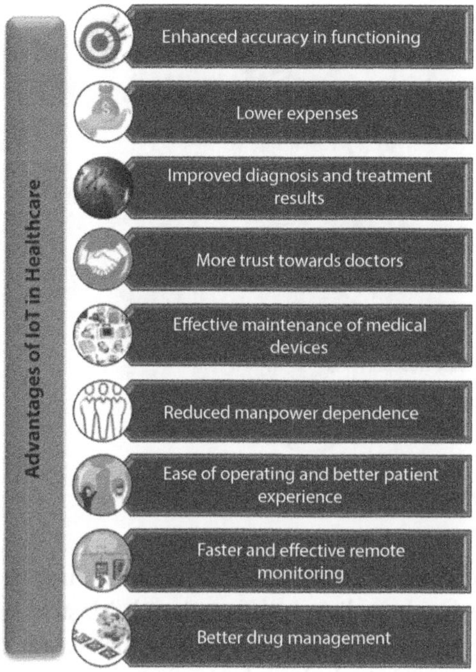

Figure 3.1 Benefits of IoT in healthcare system.

is one such technology that includes sensors for disease diagnosis, collection of physiological data from patients, monitoring and alerting health complaints and reminders for a healthy lifestyle. Significantly this IoT for healthcare encompasses a framework for various healthcare related services in preserving medical data and providing secured data access with privacy. This specialized electronic health (e-health) service also includes remote monitoring systems, easier virtual interaction between patient and healthcare professionals converting the entire healthcare regime into an easier and effective experience [2]. This is done by various IoT-facilitated services, where the entire technology operation and service rendering is channelized. This enables the electronic transfer of medical information and services from hospitals and laboratories to reach the individual families or remote patients with utmost security and accuracy [3, 4]. This remote integration is possible due to the Wireless Fidelity (Wi-Fi) commonly used for the integration and transfer of data between the intended devices and locations. This system helps in connecting the medical resources among the hospitals, laboratories, medical equipment, medical services and rehabilitation centers for patients [5].

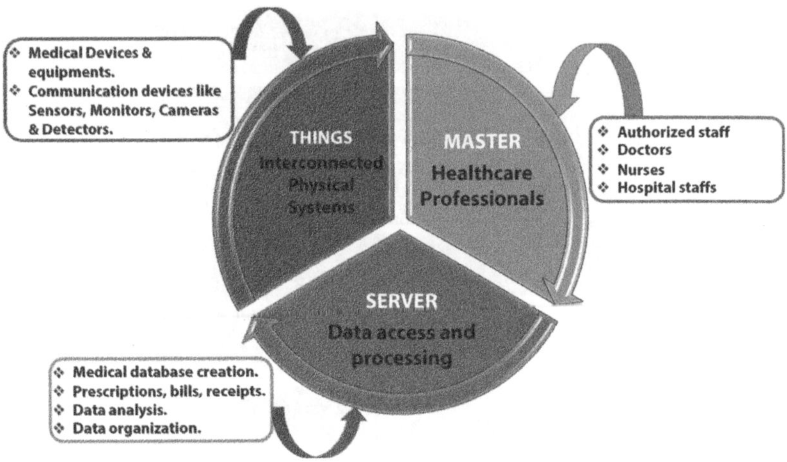

Figure 3.2 Functionality of healthcare based IoT technology.

The entire technology of IoT revolves around three major components that keep the technology live and functional: Master, Server and Things as shown in Figure 3.2. The primary part is the master that comprises of healthcare professionals including doctors, nurses, hospital staffs who own the access to authorized systems with the end user products or devices like Computers, Mobiles, Biometric accessible devices etc. The secondary part is the server which is the central dogma and the most significant part of the medical system. This includes important functions of data access and processing like managing database creating prescriptions, billing and receipts, analyzing data and creating subsystems for data organization and maintenance (Figure 3.2). The tertiary part is the, Things, constituting physical items related to patients, hospitals and which are connected to communication technology via multimedia, WAN, SMS through wireless fidelity service [6, 7]. The healthcare IoT becomes fully functional when these components are interconnected using the following four principles: Firstly, collection of data interconnected by medical and communication devices like sensors, monitors, cameras, and detectors. Second step is the data conversion to digital form for further processing by the system and medical devices. The third principle is data storage using sophisticated frameworks like cloud storage. The final principle is data processing and transfer using analytical and technical systems and ultimately the transfer to the end user with requisite information for further decision making and treatments.

This is instant and data is continuous and effective. This saves a lot of time, making the entire interaction easier and more informative [8–10].

This chapter thus summarizes the role and developments of IoT in healthcare and hygiene systems. It comprises of the following sections. Section 3.2 explains the applications of IoT in healthcare and the recent developments and scope for future advancements. It reviews the state-of-the-art services, its uses and the current developments in IoT based healthcare applications. This is followed by section 3.3, which encompasses the hygiene practices and developments enabled by Healthcare IoT (HIoT). In addition to it, Section 3.4 traverses through some of the challenges of the technology like security and privacy issues that the service providers and the end users need to focus on and the ways of confronting them for an efficient solution. In section 3.5, the chapter concludes with a summary of the various uses of Internet of Things (IoT) in health care industry along with the key highlights of the advantages and scope for further improvement.

3.2 IoT in Healthcare Applications

The current scenario of widespread infections, pandemic situations, recurrence of different types of diseases demands for a robust and a more effective system of delivering healthcare treatments and services. The Internet of Things provides this architecture for healthcare system enabling an extensive and very convenient computer assisted technology [11]. This healthcare based IoT (HIoT) basically is the amalgamation of healthcare system with IoT for a continuous, remote monitoring, error-free and long-term service [12].

This framework represented in Figure 3.3 has four layers in its architecture namely perception, network, middleware and application or business layer [13]. Perception layer comprises of the physical or the hardware components of the IoT architecture. It has the role of data collection and signaling. Network layer interconnects all the hardware components for health data transfer and exchange. It ensures a secure data transmission from the patients to the stations like Bluetooth, Zigbee, WiFi technologies etc. The middle ware layer obtains the data from network layer and stores it in the database It mainly focusses on the collection of patient details by the application programmer's interaction with the hardware and the

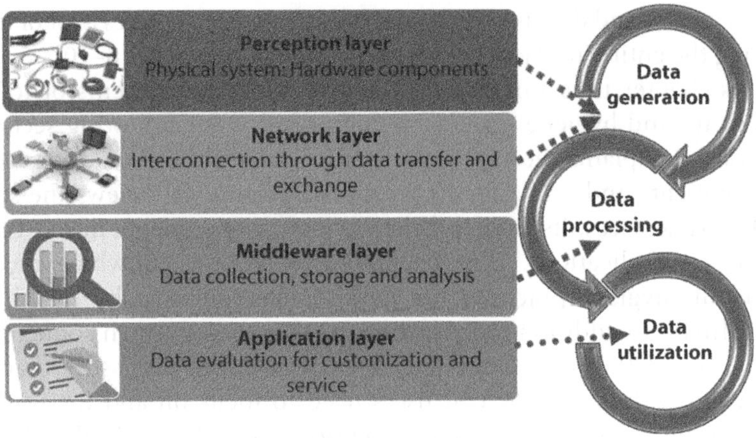

Figure 3.3 Architecture of IoT in healthcare system.

connecting networking interface. The application/business layer receives all of this information from the other layers, processes them by integrating and evaluation n the heath data. Based on this evaluated data, it provides an effective and quality healthcare service to the patents depending upon their requirements and heath record [14].

It is further understood that the entire workflow in a healthcare system does three major functions. These steps include generation of data, processing of data and data utilization [12, 14]. The first phase of data generation is enabled by various physical systems like the medical devices, sensors or even information obtained directly from the patients. This phase corresponds to the perception layer in its operation, where data is obtained from the perception layer through the network layer. Data processing comprises of analysis tools, and other machine learning methods and mechanisms for the analysis and evaluation of the generated data performed through the middle layer. The analyzed data is then utilized in the information consuming step which assists in making the appropriate decision for treatments and related health services. This evaluated information is also used for customizing and activating the devices and integral actuators. This entire operation is performed through the application/business layer.

A detailed list of the recent developments and utilization of IoT based solutions are represented in Table 3.1.

Table 3.1 List of developments in IoT enabled healthcare solutions.

S. no.	Application field	Evaluation	Reference
1	Wearable tracking devices	Effective tracking of the exercise records and collecting health details.	[15]
2	Multiple disease monitoring	Cost effective and accuracy in diagnosis using Cisco packet tracer tool for monitoring hypertension, glaucoma, and chronic obstructive pulmonary disease	[16]
3	Authentication, Access Control and Ownership	Efficient and more secure to use LACO protocol in e-health systems.	[17]
4	Early Disease diagnosis	Accurate identification of critical situations using sensors for biological data, Utilization of data mining method.	[18]
5	Security and privacy in biomedical Applications	Safe data transmission- Protocols for the transmission of the patient's data from numerous sensors and medical devices to a given healthcare network.	[19]
6	Supervise the chronic patients for long-term care	Increased accuracy in prediction using type-2 Fuzzy Logic (T2FL) and the fuzzy ontology of a patient's condition, better medical and food management.	[20]

(*Continued*)

Table 3.1 List of developments in IoT enabled healthcare solutions. (*Continued*)

S. no.	Application field	Evaluation	Reference
7	Urine-based diabetes prediction	Enhanced results in terms of temporal delay, classification efficiency, prediction efficiency, reliability and stability	[21]
8	Behavior monitoring for patients at home	Enhanced effectives of SPHERE multi modal platform by Implementation of IEEE 802.15.4 network for monitoring of behavior in residential environments	[22]
9	Early prediction chronic kidney disease (CKD)	A diagnostic prediction model for CKD and its severity produces 97% accuracy, 99% sensitivity and 95% specificity via applying decision tree (J48) classifier	[23]
10	ECG based privacy protection	Reliable authentication solution- Utilizes online algorithms to remove noises from the signals.	[24]
11	Disease diagnosis	Implementation of machine learning techniques improved interactivity between patients and doctors. 97.26% accuracy- Utilizes the method of Random Forest machine learning.	[25]

(*Continued*)

Table 3.1 List of developments in IoT enabled healthcare solutions. (*Continued*)

S. no.	Application field	Evaluation	Reference
12	Wearable sensor for disease prediction	96% in the rate of prediction and 96.33% accurate: reliable prediction model for patient suffering from colorectal diseases - Utilizes ensemble learning method.	[26]
13	Self-Recoverable application for sensor networks in medical applications.	NS2 network tool-based sensor networks for healthcare IoT showed better self-recovery, accuracy and clock drift compensation.	[27]
14	Model for identification and isolation of infected person.	Model highlights: moving objects can be tracked using proof-of-concept RFID transceiver and storing the information on the block chain to preserve the owner's privacy until required.	[28]
15	Sensor embedded patch for Blood Pressure monitoring	Sensor patch consisting of ECG and PPG sensors integrated with the same device to estimate blood pressure (BP) continuously based on the pulse arrival time (PAT) without extra wires and devices.	[29]

(*Continued*)

Table 3.1 List of developments in IoT enabled healthcare solutions. (*Continued*)

S. no.	Application field	Evaluation	Reference
16	Data quality and data transfer using oneM2M application in personal healthcare devices	Application oriented oneM2M-based IoT system-Personal Healthcare Device - two gateway faults occurred at the same time can be recovered-performs effectively and the conversion process does not cause degradation of performance.	[30]
17	Glucose monitoring technology	Mobile Medical Applications (MMAs)- Effective-non-invasive technique-optical and transdermal approaches are most efficient	[31]
18	Optical method in detecting glucose level	Non-invasive and non-infective optical method -advanced technique-sensor circuit consists of IR LEDs of wavelength 650–2500nm for optical blood glucose measurement and NIR photodiodes (InGaAs) to receive the reflected light from body parts to determine the glucose level.	[32]
19	Real time identification of core body temperature	Standalone functionality-more accurately detects a person's core body temperature, by using infrared sensors to track the temperature of the tympanic membrane	[33]

(*Continued*)

Table 3.1 List of developments in IoT enabled healthcare solutions. (*Continued*)

S. no.	Application field	Evaluation	Reference
20	Remote condition detection of body temperature and heart rate	Effective method for unlimited distance monitoring by utilizing the internet as a medium for sending the data.	[34]
21	Body temperature detection in infants	Small and lightweight wearable device-accurate and efficient in performance in alerting parents during temperature rise.	[35]
22	Cuffless wearables for recording blood pressure	The software prototype continuous non-invasive arterial blood pressure monitoring (CNAP2GO) showed excellent results in 42 patients having surgery	[36]
23	Non-invasive method of monitoring blood glucose and blood pressure	Increased performance in transmitting and storing the massive raw Photoplethysmogram (PPG) signals using adaptive IoT model (cloud, fog and hybrid computing) for BP and blood glucose monitoring.	[37]
24	Sensor for detecting the level of aldehyde, an airway irritant in asthma patients.	Effective and continuously monitors the aldehyde exposure level of asthma patients over time-Miniaturized, low powered electronics-longer battery retention	[38]

(*Continued*)

Table 3.1 List of developments in IoT enabled healthcare solutions. (*Continued*)

S. no.	Application field	Evaluation	Reference
25	In-home healthcare services - (iMedBox)- intelligent medical box	Improved user experience and service efficiency with enhanced connectivity and interchangeability for the integration of devices and services	[39]
26	Smart phone application for diabetes self-care and management	Real time monitoring, ease and comfort in measurement, alert systems and effective for remote applications.	[40]
27	Smart phone integrated -wristband device for detecting pulse and physical movements, monitoring blood oxygen and blood pressure.	Easy to wear, accurate to detect, and easy to operate.	[41]
28	Detection of falls using android application enables with accelerometer data	Easily adapted for the collection and analysis of data, remote monitoring and accuracy in measurement.	[42]
29	Sensors for decision making, deep learning and effective communication	Better accuracy than state-of-the-art systems, improved quality of healthcare service, time saving and cost effective.	[43]

(*Continued*)

Table 3.1 List of developments in IoT enabled healthcare solutions. (*Continued*)

S. no.	Application field	Evaluation	Reference
30	Wearable sensors in body for transferring physiological signals to a nearby gateway instead of the cloud service.	Possess better functionality, lesser consumption of energy using multicore processors.	[44]
31	Blood glucose monitoring and Insulin dosage management using sensors	Energy efficient, accurate and lesser expenditure.	[45]
32	Sensor for real-time glucose level measurement, detecting body temperature and contextual data.	Effective monitoring remotely in real-time, energy harvesting system with management of power and energy saving.	[46]
33	Vocal disorder detection using auditory mechanism in human.	accurate and reliable, effective in diagnosis of remote patients.	[47]
34	Sensor for remote gait impairment monitoring	Wearable devices using remote gait impairment monitoring-significantly higher performance and more feasible.	[48]
35	Wrist sensor for monitoring heart conditions	Effective and real time monitoring for a long term, lower power consumption and more accuracy.	[49]

(*Continued*)

Table 3.1 List of developments in IoT enabled healthcare solutions. (*Continued*)

S. no.	Application field	Evaluation	Reference
36	Body weight management	Completely home centric model, performs with low operational cost and lower work intensity feature and increases reliability.	[50]
37	Contact-less and free of label method for tumor surgery	Operating surgeon enabled controlled *in vivo* Identification of Glioblastoma Tumor.	[51]
38	Disease diagnosis using IoT	99% accuracy, effective and reliable than the traditional methods.	[52]
39	Non-invasive method "Cavitas sensors"	Stable, real-time and better management of dental patients- for monitoring glucose from saliva.	[53]
40	*In situ* perspiration analysis model - diagnostic and physiological monitoring applications.	Integrated sensor array that is flexible mechanically, proved to collect a detailed data and long-term functionality.	[54]
41	Non-invasive pacifier using the saliva of infant.	Portable, non-invasive, baby friendly, single pacifier platform, easy to use and effective.	[55]
42	Physical condition monitoring of construction workers using sensors.	Continuous error free monitoring, provides rich information on management of the workloads and physical requirement.	[56]

(*Continued*)

Table 3.1 List of developments in IoT enabled healthcare solutions. (*Continued*)

S. no.	Application field	Evaluation	Reference
43	Diagnosis of retinopathy caused by diabetes and glucose level identification using contact lenses.	Feasible, effective, accurate and non-invasive technique.	[57]
44	Detection of heart and kidney disease.	93.5% accuracy, lesser miss rate in classification.	[58]
45	Remote healthcare monitoring using an IoT-based real-time remote healthcare monitoring (IoT-RRHM) framework	Secure and effective in preventing data loss or breaching attacks-utilizes random oracle model.	[59]
46	Waste management in COVID infected patients.	Better wastage handling, improved quality of service, waste collection and routing process	[60]
47	IoT for Identification of COVID infection	Time saving, improved healthcare service and low cost of diagnosis and treatment.	[61]
48	Protection of healthcare professions prone to COVID patients using DBCMS	Significant control of infection spread, ease and promptness in operation-(Drone Based Covid-19 Medical Service)	[62]
49	IoT based people-monitoring scheme for identifying symptoms of disease and contain its further spread.	Accepted level of accuracy in prediction, effective and feasible prediction of disease transmission by tracking infected patient's movements.	[63]

(*Continued*)

Table 3.1 List of developments in IoT enabled healthcare solutions. (*Continued*)

S. no.	Application field	Evaluation	Reference
50	IoT based visualization of usage of medical tools and instruments in specific surgery procedures.	Visualization and better clarity in procedures, enhanced safety in operation, optimal usage of the surgical tools, creation of standardized procedures for surgeries.	[64]

3.3 IoT Accelerating the Integration of Healthcare and Hygiene for Medical Applications

The role of healthcare and hygiene are together important for a healthy and quality life. Good and efficient healthcare system ensures a disease free and healthy life [65]. Better hygiene leads to the prevention of spread of infections, diseases and is responsible for maintaining the quality of healthcare system. Advancements in IoT technology has provided promising solutions in hygiene related issues [66]. As much as healthcare has been influenced by IoT smart technology, hygiene practices and monitoring has also been greatly impacted. An intelligent system enabled by IoT includes monitoring cleanliness in hospitals and public gathering places, developments of sensors in commonly used prime points like door handles, knobs, seatings, handrails, dispensers, wash areas and accessories [67]. Another important factor in hygiene is the monitoring of dust level and air quality. The sensor deployed in the prime points in hospital premises and the IoT technology gather data. This collected data is then analyzed and a report is then generated for deciding on the action and practices to be performed. This approach plays an important role especially during emergencies, and prevents spread of infections to the people in the hospital [68]. A typical air quality monitoring consists of different types of sensors and their deployments at selected prime points, a centralized controlled and unit of remote monitoring as shown in Figure 3.4 [68]. This system integrates the sensors for dust monitoring, air quality monitoring and cleanliness monitoring to produce a final report for each parameter [68]. The framework performs on the following steps for each parameter monitoring namely,

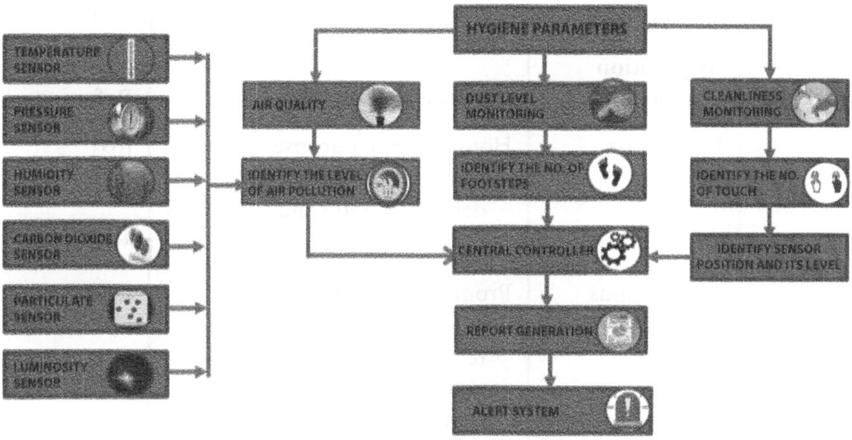

Figure 3.4 Framework of hygiene monitoring system.

- Deployment of sensors for
  - Touch count measurement and monitoring using sensor deployment at commonly used points (prime points).
  - Count of people inflow in hospital premises using sensors in door handles or knobs.
  - Air monitoring in specific places of hospital
- Measurement and data collection
  - Reading touch data for cleanliness and Reading number of footsteps data for dust level
    - If a particular pre-set threshold level is reached, the identity and location is read and collected.
    - Organized information of the various sensor identities and locations is prepared.
    - Implementation of alerts using alarm system for collecting data in the concerned zone by the zone in charge.
  - Reading level of pollutant gases (CO_2 and NO_2) for air quality
  - Check if the maximum permissible level is reached and identify the factors causing the contamination.
  - Perform measures to reduce the level of gas by alarm generation for ventilation and cleaning the surrounding air.
- Generation of report on daily basis and analysis for further action and improvements.

Some of the examples of commercial healthcare applications supporting health and hygiene are tabulated below (Table 3.2).

Table 3.2 Commercially available hygiene supporting healthcare applications.

S. no.	Application area	Purpose and outcome	Reference
1	Floorbotics	Housekeeping purposes & sanitized cleaning, assists delivery of food and medicines to the infected patients	[69]
2	Clean Hands Safe Hands	Promote fitness and safety through the usage of Wi-Fi technology, sensor-activated stations and sanitation reminders.	[70]
3	Differential Pressure Transmitter	Entrap pathogens using negative air pressure to prevent the spread of the virus into the hallway and beyond	[71]
4	Washroom/ Restroom Management System	controls restroom cleanliness and enhances restroom service, plenty like kitchen or restroom management. observe wetness, allow visits with a special ID, deploy touchscreens to document cleanliness complaints, screen air quality, remote control temperature, and light, optimize and monitor the use of toiletries, send vacancy alerts,	[72]
5	Automated visitor management system	permits monitoring and recording of visitor information, establishes a touch-free environment, facilitates booking or reservations based on workplace occupancy, and timely isolation of a person with the potential to transmit illness	[73]

Hence it is always important to realize that practicing hygiene on daily basis is of utmost importance, and it is now more important than ever since the COVID-19 epidemic has captured the attention of the entire globe. The Internet of Things offers the right capabilities at the right moment for no-contact applications and remote connectivity, all of which enable more hygienic health management.

3.4 Challenges in IoT Enabled Healthcare

IoT has an enormous potential in revolutionizing and enhancing technology with manyfold-benefits improving results in various applications. Nevertheless, it is also equally essential in analyzing the pitfalls associated to these IoT based healthcare services. Most importantly intended users should have availability of the IoT service in terms of accessibility, cost-effectiveness in owning the personalized devices, awareness and familiarity with the operational interface along with an uninterrupted broadband network. Further, the interoperability and the robustness of the IoT solution are also essential in recommending the solution for implementation. Similarly planning for any IoT app development for healthcare solution also comes with decision on the costs of availing and maintain the personalized systems. This would prove worthy considering the effectiveness of the solution and the service provided. Some of the issues to be addressed are represented in Figure 3.5 and discussed below.

3.4.1 Data Security, Privacy and Quality

Medical data are confidential and personal. These data are more vulnerable to breaching and are susceptible to loss due to hackers, malicious and technical reasons. Since data are captured in real time, many lack adherence to the standards and protocol of data. A lot of ambiguity persists on the data regulation and ownership and hence are prone to thefts and exposed to cybercriminals [74]. Similarly, data quality due to noise can be affected during data transmission. Efficient noise elimination methods and better architecture can help in resolving these issues.

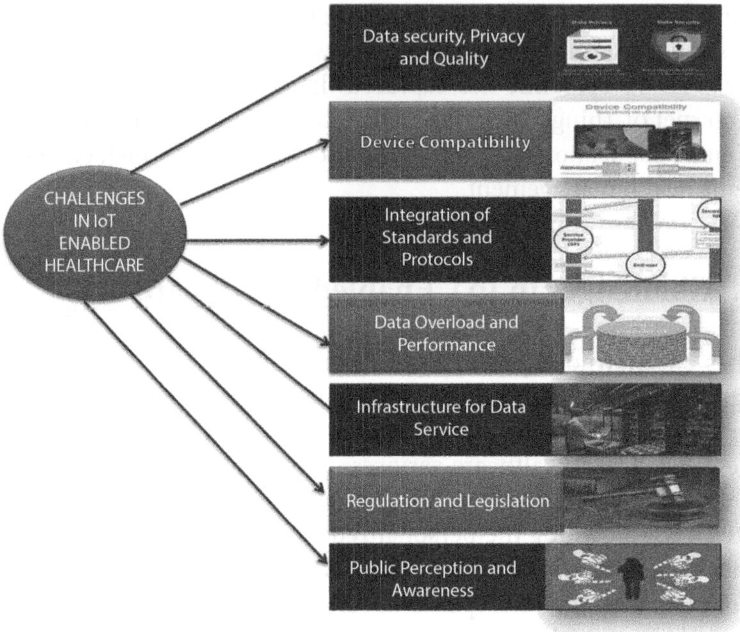

Figure 3.5 Challenges in IoT-based healthcare solutions.

3.4.2 Device Compatibility and Integration of Standards and Protocols

Operation of several devices requires device compatibility which otherwise could lead to performance issues and compromise on the security features. Moreover, interconnection and operation of devices would be effective only with a proper communication standards and synchronous protocol for operation and data collection. These deviations and non-uniformity in the performance will reduce the accuracy of the results and the further expansion of the IoT service gets limited [75].

3.4.3 Data Overload and Performance

IoT collects large and important data from several sources in real time. Data aggregation without an appropriate protocol for data collection, architecture for data segregation, processing and analysis can lead to accumulation of huge data leading to overloading. In the long run, this unsegregated data masses will hamper the decision making in healthcare, can cause delays in the patient treatments and services and would lead to the failure of the IoT solution [76].

3.4.4 Infrastructure Requirements for Data Service

IoT platforms are vast and have several softwares and hardwares as the functional units. The IoT ecosystem requires connectivity to enable communication between the devices and the interface of the technology is the web-based application of the IoT System. Cloud computing for data storage and access is again an integral part of the Internet of Things infrastructure. All of the above components operate at a very large network of locations and involve several and highly complicated web of communication channels and protocols. Establishing and maintaining such a huge infrastructure is again a question of the need of the IoT solution, its performance efficiency and outcome, the beneficiaries and the cost involved in its implementation. Moreover, the system requires higher energy consumption for its operation and processing due to the huge number of sensors and devices in the application leading to the increase in cost [77].

3.4.5 Regulation and Legislation

Any technological advancement happening must be compliant with the rules and regulation pertain to its usage and application. The risks in the data loss and misusages are again a matter of liability. The strong legislative process, extremely high security standards and protocols adhering to the regulation are a mandate for a safer technology [78].

3.4.6 Public Perception and Awareness

IoT technology is a huge and ever-growing market. The complexity in its networking and transparency plays a key role in impacting the perception of people. Clarity of the solution provider, the framework of the service, familiarity in the interface and application are important characteristics that create and modify customer opinions. The overall improvement in the patient heath and the quality of the service would help in increasing the trust on the healthcare professional and the service provider. Misleading customers can be a threat to the data security. Similarly, adherence to regular and planned response and cooperation from the end user (patient) is a must for obtaining a complete solution and better experience of the healthcare [79].

3.5 Conclusion

Modern and emerging technologies are making a huge impact in the healthcare and services domain. This chapter has reviewed the comprehensive details on the different aspects of the healthcare and hygiene based IoT systems. It provides information on the current applications of healthcare based IoT (HIoT) devices. The primary aim of this study is to demonstrate the enabling role of IoT in improving the quality and effectiveness of healthcare technology and the services to patients. The chapter has extensively covered some of the significant developments in the medical fields in terms of information and service accessibility, connectivity, ease in utilization of healthcare infrastructure, comfortable and patient-friendly experience in utilizing the health related IoT enabled medical services. Recent IoT trends on smart devices like wearables, sensors, personalized and community-based healthcare services, Mobile IoT along with cloud computing and advanced communication technology has remarkably transformed the remote monitoring of health data within shorter response times. This is a life-saving technology for people suffering from chronic illnesses, those requiring emergency life-saving treatment and the elderly healthcare industry, where the technology has alert systems for availing medical assistance and self-monitoring features and reminders to maintain and surveillance for a healthy lifestyle. A strong emphasis on hygiene along with healthcare has been laid which together would synchronously improve the overall healthcare system. The fact that both healthcare and hygiene could harness the benefits in terms of effective treatment outcomes, sustained and reliable health care has been reviewed with several real time examples of IoT based solutions.

This chapter also discusses the scope for future research in the technology focusing on the major challenges of the Healthcare based IoT (HIoT) technology. The need to address the various security issues, establishing standards and protocols for data collections and transmission would pave way for a safer and secured medical system. These lacunae will form the basis of research focus and further developments in future. The content gives an in-depth understanding and profound insights of HIoT devices, operation and various smart IoT platforms and architectures and explored the impact and significance of these technical solutions in bring into existence of a smart healthcare facility enabled with improved diagnosis and proactive treatment plans, increased accuracy and better treatment outcomes, accessibility to one's medical information and patient friendly framework.

References

1. Devendra, S., Himanshu, P., Virendra, S., Devandra, P., The Role of IoT in Healthcare Services: An extensive Review, in: *Internet of Things and Data Mining for Modern Engineering and Healthcare Applications*, B. Ankan (Ed.), pp. 1–51, CRC Press-Taylor and Francis, Chennai, 2023.
2. Haipeng, P., Ye, T., Jurgen, K., Lixiang, L., Yixian, Y., Daoshun, W., Secure and energy-efficient data transmission system based on chaotic compressive sensing in body-to-body networks. *IEEE Trans. Biomed. Circuits Syst.*, 11, 3, 558–573, 2017.
3. Singh, A., Chatterjee., Securing smart healthcare system with edge computing. *Comput. Secur.*, 108, 102353, 2021.
4. Lisetti, C., Nasoz, F., LeRouge, C., Ozyer, O., Alvarez, K., Developing multimodal intelligent affective interfaces for tele-home health care. *Int. J. Hum.-Comput. Stud.*, 59, 1-2, 245–255, 2003.
5. Yin, Y.H. and Xing, C., Bioelectrochemical control mechanism with variable-frequency regulation for skeletal muscle contraction - Biomechanics of skeletal muscle based on the working mechanism of myosin motors (II). *Sci. China Technol. Sci.*, 55, 2115–2125, 2012.
6. Sadat, S., Fardis, M., Geran, F., Dadashzadeh, G., Hojjat, N., Roshandel, M., A compact microstrip square-ring slot antenna for UWB applications. *IEEE Antennas Propag.*, 67, 4629–4632, 2006.
7. Javaid, M. and Khan, I.H., Internet of Things (IoT) enabled healthcare helps to take the challenges of COVID-19 Pandemic. *J. Oral. Biol. Craniofac Res.*, 11, 2, 209–214, 2021.
8. Psiha, M.M. and Panayiotis, V., IoT applications with 5G connectivity in medical tourism sector management: third-party service scenarios. *Adv. Exp. Med. Biol.*, 989, 141–154, 2017.
9. Siddique, L., Junaid, Q., Shahzad, F., Muhammad, A.I., How 5G wireless (and concomitant technologies) will revolutionize healthcare? *Future Internet*, 9, 93, 2017.
10. O'Brolcháin, F., de Colle, S., Gordijn, B., The ethics of smart stadia: a stakeholder analysis of the Croke Park project. *Sci. Eng. Ethics*, 25, 3, 737–769, 2019.
11. Bikash, P., Saugat, B., Kunal, P., IoT-Based Applications in Healthcare Devices. *J. Healthcare Eng.*, 2021, 18, 2021.
12. Yan, Y., Qi, L., Heping, L., Xuejun, Z., Lei, W., A home-based health information acquisition system. *Health Inf. Sci. Syst.*, 1, 12, 2013.
13. Qi, J., Yang, P., Min, G., Amft, O., Dong, F., Xu, L., Advanced internet of things for personalised healthcare systems: a survey. *Pervasive Mob. Comput.*, 41, 132–149, 2017.
14. Kashani, M.H., Madanipour, M., Nikravan, M., Asghari, P., Mahdipour, E., A systematic review of IoT in healthcare: Applications, techniques, and trends. *J. Netw. Comput. Appl.*, 192, 103164, 2021.

15. Wang, H., Kadry, S.N., Raj, E.D., Continuous health monitoring of sportsperson using IoT devices based wearable technology. *Comput. Commun.*, 160, 588–595, 2020.
16. Abdul, A.A.G., Mostafa, S.M., Ammar, A., Tarek, S., Elhadi, M.S., Internet of Things based multiple disease monitoring and health improvement system. *J. Ambient Intell. Humaniz. Comput.*, 11, 1021–1029, 2020.
17. Seyed, F.A., Hamid, M., Mohammad, S., Periz-Lopez, P., LACO: Lightweight Three-Factor Authentication, Access Control and Ownership Transfer Scheme for E-Health Systems in IoT. *Future Gener. Comput. Syst.*, 96, 410–424, 2019.
18. Akhbarifar, S., Javadi, H.H.S., Rahmani, A.M., Mehdi, H., A secure remote health monitoring model for early disease diagnosis in cloud-based IoT environment. *Pers. Ubiquit Comput.*, 27, 697–713, 2020.
19. Faruk Aktas, C.C., IoT-Based Healthcare Framework for Biomedical Applications. *J. Med. Biol. Eng.*, 38, 966–979, 2018.
20. Farman Ali, S.R.-J., Type-2 fuzzy ontology–aided recommendation systems for IoT–based healthcare. *Comput. Commun.*, 119, 138–155, 2018.
21. Munish Bhatia 1, S.K., Internet of things-inspired healthcare system for urine-based diabetes prediction. *Artif. Intell. Med.*, 107, 101913, 2020.
22. Elsts, A., Fafoutis, X., Woznowski, P., Tonkin, E., Oikonomou, G., Robert Piechocki, I.C., Enabling Healthcare in Smart Homes: The SPHERE IoT Network Infrastructure. *IEEE Commun. Mag.*, 1, 164–170, 2018.
23. Mehdi Hosseinzadeh, J.K., A diagnostic prediction model for chronic kidney disease in internet of things platform. *Multimed. Tools Appl.*, 80, 16933–16950, 2021.
24. Huang, P., Guo, L., Li, M., Fang, Y., Practical Privacy-Preserving ECG-Based Authentication for IoT-Based Healthcare. *IEEE Internet Things J.*, 2929087, 9200–9210, 2010.
25. Pavleen, K., Ravinder, K., Munish, K., A healthcare monitoring system using random forest and internet of things (IoT). *Multimed. Tools Appl.*, 78, 19905–19916, 2019.
26. Bala, A.M., Sivaparthipan, C.B., Manogaran, G., Sundarasekar, R., Seifedine, K., Shanthini, A., Antony, D., IOT based wearable sensor for diseases prediction and symptom analysis in healthcare sector. *Peer Peer Netw. Appl.*, 13, 2123–2134, 2020.
27. Qiu, T., Liu, X., Han, M., Li, M., Zhang, Y., SRTS: A Self-Recoverable Time Synchronization for sensor networks of healthcare IoT. *Comput. Networks*, 129, 481-492, 2017.
28. Garg, L., Chukwu, E., Nasser, N., Chakraborty, C., Garg, G., Anonymity Preserving IoT-Based COVID-19 and Other Infectious Disease Contact Tracing Model. *IEEE Access*, 4, 159402–159414, 2020.
29. Wu, T., Wu, F., Qiu, C., Redouté, J.M., Yuce, M.R., A Rigid-Flex Wearable Health Monitoring Sensor Patch for IoT-Connected Healthcare Applications. *IEEE Internet Things J.*, 7, 6932–6945, 2020.

30. Min, W.W., Lee, J.W., Park, K.H., A reliable IoT system for Personal Healthcare Devices. *Future Gener. Comput. Syst.*, 78, 626–640, 2018.
31. Sargunam, B. and Anusha, S., IoT based mobile medical application for smart insulin regulation. *International Conference on Electrical, Computer and Communication Technologies (ICECCT)*, Coimbatore, India, 20 Feb, 2019, IEEE, pp. 1–5.
32. Sunny, S. and Swapna, K.S., Optical based non-invasive glucometer with IoT. *International Conference on Power, Signals, Control and Computation (EPSCICON)*, Thrissur, India, 14 June, 2018, IEEE Xplore, pp. 1–3.
33. Ota, H., Chao, M., Gao, Y., Wu, E., Li-Chia, T., Chen, K., Matsuoka, Y., Iwai, K., Fahad, H.M., Gao, W., Nyein, H.Y.Y., Lin, L., Javey, A., 3D printed "Wearable" smart devices for real-time detection of core body temperature. *ACS Sens.*, 2, 990–7, 2017.
34. Gunawan, I.P.C., Andayani, D.H., Triwiyanto, T., Yulianto, E., Rahmawati, T., Soetjiatie, L., Musvika, S.D., Design and development of telemedicine-based heartbeat and body temperature monitoring tools. *IOP Conference Series: Materials Science and Engineering*, vol. 850, p. 012018, 2020.
35. Zakaria NA, S.F., IoT (Internet of Things) based infant body temperature monitoring. *2nd international conference on biosignal analysis, processing and systems (ICBAPS)*, Kuching, Malaysia, 24 July, 2018, IEEE, pp. 148–153.
36. Xin, Q. and Wu, J., A novel wearable device for continuous, non-invasion blood pressure measurement. *Comput. Biol. Chem.*, 69, 134–7, 2017.
37. Guntha, R., IoT architectures for noninvasive blood glucose and blood pressure monitoring. *9th International Symposium on Embedded Computing and System Design*, Kollam, India, 13 December, 2019, IEEE, pp. 1–5.
38. Li, B., Dong, Q., Downen, R.S., Tran, N., Jackson, J.H., Pillai, D., Zaghloul, M., Li, Z., A wearable IoT aldehyde sensor for pediatric asthma research and management. *Sens. Actuators, B.*, 287, 584–94, 2019.
39. Yang, G., Li, X., Matti, M., Zhou, X., Pang, Z., Xu, L.D., Kao-Walter, S., Chen, Q., Li-Rong, Z., A health-IoT platform based on the integration of intelligent packaging, unobtrusive bio-sensor, and intelligent medicine box. *IEEE Trans. Ind. Inf.*, 10, 4, 2180–91, 2014.
40. Istepanian, R.S., Casiglia, D., Gregory, J.W., Mobile health (m-Health) for diabetes management. *Br. J. Health Care Manage.*, 23, 102–8, 2017.
41. Zhang, Y., Cui, J., Kai, M., Chen, H., Zhang, J., A wristband device for detecting human pulse and motion based on the internet of things. *Measurement*, 163, 108036, 2020.
42. Mauldin, T.R., Canby, M.E., Metsis, V., Anne, H.H.N., Rivera, C.C., SmartFall: A smartwatch-based fall detection system using deep learning. *Sensors*, 18, 3363, 2018.
43. Amin, S.U., Hossain, M.S., Muhammad, G., Alhussein, M., Rahman, A., Cognitive smart healthcare for pathology detection and monitoring. *IEEE Access.*, 7, 10745–53, 2019.

44. Hamza, D., Desi, M.A., Issam, B., Amira, A., Bensaali, F., Christos, K., Politi, E., Mara, N., George, D., Real-time ECG monitoring using compressive sensing on a heterogeneous multicore edge-device. *Microprocess. Microsyst.*, 72, 102839, 2020.
45. Gia, T.N., Imed, B.D., Ali, M., Amir, M.R., Tomi, W., Pasi, L., Hannu, T., Energy efficient fog-assisted IoT system for monitoring diabetic patients with cardiovascular disease. *Future Gener. Comput. Syst.*, 93, 198–211, 2020.
46. Gia, T.N., Ali, M., Imed, B.D., Amir, M.R., Tomi, W., Pasi, L., Hannu, T., IoT-based continuous glucose monitoring system: A feasibility study. *Proc. Comput. Sci.*, 109, 327–334, 2017.
47. Ali, Z., Hossain, M.S., Ghulam, M., Arun, K.S., An intelligent healthcare system for detection and classification to discriminate vocal fold disorders. *Future Gener. Comput. Syst.*, 85, 19–28, 2018.
48. Matthew, A.D. and Brodie, M.J., Wearable pendant device monitoring using new wavelet-based methods show daily life and laboratory gaits are different. *Med. Biol. Eng. Comput.*, 54, 663–674, 2015.
49. Shi, W.Y. and Chiao, J.-C., Neural network based real-time heart sound monitor using a wireless wearable wrist sensor. *IEEE Dallas Circuits and Systems Conference (DCAS)*, pp. 1–4, 2016.
50. Alturki, R., Alharbi, A., II, AlQahtani, S.S., Khan, S., Hoang, V.T., A Proposed Application for Controlling Overweight and Obesity within the Framework of the Internet of Things, in: *Intelligent Data Analytics for Internet of Things-Based Applications*, pp. 1–9, 2019.
51. Fabelo, H., Halicek, M., Ortega, S., Shahedi, M., Szolna, A., Piñeiro, J.F., Sosa, C., O'Shanahan, A.J., Bisshopp, S., Espino, C., Márquez, M., Hernández, M., Carrera, D., Morera, J., Callico, G., Sarmiento, R., Fei, B., Deep learning-based framework for *in vivo* identification of glioblastoma tumor using hyperspectral images of human brain. *Sensors*, 19, 4, 920, 2019.
52. Alotaibi, M. and Alotaibi, S.S., Optimal disease diagnosis in the internet of things (IoT) based healthcare system using energy efficient clustering. *Appl. Sci.*, 12, 8, 3804, 2022.
53. Takahiro., A., Yusuke, K., Hiroki, N., Prem, C., Koji, T., Shin-ichi, S., Shuhei, T., Toshiak, S., Kazunari, A., Shunsuke, M., Kohji, M., Mouthguard biosensor with telemetry system for monitoring of saliva glucose: A novel cavitas sensor. *Biosens. Bioelectron.*, 84, 106–111, 2016.
54. Gao, W., Emaminejad, S., Nyein, H.Y.Y., Challa, S., Chen, K., Peck, A., Fahad, H.M., Ota, H., Shiraki, H., Kiriya, D., Lien, D.H., Brooks, G.A., Davis, R.W., Javey, A., Fully integrated wearable sensor arrays for multiplexed *in situ* perspiration analysis. *Nature*, 529, 7587, 509–514, 2016.
55. Carmona, L.G., Martin, A., Sempionatto, J.R., Escarpa, A., P. Biosensor: Toward Noninvasive Saliva Biomarker Monitoring. *Anal. Chem.*, 91, 13883–13891, 2019.
56. Hwang, S. and Lee, S., Wristband-type wearable health devices to measure construction workers' physical demands. *Autom. Constr.*, 83, 330–340, 2017.

57. Keum, D.H., Kim, S.K., Koo, J., Lee, G.H., Jeon, C., Mok, J.W., Mun, B.H., Lee, K.J., Kamrani, E., Joo, C.K., Shin, S., Sim, J.Y., Myung, D., Yun, S.H., Bao, Z., Hahn, S.K., Wireless smart contact lens for diabetic diagnosis and therapy. *Sci. Adv.*, 6, 17, 1–12, 2020.
58. Malibari, A.A., An efficient IoT-Artificial intelligence-based disease prediction using lightweight CNN in the healthcare system. *Meas.: Sens.*, 26, 100695, 2023.
59. Krittibas Parai, S.H., IoT-RRHM: Provably secure IoT-based real-time remote healthcare monitoring framework. *J. Syst. Archit.*, 138, 102859, 2023.
60. Krittibas, P. and Hafizul Islam, S.K., IoT based smart waste management system in aspect of COVID-19. *J. Open Innov. Technol. Market Complexity*, 138, 100048, 2023.
61. Singh, R., Javaid, M., Haleem, A., Suman, R., Internet of things (IoT) applications to fight against COVID-19 pandemic. *Diabetes Metab. Syndr.*, 14, 4, 521–524, 2020.
62. Mohit, A., Manju, B., Sukhvinder, S.B., Rajbir, K., Prabhdeep, S., An internet of things assisted drone-based approach to reduce rapid spread of COVID 19. *J. Saf. Sci. Resilience*, 1, 1, 31–35, 2020.
63. Said, O., A Large-Scale IoT-Based Scheme for Real-Time Prediction of Infectious Disease Symptoms. *Mobile Netw. Appl.*, 28, 1–19, 2023.
64. Ushimaru, Y., Takahashi, T., Souma, Y., Yanagimoto, Y., Nagase, H., Tanaka, K., Miyazaki, Y., Makino, T., Kurokawa, Y., Yamasaki, M., Mori, M., Doki, Y., Nakajima, K., Innovation in surgery/operating room driven by Internet of Things on medical devices. *Surg. Endosc.*, 33, 10, 3469–77, 2019.
65. Matthew, C., Freeman, M., Cumming, O., Jeandron, A., Higgins, J.P.T., Wolf, J., Prüss-Ustün, A., Bonjour, S., Hunter, P.R.,., Fewtrell, L., Curtis, V., Systematic review: Hygiene and health: systematic review of handwashing practices worldwide and update of health effects. *Trop. Med. Int. Health*, 19, 8, 916, 2014.
66. Bal, M. and Abrishambaf, R., A system for monitoring hand hygiene compliance based-on Internet-of-Things. *IEEE International Conference on Industrial Technology (ICIT)*, pp. 1348–1353, 2017.
67. Lenglet, A., Deursen, B., Viana, R., Abubakar, N., Hoare, S., Murtala, A., Keller, S., Inclusion of Real-Time Hand Hygiene Observation and Feedback in a Multimodal Hand Hygiene Improvement Strategy in Low-Resource Settings. *JAMA Netw. Open*, 2, 8, e199118–e199118, 2018.
68. Bevish, J.Y., Joshua, T.J., Priestly, S.B., Internet of Things Enabled Approach for Hygiene Monitoring in Hospitals. *4th International Conference on Computer, Communication and Signal Processing (ICCCSP)*, Chennai, India, 29 September 2020, IEEE Xplore, pp. 1–5.
69. Canedo, D., Fonseca, P., Georgieva, P., Neves, A.J.R., An Innovative Vision System for Floor-Cleaning Robots Based on YOLOv5. In: Pinho, A.J., Georgieva, P., Teixeira, L.F., Sánchez, J.A. (eds) Pattern Recognition and Image Analysis, 13256, 378-389, 2022.

70. Fox, C., Wavra, T., Drake, D., Mulligan, D., Bennett, Y., Carla, N., Kirkwood, P., Louise, J., Bader, M.K., Use of a Patient Hand Hygiene Protocol to Reduce Hospital-Acquired Infections and Improve Nurses' Hand Washing. *American Journal of Critical Care : an official publication, American Association of Critical-Care Nurses*, 24, 216-224. 2015.
71. Xuanrui, C., Li, C., Ma, X., Shao, X., Differential pressure control method for pharmaceutical cleanrooms under variable air supply conditions. *Build. Environ.*, 213, 108849, 2022.
72. Mohammad, M.R., Gahangir, H., Rajab, C., Maher, R., iRestroom: A smart restroom cyber infrastructure for elderly people. *Internet Things*, 19, 100573, 2022.
73. Jose Naldrix, D. and Rivera, V.M.S., Support: A mobile-based support to computerized visitor management system. *Software Impacts*, 8, 100056, 2021.
74. Sun, W., Cai., Z., Li., Y., Liu, F., Fang, S., Wang., G., Security and privacy in the medical internet of things: A review. *Secur. Commun. Netw.*, 2018, 1–9, 2018.
75. Catarinucci, L., An IoT-Aware architecture for smart healthcare systems. *IEEE Internet Things J.*, 2, 6, 515–526, 2015.
76. Thilakarathne, N., Mohan, K.K., Thippa, R.G., The Role of the Internet of Things in Health Care: A Systematic and Comprehensive Study. *Int. J. Manage. Sci. Eng. Manage.*, 10, 4, 145–59, 2020.
77. Ziegeldorf, J.H., Morchon, O.G., Wehrle, K., Privacy in the internet of things: Threats and challenges. *Secur. Commun. Netw.*, 7, 12, 2728–2742, 2013.
78. Mitchell, M. and Kan, L., Digital technology and the future of health systems. *Health Syst. Reform.*, 5, 2, 113–20, 2019.
79. Kelly, J.T., Campbell, K.L., Gong, E., Scuffham, P., The Internet of Things: Impact and Implications for Health Care Delivery. *J. Med. Internet Res.*, 22, 11, e20135, 2020.

4

Self-Powered, Flexible, and Wearable Piezoelectric Nanocomposite Tactile Sensors with IoT for Physical Activity Monitoring

Arjun Hari M.* **and Lintu Rajan**

Department of Electronics and Communication Engineering, National Institute of Calicut, Kozhikode, Kerala, India

Abstract

Self-powered, flexible, and wearable piezoelectric sensors can be applied for physical activity monitoring. Most wearable sensors now available have significant limitations: they need continuous power sources and regular maintenance. Piezoelectric self-powered sensors can be used; however, they are ineffective because of their intrinsic non-polar phase, requiring a high-voltage poling process. This chapter investigates the piezoelectric enhancement of PVDF functional material for wearable sensors by adding different nanoparticles, which act as a self-polarization technique. Incorporating nanoparticles can help functional materials to enhance the piezoelectric characteristics of PVDF. The composite layers were then characterized using SEM, EDS, FTIR, and DC-EFM to evaluate the structure, morphology, thermal and piezoelectric properties. Wearable sensors with sandwich structures were fabricated using thin-film technologies due to their low cost, easy fabrication, and adaptability. After a separate experimental investigation of the mechanical properties to match the human skin, a PDMS packaging layer was introduced on the sensor surface for protection. The data collected can be transmitted to faraway locations using Internet of Things (IoT) technology. The technological advancement of the IoT has made it possible to monitor health conditions and wirelessly communicate the real-time status of patients to clinical professionals. Thus, the IoT strategy has developed a new category of piezoelectric composite materials, stretchable devices, integration strategies, and wireless communication

**Corresponding author*: a.arjunhari@gmail.com

Hari Murthy, Marta Zurek-Mortka, Vinay Jha Pillai and Kukatlapalli Pradeep Kumar (eds.) Internet of Things in Bioelectronics: Emerging Technologies and Applications, (69–88) © 2024 Scrivener Publishing LLC

mechanisms for intelligent healthcare monitoring systems. With the improvement of self-powered sensor characteristics, the proposed system allows clinical practitioners to regularly check on health, vital signs, and bodily functions without physically interacting with them.

***Keywords*:** Wearable tactile sensors, piezoelectric sensors, PVDF composites, IoT, healthcare management, physical activity monitoring

4.1 Introduction

Physical activity (PA) monitoring is a leading health indicator crucial for healthcare management among individuals with chronic health conditions. Continuous monitoring of the health status is essential, even when the patients are in their remote environment. Such regular monitoring, aggregation, and effective analysis can bring positive health transformation and promote a healthier lifestyle, improving the quality of life of the affected individual [1]. A wearable and intelligent tactile sensing system that can detect and monitor physiological parameters and real-time physical activities is thus essential in the context mentioned above. Wearable sensor systems comprise sensor elements, data acquisition units, transmission, and analysis modules. Thus, a low-cost, non-invasive wearable sensor could be developed for recording the electrophysiological information produced by humans [2].

Advances in information and communication technologies have opened up possibilities that allow transmission of the detected data through the Internet, providing more data interoperability options. Thus, the development of a flexible wearable sensing system requires the integration of several disciplines, including biomedicine, materials science, control science, and communication technology. The power consumption, biocompatibility, and sensitivity-related problems have significantly hampered the widespread acceptance of flexible and wearable sensors [3]. Impaired manual dexterity is one of the most displayed unhealthy physical symptoms. A thorough investigation of contact and bending forces while holding and grasping is carried out for detection and monitoring. Physiological measurements that can be interfaced with skin surfaces or human body organs have been of interest over decades, as evidenced by the increasing research and development effort in this area [4]. Wearable and flexible technological devices are sensitive and robust, attracting much research interest in IoT-based healthcare systems. Flexible, stretchable, repeatable, robust, self-powered, and lightweight wearable sensors are required for the application [5]. Wearable technology provides a non-intrusive technique incorporating sensor elements into wearable human accessories like clothing, bracelets, and shoes [6]. Arruda *et al.* used textile sensors in the healthcare sector for physical activity monitoring. A conductive ink is used for the electrodes, which passes information on the physical activity details of the body [7].

The Internet of Things (IoT) can be utilized in the healthcare sector to enhance the lives of numerous individuals. The introduction of IoT enhances treatment by lowering the likelihood of human error. The IoT has the potential to enable a variety of medical applications, such as remote wellness tracking, training regimens, controlling chronic illnesses, and elderly support. Compliance with therapy and medication at home and by healthcare providers is another significant prospective of IoT applications [8–10]. As a result, various sensor elements, medical tools, and detection and imaging instruments can be used as smart devices or products that are critical components of the IoT-based system. IoT-based healthcare monitoring aids medical professionals in both early diagnosis and the entire course of treatment. Recent developments in the IoT sector have made it possible to track the physical activity of patients in real-time situations, which was not at all possible just a few years ago. This development also allows efficient doctors to serve more patients concurrently and cost-effectively. A significant number of advancements in cloud computing have also increased the effectiveness of this IoT-based physical activity monitoring system. Healthcare services based on IoT are expected to reduce treatment costs with improved quality [11].

Despite the advantages indicated above, the IoT-based healthcare system has several areas for improvement. The most noted challenges include performance, quality, repeatability, and robustness of the sensor elements, power consumption and system maintenance, and data security of the cloud network [12]. Flexible and wearable technology can be employed in healthcare management systems to track physical activity and manage various health concerns effectively. Technological improvements over the years have made the development of flexible and wearable tactile sensor devices with improved sensing mechanisms. Several sensing mechanisms, device and material structures, and their preparation methodologies were optimized for further development. Several principles have been adopted, like capacitive, piezo resistive, piezoelectric, and optoelectronic methods. However, most of these wearable devices are mainly powered by an external source, creating additional challenges such as limited sensor competence, higher power consumption, frequent power checks, replacements, and increased structural complexity [13].

Piezoelectric and triboelectric wearable sensors are drawing massive attention due to their self-powering nature, which makes the sensing units work independently without the help of external power sources, and thus operational longevity can be improved further [14]. The triboelectric effect is especially prone to device sensitivity concerns induced by static electricity and heat changes. As a result, the piezoelectric technique, which creates a voltage in reaction to applied external forces, may be a preferable option in sensors for human interaction.

Polyvinylidene fluoride (PVDF) is an ideal piezoelectric material for developing wearable sensors primarily due to its excellent thin film-forming capability. PVDF has a significantly more flexible structure with a carbon chain as its basic skeleton and can be used in areas where twisting and bending are required [15]. Also, PVDF is chemically and thermally stable with low permittivity and wide frequency response as a sensing element for tactile sensing due to its low cost, flexibility, and bio-compatibility. Even though PVDF possesses five different phases, the β-phase with all-trans conformation is suitable for wearable sensor applications. When developed, PVDF will remain in its non-piezoelectric α-phase and requires extra transformation steps to convert into β-phase. A nanoparticle-involved β-phase transformation mechanism enables the selection of PVDF as the priority functional material for wearable sensors [16]. Mahanty *et al.* [17] developed a PVDF-based IoT system for healthcare monitoring. The PVDF was doped with MWCNTs, and then a high-level mechanical stretching was performed to improve piezoelectric properties. Dai *et al.* [18] developed a multifunctional sensor system with PVDF in combination with gold (Au) and polyethylene naphtalate (PAN) for IoT systems. The system was able to deliver a stable performance with stable response and operation.

Proper selection of nanoparticles and their preparation methods are to be considered while fabricating wearable sensors using PVDF-based nanocomposites. The initial section of this chapter investigates the piezoelectric enhancement while adding various nanocomposites to the PVDF. The later section evaluates the influence of particle size on the polar phase enhancement of the nanocomposite materials. The nanoparticles in the PVDF act as nucleating centers of a crystalline phase, enhancing the PVDF piezoelectric properties [19]. The addition of a large weight fraction of fillers into the PVDF matrix is usually done to improve the piezoelectric coefficient, but it affects the uniform distribution and flexibility [20]. Effective particle size reduction can avoid the complex poling process and opens the way for designing advanced and susceptible tactile sensor arrays using low-cost micro-fabrication techniques [21].

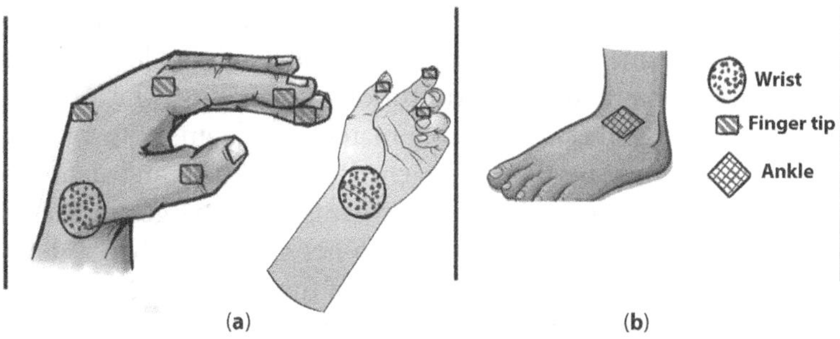

Figure 4.1 Schematic of wearable sensors at (a) hand (b) limb for physical activity monitoring.

Electrical, thermal, and piezoelectric properties of the sensor films with different nanoparticles are conducted, and the film with the optimized parameters and piezoelectric properties is selected for sensor fabrication. After the sensor film optimization, a separate study on the mechanical properties of the encapsulation layer is conducted. The encapsulation of the wearable sensor is equally important as it acts as a protective layer that prevents the sensor from deviating from its original working condition. In addition, the encapsulation layer should be robust, flexible, and biocompatible [22]. PDMS has the properties mentioned above with excellent adhesion and can be glued to any material for support. PDMS structure and softness are similar to human tissues with low Young's modulus value [23].

In this chapter, a comprehensive analysis was performed to fine-tune the sensitivity of the PVDF-nanocomposite-based wearable sensors for physical activity monitoring. In addition, the sensitivity variation of sensor films with the particle size variation of filler materials was also explored. The optimized wearable sensor elements can be attached to the body parts (as shown in Figure 4.1), and the physical activity data can be monitored through IoT. Thus, a flexible self-powered wearable sensor for physical activity monitoring was developed for IoT-based healthcare systems. The improvements presented in this chapter help the researchers working in this area to adapt for further application.

4.2 PVDF-Based Nanocomposites for Tactile Sensing

PVDF is a non-toxic semi-crystalline polymer material widely used for wearable sensors due to its mechanical and piezoelectric properties of thin films, like flexibility, chemical resistance, and bio-compatibility. The dielectric's large value keeps the signal-to-noise ratio as low as possible. The material also has a low glass transition temperature. The low value of glass transmission makes it a flexible material at room temperature. The wearable sensors may be tightly attached to the body, and deformation happens to the film due to body movements. The charges in the PVDF materials are in a balanced state, with no net charges. When a deformation happens on the material, the balance of the charges gets affected, and hence, a net charge will appear on the sides of the crystals. Thus, a voltage is generated by any mechanical action on the PVDF material. A polarization shift happens inside the PVDF material due to the geometric deformation; thus, a charge is created on the material surface. The amount of charge generated depends on the deformation, and using this principle, PVDF can be employed in thin-film-based wearable sensors. Depending upon the chain conformations, PVDF exhibits five different crystalline phases referred to as α (TGTG|), β (TTTT), γ (TTTGTTTG|), ε and ε. Among the five crystalline phases, the β-phase shows the maximum amount of piezoelectricity due to the largest moment of dipoles. The phase content should be improved for applying PVDF material in wearable sensing scenarios. PVDF materials are in the non-polar phase in their pure form.

The external transformation technique is often required to convert the PVDF material from non-polar α to polar β-phase. It effectively develops the piezoelectric nature by creating nucleation sites in the host polymer matrix (PVDF). Mechanical stretching, high-temperature annealing, high-voltage electrical polling, and nanoparticle addition are the various methods for phase improvement. Among the available phase transformation methods, nanoparticle addition can be effectively used for phase transformation, as it does not involve any complex procedures that destroy the material. All other phase transformation process possesses a risk factor of losing the quality of film even after the complete fabrication.

Over the years, various methods of including nanoparticles have been explored to improve the piezoelectric nature and to optimize the nanocomposites for improved sensitivity and power. Research has been developing PVDF-based nanocomposites with various nanoparticles like lead zirconate (PZT), barium titanate ($BaTiO_3$), titanium oxide (TiO_2), zinc oxide (ZnO), and nano-silica (SiO_2). The presence of lead in the PZT makes it unusable for biomedical applications. The preparation methods for the nanocomposite thin films also affect the piezoelectric improvement. Therefore, careful selection of preparation should be adopted for the fabrication.

4.3 Internet of Things (IoT) for Health Care: System Architecture

The Internet of Things (IoT) is a concept that depicts a networked collection of everyone at any moment, at any place, and on any network. Among the most exciting IoT applications are those related to medicine and healthcare services. The system architecture for healthcare monitoring systems using IoT includes a data acquisition, data transmission, and cloud processing unit. The arrangement of the system is shown as a block diagram (Figure 4.2). The Data acquisition unit contains the wearable piezoelectric tactile sensing unit that can sense body movements. With the wearable sensor tightly tied to human bending joints or knees, a stretch-induced voltage generation happens, and the data could be shared with the controller unit. The tactile data from various body movements have specific voltage patterns with a representative range. These data are communicated to a microcontroller unit, and the controller acts as the intelligent unit that controls the whole system. Arduino UNO microcontroller is used, and the data transmission unit sends the acquired tactile data to the cloud server through the ESP-8266 Wi-Fi module. ESP-8266 contains an inbuilt SOC and works on TCP/IP protocol to send the tactile information to the cloud server through the Internet. The cloud processing unit consists of a storage unit that stores the data received over the Internet from the sensor unit [24]. Thing Speak open IoT cloud platform is selected to store and transmit the data to healthcare professionals at remote locations [25].

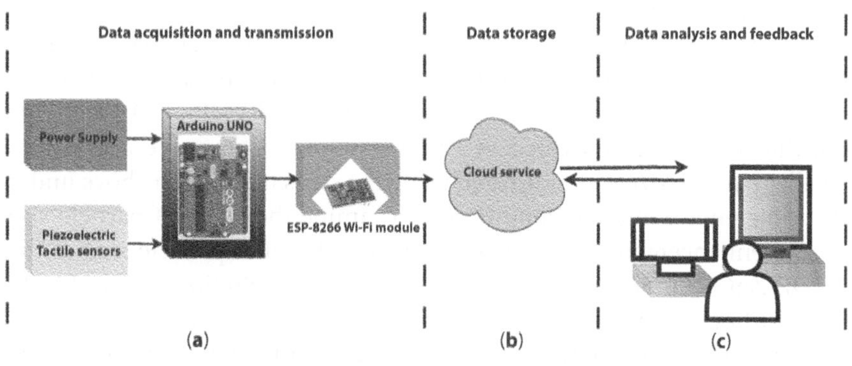

Figure 4.2 Block schematic of piezoelectric tactile sensor-based physical activity monitoring system using IoT.

4.4 Experiments

The wearable tactile sensors are connected to the human body, and the data can be observed through the oscilloscope. A piezoelectric PVDF nanocomposite layer layered between copper electrodes and sealed inside a PDMS layer serves as a single sensor element of the wearable sensor. The piezoelectric sensor layer deforms when a contact force changes the polarization of the surface. This leads to a voltage being induced on the film under the applied external pressure or twist, and the acquired tactile data is communicated to distant locations over the Internet.

4.4.1 Sensor Film Fabrication

PVDF-based nanocomposite films were fabricated by the solvent casting method. PVDF in its powder form (Alfa Assar-Fischer Scientific) and N, N dimethyl formamide (Sigma Aldrich) as solvent were used to create the solution. Nano silica (SiO_2), Titanium dioxide (TiO_2), and Zinc Oxide (ZnO) nanoparticles were selected and added separately into the PVDF mixture to develop nanocomposite sensor films. The sensor film fabrication starts with mixing nanopowder (3 wt%) with the DMF, followed by probe sonication for around 10 minutes. The sonication is done for the uniform spread of nanoparticles in the solvent.

Further, the PVDF powder (10 wt%) was added into the solution accordingly and then bath sonicated for around 30 minutes. The mixture is then kept for magnetic stirring at room temperature for around three hours. This step will prevent agglomeration of the particles in the solution, as agglomeration may affect the flexibility of the sensor. Then, the nanocomposite solution is poured into the glass mold with the utmost care, vacuum-dried for four hours at 60° C, and kept overnight in a vacuum. The dried film was then separated from the mold and then annealed at 120° C for two hours to improve piezoelectric properties. Thus, the nanocomposite sensor films (PVDF- SiO_2, PVDF-ZnO, and PVDF- TiO_2) with 100 μm thickness were fabricated. A PVDF-ZnO nanocomposite film with a smaller particle size was fabricated using the steps mentioned above under the same environmental conditions to examine the effect of particle size on the enhancement of piezoelectric properties. The particle size of the PVDF-ZnO composite was selected as 20 nm. In addition, a neat PVDF film (without any nanofiller) was also fabricated later for comparison purposes without nanoparticle addition. The schematic of the nanocomposite sensor film solution preparation is shown in Figure 4.3.

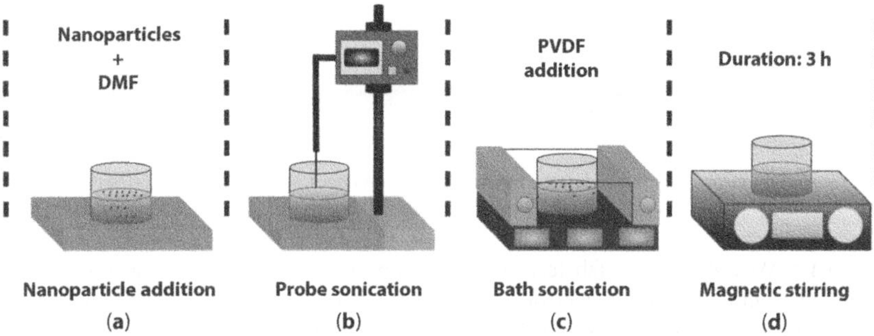

Figure 4.3 Schematic of nanocomposite solution preparation for sensor film fabrication (a) nanoparticles are mixed with DMF solvent (b) probe sonication for 10 minutes (c) PVDF addition into the solution and bath sonication for 30 minutes (d) magnetic stirring for 3-hour duration at room temperature.

a. Packaging Layer Preparation

The packaging layer should be introduced above the PVDF nanocomposite layer for protection from external environmental variations. The packaging layer selection should not affect the overall flexibility of the sensor array. The layer should be compatible with PVDF and offer robustness to the design. The proportion of the base with the curing agent should be carefully selected to match human skin's properties. The proportion of the mixture was varied and selected based on the results presented in Table 4.1. The solution preparation starts with mixing the base and curing agent in a glass beaker, followed by the solution's degassing and then drying.

b. Tactile Sensor Assembly and Packaging

Sensor assembly starts with dicing the PVDF nanocomposite layer with the required dimensions. Bendable copper sheets were thoroughly cleaned and, dried and attached tightly with the sensor film. The sensor assembly was then kept in a mold, and the PDMS mixture was poured onto the sensor surface. Degassing of the mixture was performed in a vacuum for around 25-30 minutes to remove any air bubble traps. The curing was then done at 120° C for 30 minutes. A transparent and flexible packaged layer

Table 4.1 Tensile properties of packaging PDMS layer.

Ratio	10.0.5	10.0.7	10.1
Elastic Modulus (MPa)	0.385	0.853	1.373

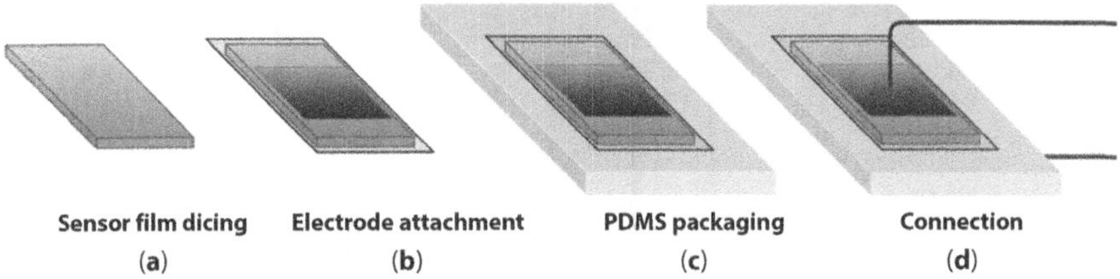

Figure 4.4 Wearable sensor fabrication steps and packaging using PDMS layer (a) dicing of the sensor film (b) copper electrode attachment to the sensor film (c) packaging the sensor using PDMS layer (d) establishing external connection leads.

was thus created using the PDMS layer. The sensor fabrication and fabrication steps are presented in the Figure 4.4.

c. Sensor Characterization

The morphological features of the PVDF nanocomposites were analyzed and characterized using field emission scanning electron microscopy (FESEM-SU 6600). The uniform distribution of the particles was confirmed with EDS mapping. The information on the polar phase transition can be observed through the Fourier transform infrared (FTIR) spectroscopy (Jasco-4700). Thermal properties of the film were characterized using Differential Scanning Calorimetry (DSC) (DSC Q20 TA) instrument. Enhancement of piezoelectricity was studied using Atomic Force Microscopy (AFM) in the Dynamic Contact Electrostatic Force Microscopy (DC-EFM) mode. The piezoelectric properties of the sensor placed at different joints were analyzed using a mixed signal oscilloscope connected to the sensor module. A tapping force analysis was performed using a vibration apparatus, and the force measurement was calculated using a force-sensitive resistor (FSR) connected to an Arduino UNO board.

d. IoT-Enabled Sensor System Design and Implementation.

The wearable health tracking system consists of the PVDF nanocomposite tactile sensor unit, Arduino UNO microcontroller unit, and Wi-Fi module (ESP-8266) for transmitting data over the Internet. In order to transmit the data through the Internet, a Wi-Fi module is used, which uses TCP/IP protocol to send the acquired sensor data and store it in the cloud storage. The sensor system is attached to the analog pin of Arduino and programmed to perform according to the tactile data received from the PVDF-based sensor units. The microcontroller unit itself powers the Wi-Fi module. The data stored in the cloud storage can be retrieved at any remote location through an open-source cloud storage and management system.

4.5 Results and Discussion

FESEM reveals the structural properties of the PVDF-based composite films (Figure 4.5). The neat PVDF gives a spherulite structure, which is affected by the inclusion of nanoparticles. The composite films exhibit a porous structure with increased surface roughness. The improved surface roughness is due to the nanoparticle addition into the PVDF matrix. The nanoparticle addition creates nucleation sites. A reduced spherulite was observed for PVDF-ZnO with reduced nanoparticle size due to the ability of the fillers to generate more nucleation sites with the reduction of filler size. Thus, the polar phase can be improved using ZnO nanoparticles with reduced size in the PVDF matrix. The integrated EDS mapping confirmed the uniform distribution of the particles in the polymer. The non-uniform distribution of the particles causes the agglomeration of nanoparticles in the polymer and thus reduces the flexibility of the sensor. SEM images of the ZnO nanopowders were also analyzed to observe the particle size variation.

FTIR in the ATR-IR mode was used to analyze the piezoelectric phase improvement of the different nanoparticles. The piezoelectric enhancement was analyzed by observing the β–phase peaks in the FTIR plot corresponding to 840, 1073, 1232, and 1400 cm^{-1}. The symmetric stretching of CF_2 causes the rise in peaks at 840 cm^{-1} and 1073 cm^{-1}, whereas the peak at 1400 cm^{-1} indicates the parallel alignment of dipoles in the composite films. Thus, FTIR results can be used to observe and compare the piezoelectric

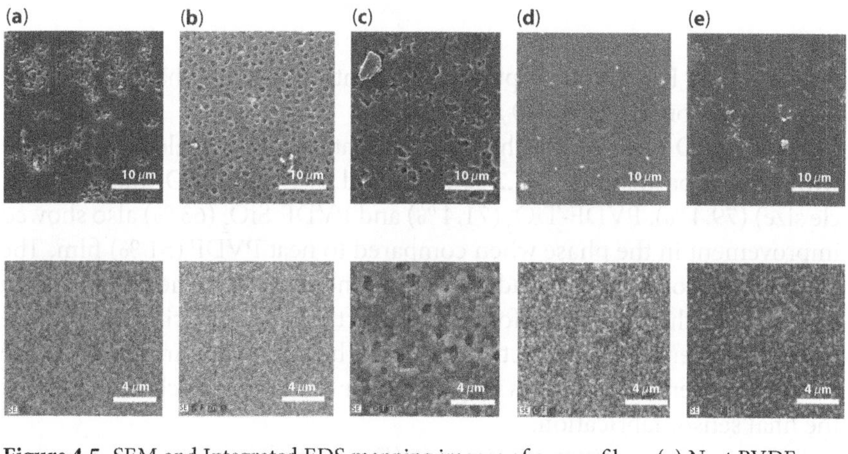

Figure 4.5 SEM and Integrated EDS mapping images of sensor films. (a) Neat PVDF (b) PVDF-ZnO (higher particle size) (c) PVDF-TiO_2 (d) PVDF-ZnO (lower particle size) (e) PVDF-ZnO.

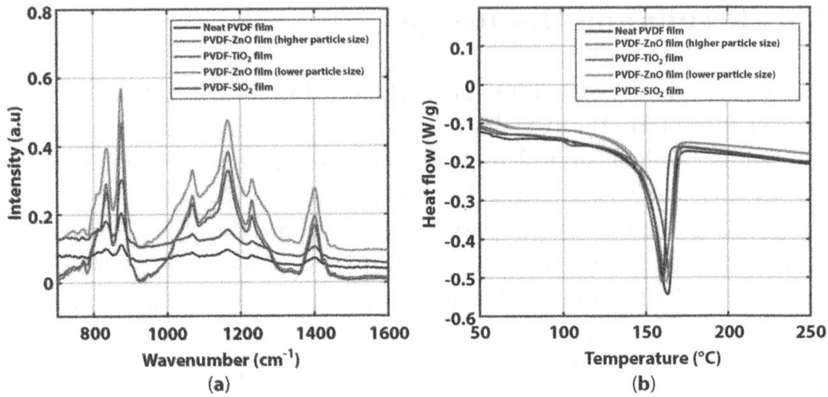

Figure 4.6 (a) ATR-IR spectra showing the piezoelectric improvement with the nanoparticle addition into the PVDF material and (b) DSC curve showing the thermal characteristics.

phase enhancement. The results shown in Figure 4.6 (a) show that the ZnO nanoparticles have an improved piezoelectric phase. Further improvement of the piezoelectric phase was observed by adding ZnO nanoparticles with reduced particle size (20 nm). The content of piezoelectric phase content in the films was analyzed with the equation below [26].

$$F(\beta)=\frac{X_\beta}{X_\alpha+X_\beta}=\frac{A_\beta}{\left(\frac{K_\beta}{K_\alpha}\right)A_\alpha+A_\beta} \tag{4.1}$$

where, K_α and K_β = the absorption coefficients of α and β-phase and A_α and A_β = absorption bands at 740 and 840 cm^{-1}.

PVDF-ZnO showed the highest percentage of piezoelectric β-phase with a lower particle size (87.2 %), followed by PVDF-ZnO (higher particle size) (79.4 %). PVDF-TiO_2 (71.4 %) and PVDF-SiO_2 (63 %) also showed improvement in the phase when compared to neat PVDF (51 %) film. The FTIR results confirmed that adding ZnO nanoparticles to the PVDF matrix can improve the phase transformation effectively. By reducing the particle size of the filler, the piezoelectric phase can be improved further. Thus, the FTIR characterization results help us decide the nanoparticle selection for the final sensor fabrication.

Differential scanning calorimetry (DSC) studies were performed to obtain the thermal properties, and the influence of filler particles on the crystallization was observed. The DSC results are plotted in Figure 4.6(b), and Table 4.2 shows the crystallization values. The variation in melting point originates from the nanoparticle addition, and the melting point variation helps in the improvement of the piezoelectric properties of PVDF nanocomposites. DC-EFM magnitude and phase spectrum were plotted to ensure the improvement obtained during the earlier-mentioned studies (Figure 4.7). The characteristic butterfly diagram was plotted for amplitude, and the amplitude loop shows the piezoelectricity enhancement. The highest amplitude was obtained for ZnO with a smaller particle size, which confirms the result obtained with the other characterization methods. The phase plot of the DC-EFM reveals the polarization reversibility at different

Table 4.2 DSC analysis results of PVDF composite film.

Film	Melting enthalpy (J/g)	Crystallinity (%)
Neat PVDF	50	47.75
PVDF-ZnO (higher particle size)	60.96	60.77
PVDF-TiO_2	51.80	49.97
PVDF-ZnO (lower particle size)	71.06	70.80
PVDF-SiO_2	51.26	48.90

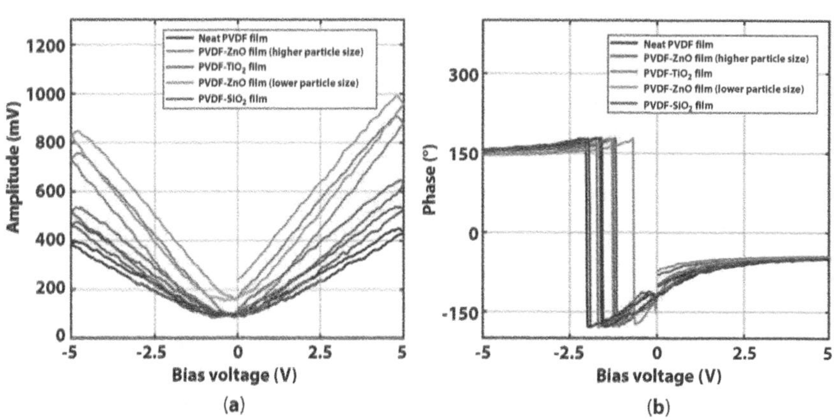

Figure 4.7 DC-EFM (a) amplitude plot showing the butterfly loop (b) phase plot results of nanocomposite films.

bias voltages. The polarization reversibility was observed at 180° for both applied voltage polarities.

From the characterization results, the enhancement of the piezoelectric nature of the nanocomposite sensor films was confirmed, and the fabrication of the sensor was done with the PVDF-ZnO (20 nm) composite, which showed the highest improvement. The mechanical properties of the PDMS layer were examined using the H10KS instrument to identify the close match with human skin (0.42 to 0.85 MPa). Based on the characterization results, a 10:0.7 ratio opted for packaging. The characterization results are plotted in Figure 4.8(a). Universal vibration equipment was used to exert dynamic forces on the top of the developed sensors to evaluate the experimental sensors. A force-sensitive resistor (FSR-402) coupled to an Arduino board was implemented to measure the applied force. For force ranges from 1N to 10 N, the response to tapping forces was recorded and analyzed. When pressure is applied to the sensor surface, dimensional changes occur, causing the material to generate a force-proportional amount of voltage. The generated voltage was observed through a mixed signal oscilloscope (MSO-MSOX3014T). The sensors exhibited a linear response with good repeatability for 400 cycles. The current measurements showed the values in the nA range, which was also improved with the nanoparticle inclusion to the PVDF. The calculated sensitivity of the nanocomposite-based sensor was 123 mV/N for nanocomposite with less particle size. When particle size decreases, the surface area to volume ratio becomes high, and hence, the sensor may give higher sensitivity values. The sensitivity of the device to bending actions was also characterized by

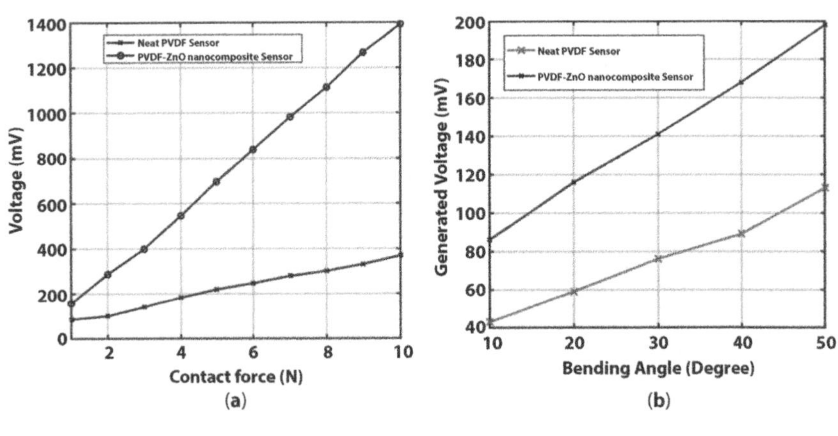

Figure 4.8 Characterization of the sensor for (a) tapping force from 1N to 10 N (b) bending action.

attaching the sensor tightly to the glove. The bending angle was up to 90°, and sensors were characterized for normal and bending actions. The sensitivity of 29 mV/° was obtained for the sensor, and the results are plotted in Figure 4.8 (b). The sensor output to various physical activities are shown in Figure 4.9. The performance of the wearable sensors was compared to that of existing sensors, and a significant improvement in the sensitivity of the sensors reported in this work was observed. Table 4.3 shows a comparison of the outcomes. The piezoelectric enhancement was obtained in PVDF

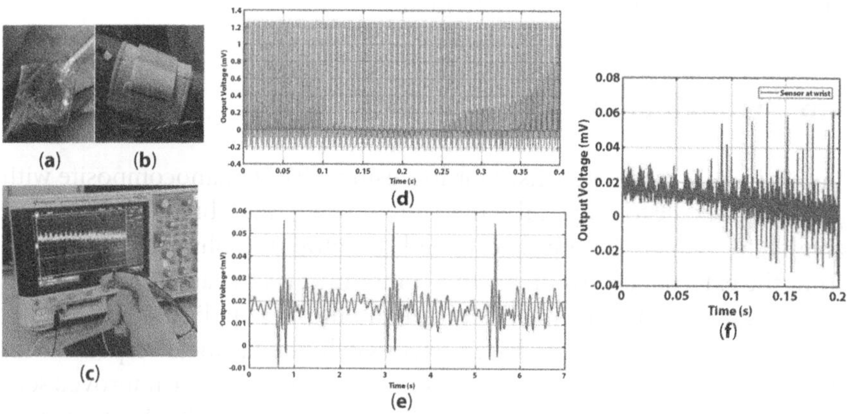

Figure 4.9 (a) Fabricated sensor (b) sensor attached to the body for movement detection (c) finger bending detection (d) tapping response showing repeatability (e) response of wrist movement (f) response of wrist movement.

Table 4.3 Comparison of our work with earlier reported piezoelectric wearable sensors.

Sensor film with concentration	Filler	Filler concentration	Sensitivity	Reference
PVDF (25 wt.%)	$BaTiO_3$	6 wt.%	6 mV/N	[27]
PVDF (17 wt.%)	Ag NM's+ MWCNT's	1.9 wt.% + 2 wt.%	24 mV/N	[28]
PVDF (12 wt.%)	Graphene oxide	0.5 wt.%	38.8 mV/N	[29]
PVDF (16 wt.%)	PAN	64 wt.%	42 mV/KPa	[30]
PVDF (10 wt.%)	ZnO higher particle size	3 wt.%	103 mV/N	This work
PVDF (10 wt.%)	ZnO lower particle size	3 wt.%	123 mV/N	This work

without any electric polling process, and thus, the addition can be considered an effective self-polarization technique.

The wearable sensor system is connected to the Arduino UNO board, and the data generated due to the physical activity like bending/twisting/moving is transmitted to open-source cloud storage through the Internet via the ESP 8266 Wi-Fi module. Thing Speak, an open-source IoT platform, is used for cloud storage, and healthcare professionals can retrieve and analyze data from anywhere in the world. Thus, the PVDF-nanocomposite-based IoT system allows the effective and efficient monitoring and feedback of the physical activity of the individual.

4.6 Conclusion

In this work, a wearable sensor for IoT using a PVDF nanocomposite with a PDMS package for physical activity monitoring was fabricated. The wearable tactile sensor system detects and monitors the physical parameters from the external environment and communicates the acquired data with remote stations in real-time healthcare monitoring applications. The low-cost PVDF-nanocomposite-based sensors exhibited a linear response with high sensitivity for 400 cycles with minimum variations. The improved sensitivity is due to the incorporation of nanoparticles into the PVDF matrix. Using the PDMS layer, the device packaging gives the required protection and enhances the life cycle. Implementing IoT technology for transmitting sensor data to remote locations enabled healthcare professionals to monitor the condition of the patient continuously. As demonstrated, the cutting-edge wearable sensor system with PVDF-nanocomposite expands the potential for self-powered mechanisms. It offers an efficient and practical technique for monitoring physical activities remotely for IoT systems. However, the information security in the cloud network still needs to be fixed. Implementing secure cloud data storage can increase the confidentiality of the data that is being stored. Finally, a highly sensitive wearable sensor system using PVDF-ZnO nanocomposite was fabricated for physical activity monitoring for IoT.

References

1. Qi, J., Yang, P., Waraich, A., Deng, Z., Zhao, Y., Yang, Y., Examining sensor-based physical activity recognition and monitoring for healthcare using Internet of Things: A systematic review. *J. Biomed. Inf.*, 87, 138–53, 2018 Nov 1.

2. Bleser, G., Steffen, D., Reiss, A., Weber, M., Hendeby, G., Fradet, L., Personalized physical activity monitoring using wearable sensors, in: *Smart health: Open problems and future challenges*, pp. 99–124, 2015.
3. Hari, M.A. and Rajan, L., Advanced materials and technologies for touch sensing in prosthetic limbs. *IEEE Trans. Nanobiosci.*, 20, 3, 256–70, 2021 Apr 13.
4. Shores, J.T., Brandacher, G., Lee, W.A., Hand and upper extremity transplantation: an update of outcomes in the worldwide experience. *Plast. Reconstr. Surg.*, 135, 2, 351e–60e, 2015 Feb 1.
5. Nasiri, S. and Khosravani, M.R., Progress and challenges in the fabrication of wearable sensors for health monitoring. *Sens. Actuators, A*, 312, 112105, 2020 Sep 1.
6. Zhang, Y., Cui, J., Ma, K., Chen, H., Zhang, J., A wristband device for detecting human pulse and motion based on the Internet of Things. *Measurement*, 163, 108036, 2020 Oct 15.
7. Arruda, L.M., Design and Testing of a Textile EMG Sensor for Prosthetic Control, in: *Proceedings of the EAI International Conference on IoT Technologies for HealthCare*, Braga, Portugal, pp. 47–61, December 2019.
8. Kashani, M.H., Madanipour, M., Nikravan, M., Asghari, P., Mahdipour, E., A systematic review of IoT in healthcare: Applications, techniques, and trends. *J. Netw. Comput. Appl.*, 192, 103164, 2021 Oct 15.
9. Nazir, S., Ali, Y., Ullah, N., García-Magariño, I., Internet of things for healthcare using effects of mobile computing: a systematic literature review. *Wirel. Commun. Mobile Comput.*, 2019, 1–20, 2019 Nov 14.
10. Krishnamoorthy, S., Dua, A., Gupta, S., Role of emerging technologies in future IoT-driven Healthcare 4.0 technologies: A survey, current challenges, and future directions. *J. Ambient Intell. Hum. Comput.*, 14, 1, 361–407, 2023 Jan.
11. Islam, S.R., Kwak, D., Kabir, M.H., Hossain, M., Kwak, K.S., The Internet of things for health care: a comprehensive survey. *IEEE Access.*, 3, 678–708, 2015 Jun 1.
12. Lopez Martinez, A., Gil Pérez, M., Ruiz-Martínez, A., A Comprehensive Review of the State-of-the-Art on Security and Privacy Issues in Healthcare. *ACM Comput. Surv.*, 55, 12, 1–38, 2023 Mar 28.
13. Ates, H.C., Nguyen, P.Q., Gonzalez-Macia, L., Morales-Narváez, E., Güder, F., Collins, J.J., Dincer, C., End-to-end design of wearable sensors. *Nat. Rev. Mater.*, 7, 11, 887–907, 2022 Nov.
14. Chorsi, M.T., Curry, E.J., Chorsi, H.T., Das, R., Baroody, J., Purohit, P.K., Ilies, H., Nguyen, T.D., Piezoelectric biomaterials for sensors and actuators. *Adv. Mater.*, 31, 1, 1802084, 2019 Jan.
15. Li, J., Zhou, G., Hong, Y., He, W., Wang, S., Chen, Y., Wang, C., Tang, Y., Sun, Y., Zhu, Y., Highly sensitive, flexible and wearable piezoelectric motion sensor based on PT promoted β-phase PVDF. *Sens. Actuators, A*, 337, 113415, 2022 Apr 16.

16. Cao, X., Ma, J., Shi, X., Ren, Z., Effect of TiO2 nanoparticle size on the performance of PVDF membrane. *Appl. Surf. Sci.*, 253, 4, 2003–10, 2006 Dec 15.
17. Mahanty, B., Ghosh, S.K., Maity, K., Roy, K., Sarkar, S., Mandal, D., All-fiber pyro-and piezoelectric nanogenerator for IoT based self-powered healthcare monitoring. *Mater. Adv.*, 2, 13, 4370–9, 2021.
18. Dai, Y., Chen, J., Tian, W., Xu, L., Gao, S., A PVDF/Au/PEN multifunctional flexible human-machine interface for multidimensional sensing and energy harvesting for the Internet of Things. *IEEE Sens. J.*, 20, 14, 7556–68, 2020 Feb 14.
19. Devi, P.I. and Ramachandran, K., Dielectric studies on hybridised PVDF–ZnO nanocomposites. *J. Exp. Nanosci.*, 6, 3, 281–93, 2011 Jun 1.
20. Karumuthil, S.C., Rajeev, S.P., Varghese, S., Poly (vinylidenefluoride-trifluoroethylene)-zno nanoparticle composites on a flexiblepoly (dimethylsiloxane) substrate for energy harvesting. *ACS Appl. Nano Mater.*, 2, 7, 4350–4357, 2019.
21. Hari, M.A., Rajan, L., Subash, C.K., Varghese, S., Effect of nanoparticle size on the piezoelectric properties of PVDF based nanocomposite thin films. *Mater. Today Proc.*, 46, 5781–4, 2021 Jan 1.
22. Panahi, A., Hassanzadeh, A., Moulavi, A., Design of a low cost, double triangle, piezoelectric sensor for respiratory monitoring applications. *Sens. Bio-Sens. Res.*, 30, 100378, 2020 Dec 1.
23. Pawlaczyk, M., Lelonkiewicz, M., Wieczorowski, M., Age-dependent biomechanical properties of the skin. *Adv. Dermatol. Allergol. Postepy Dermatol. Alergol*, 30, 5, 302, 2013.
24. Hassanalieragh, M., Page, A., Soyata, T., Sharma, G., Aktas, M., Mateos, G., Kantarci, B., Andreescu, S., Health monitoring and management using Internet-of-Things (IoT) sensing with cloud-based processing: Opportunities and challenges, in: *2015 IEEE international conference on services computing*, IEEE, pp. 285–292, 2015 Jun 27.
25. Kulkarni, M.B., Goyal, S., Dhar, A., Sriram, D., Goel, S., Miniaturized and IoT enabled continuous-flow-based microfluidic PCR device for DNA amplification. *IEEE Trans. Nanobiosci.*, 21, 1, 97–104, 2021 Jun 25.
26. Parangusan, H., Ponnamma, D., AlMaadeed, M.A.A., Flexible tri-layer piezoelectric nanogenerator based on pvdf-hfp/ni-doped zno nanocomposites. *RSC Adv.*, 7, 79, 50 156–50 165, 2017.
27. Kalani, S., Kohandani, R., Bagherzadeh, R., Flexible electrospun PVDF–$BaTiO_3$ hybrid structure pressure sensor with enhanced efficiency. *RSC Adv.*, 10, 58, 35090–8, 2020.
28. Sang, M., Wang, S., Liu, S., Liu, M., Bai, L., Jiang, W., Xuan, S., Gong, X., A hydrophobic, self-powered, electromagnetic shielding PVDF-based wearable device for human body monitoring and protection. *ACS Appl. Mater. Interfaces*, 11, 50, 47340–9, 2019 Nov 19.

29. Chen, G., Chen, G., Pan, L., Chen, D., Electrospun flexible PVDF/GO piezoelectric pressure sensor for human joint monitoring. *Diamond Relat. Mater.*, 129, 109358, 2022 Nov 1.
30. Mu, J., Xian, S., Yu, J., Zhao, J., Song, J., Li, Z., Hou, X., Chou, X., He, J., Synergistic enhancement properties of a flexible integrated pan/pvdf piezoelectric sensor for human posture recognition. *Nanomaterials*, 12, 7, 1155, 2022 Mar 31.

5

Securing Electronic Health Records (EHRS) in Internet of Things (IoT)-Based Cloud Networking Using Elliptic Curve Cryptography (ECC) with ECIES Algorithm

J. Shyamala Devi[1] and Selvanayaki Kolandapalayam Shanmugam[2]*

[1]*Department of Computer Science and Business Systems, Rajalakshmi Institute of Technology, Chennai, India*
[2]*Department of Mathematics and Computer Science, Ashland University, Ashland, Ohio, USA*

Abstract

The current life of society is revolutionized by the Internet of Things (IoT) by its nature portable, wearable, and implantable and which makes life easier to process any information that can make a huge impact in everyone's life. In the health-care industry, with the increased benefit and applicability of the Internet of Things (IoT), there is a promising need for secure and efficient methods of protecting Electronic Health Records (EHRs). Electronic Health Records (EHR) are secured in IoT-based cloud networking using different basic techniques like Encryption, Authentication, Network Segmentation, Firewall, User access controls, Incident response planning, Compliance with relevant regulations, and regular monitoring and updating security measures. One such method is Elliptic Curve Cryptography (ECC), which provides strong security while requiring less computational power and memory than traditional encryption methods. This chapter aims to detail the use of Elliptic Curve Cryptography in securing Electronic Health Records stored in IoT devices. Remarkably, this chapter discusses the Elliptic Curve Integrated Encryption Scheme (ECIES) algorithm, a hybrid encryption scheme that combines the security of Elliptic Curve Cryptography with symmetric key encryption. This

**Corresponding author*: skolanda@ashland.edu

Hari Murthy, Marta Zurek-Mortka, Vinay Jha Pillai and Kukatlapalli Pradeep Kumar (eds.) Internet of Things in Bioelectronics: Emerging Technologies and Applications, (89–106) © 2024 Scrivener Publishing LLC

chapter acquaints the readers with an overview of Elliptic Curve Cryptography and its advantages over other encryption methods. The introduction of the Elliptic Curve Integrated Encryption Scheme algorithm, its working principles, and the advantages of using the Elliptic Curve Integrated Encryption Scheme in securing EHRs, including its resistance to quantum computing attacks, are also discussed. As the encryption could be done at various levels of Electronic Health Record storage and processing, various steps involved in key generation, encryption, and decryption using the Elliptic Curve Integrated Encryption Scheme algorithm are also detailed in this chapter. The practical implementation of the Elliptic Curve Integrated Encryption Scheme in an IOT-based Electronic Health Records system and the performance of the Elliptic Curve Integrated Encryption Scheme in terms of security, efficiency, and memory usage are also explicitly discussed. This chapter justifies or convinces the readers that Elliptic Curve Integrated Encryption Scheme is a secure and efficient method of securing Electronic Health Records in IoT devices and is well-suited for resource-constrained environments. Also, it is a promising solution for securing Electronic Health Records in resource-constrained environments, and focusing research in this domain has hypothetical chances to improve the security and efficiency of IoT-based Electronic Health Records systems.

Keywords: Internet of Things (IoT), cryptography, encryption, security, quantum computing

5.1 Introduction

Medical knowledge and record-keeping techniques were not as developed in medieval times as they are now. In the past, medical histories, physical examinations, and laboratory testing were not generally recorded in the same depth as they are now. Instead, medical professionals depended on their personal expertise and knowledge as well as that which had been passed down through the years.

The practice of medicine evolved into a profession in the later medieval era, and doctors started keeping their own records. These records, meanwhile, were still quite simple, frequently consisting only of a mention of the patient's symptoms and the remedies that had been attempted. The Tamil civilization also had a rich heritage of medicine and medical expertise during its heyday in South India and Sri Lanka between BCE and CE. Ayurvedic principles served as the foundation for the Siddha medical system, which was used by Siddhars in Tamil.

The majority of medical records were retained as palm-leaf manuscripts that were meticulously preserved and handed down through the centuries. These publications included thorough explanations of numerous medical disorders, along with information on their causes, symptoms, and treatments. The Agastya Samhita, which was written in Tamil in the first century BCE, is the first surviving medical treatise in the language. The human body, including its organs and systems, are thoroughly described in this literature, along with a number of medical interventions, such as surgical techniques and herbal medicines. Other significant Tamil medical writings include the Kural Venba, the Vaithiyam Padi, and the Pothu Marai. These works address a wider range of medical subjects, such as gynecology, pediatrics, and psychiatry [3, 13].

The fact that these medical records frequently included thorough details of the patient's lifestyle and habits in addition to their medical history is a fascinating element of them. This gave doctors the opportunity to create customized treatment programs that took into account the patient's requirements and situation. The invention of the stethoscope and other medical technologies in the 19th century facilitated the development of thorough medical records and more in-depth physical examinations. Medical records, however, were still largely paper-based and frequently challenging to access or transfer between various healthcare practitioners. The creation, storage, and sharing of medical records have changed as a result of the digital revolution in the late 20th and early 21st centuries. Electronic medical records (EMRs) have taken the role of paper-based records, enabling more accurate and efficient record-keeping as well as simpler access to patient data.

Health information exchanges (HIEs) have made it easier for healthcare practitioners to transfer patient data among various systems and locations. Patient safety has increased as a result, and care is now more organized and more efficient. Future technological developments, particularly those in the areas of artificial intelligence (AI) and machine learning (ML), will further transform the world of medical records. With the use of these technologies, healthcare professionals will be able to evaluate massive amounts of data rapidly and precisely, providing patients with efficient and individualized care [1].

5.1.1 Terms Used in Literature

- IoT: Internet of Things
- EHR: Electronic Health Record
- ECC: Elliptic Curve Cryptography
- ECIES: Elliptic Curve Integrated Encryption Scheme
- EMR: Electronic Medical Records
- HIE: Health Information Exchanges

- HIS: Healthcare Information Systems
- PHR: Patient Health Record
- AI: Artificial Intelligence
- ML: Machine Learning
- EPR: Electronic Patient Record
- IDS/IPS: Detection and Prevention Systems
- NAC: Network Access Control
- VPN: Virtual Private Network
- SSL: Secure Sockets Layer
- TLS: Transport Layer Security
- MQTT: Secure Message Queuing Telemetry Transport
- CoAP: Secure Constrained Application Protocol
- Secure SHC: Secure Health Transport
- HIPAA: Health Insurance Portability and Accountability Act
- GDPR: General Data Protection Regulation
- RSA Algorithm: Rivest, Shamir, Adleman Algorithm
- KEM: Key Encapsulation Mechanism

5.2 E-Records in Healthcare

Healthcare facilities use electronic record-keeping systems including EHR, EMR, and EPR. While these factors are similar in some respects, there are several significant differences:

Electronic Health Records (EHRs) are complete archives of a patient's health and medical background. They can contain data from several sources, such as medical records, test results, and prescription histories, and are intended to be shared among healthcare practitioners. EHRs are primarily utilized to assist coordinated treatment among various providers and to offer a complete report on a patient's health status [2].

Electronic Medical Records (EMRs) are digital archives of a patient's medical information from a single healthcare facility, like a hospital or doctor's office. They are used to assist patient care inside a single organization and contain data such as medical history, diagnosis, prescriptions, and test results. EMRs are not frequently shared among many clinicians, in contrast to EHRs [13].

Electronic Patient Records (EPRs) In the same way as electronic health records (EHRs) do, electronic patient records (EPRs) are comprehensive archives of a patient's medical history. The term "EPR" is frequently used synonymously with "EHR," despite the fact that EPRs are primarily used outside of the United States and Canada. Similar to an EMR, the word "EPR" in some countries may be used to refer particularly to a system that is employed within a single healthcare organization.

While all three systems are electronic records of a patient's health history, EHRs are comprehensive records that can be shared among different healthcare providers, EMRs are records from a single healthcare provider, and EPRs are similar to EHRs but are typically used outside of the United States and Canada.

5.3 Why Do We Need EHR? And Why Now?

In this digital world, the usage of the Healthcare Information System (HIS) in the healthcare domain is evident as electronic health or e-health. The tremendous advancement of technology in the field of Data Science, the Internet of Things (IoT), 5G Networks, Web Applications facilitates or supports patient empowerment. This makes most parts of the world digitized, and the healthcare system is not an exception. Also, this brings happiness to people because they can prioritize their needs and build transparent relationships between patients and healthcare organizations. So, digitization of healthcare starts by transferring paper-based health records into e-health records. In the healthcare system, healthcare professionals maintain all the E-Records.

The personal data of any patient, Patient Health Record (PHR), is controlled and secured by either the patient or authorized personnel nominated by the patient. An Electronic Health Record (EHR) is a patient health record stored in an organized record format using computers and computing [5]. The ability to exchange health information electronically helps both patients and healthcare providers with high-quality safety measures. EHR has limitless advantages, and a few to mention are quick/timely access to patient records, handling treatments with feasible medical work progress, fast and reliable prescribing, improved medical decision-making by having consultation possible around the globe, decreased medical expenses, expanded security of patient, etc.

The Electronic Medical Record (EMR) is the medical history of a patient maintained by a single provider, mainly used for diagnosis and treatment. But, both EMR and EHR help both patients and providers make quick decisions and diagnoses.

5.4 Securing EHR in IoT-Based Cloud Networking

The field of Computer science introduced basic security steps to secure Electronic Health Records (EHRs) in the Internet of Things (IoT) based Cloud Networking:

Encryption: EHRs should be encrypted both in rest and transit of data at to protect against unauthorized access and data breaches. This is possible by using secure protocols such as HTTPS and SFTP for data transmission [2].

Authentication: Strong authentication mechanisms should be used to access EHRs and ensure access only by authorized users. This could include multi-factor authentication methods such as biometrics or token-based systems.

Network segmentation: It is advised that network infrastructure be segmented in order to potentially prevent and reduce the consequences of security breaches. This may entail employing virtual private networks (VPNs) to encrypt connections or separating IoT devices and EHR systems on distinct networks.

Firewall: A firewall can be used to protect the network from outside threats and to regulate access to EHRs. This can entail employing Network Access Control (NAC) systems and establishing Intrusion Detection and Prevention Systems (IDS/IPS).

User access controls: Strong user access restrictions should be present in EHR systems to ensure secure access to sensitive data. This might contain capabilities for logging and auditing as well as role-based access controls.

Planning for incident response: To respond swiftly and effectively to security breaches or other incidents, organizations should have incident response strategies in place. This includes instructing staff members on incident response protocols and routinely testing incident response plans.

Compliance: Organizations need to make sure that their EHR systems abide by pertinent laws like HIPAA and GDPR.

Regularly monitoring systems and updating security measures: It is essential to preserve the security of EHRs in IoT-based cloud networks. This is because new threats and vulnerabilities require new security measures to be implemented.

5.5 Role of IoT in Electronic Health Records

Systems for electronic health records (EHRs) have the potential to be considerably improved by the Internet of Things (IoT). IoT can assist EHRs in a number of ways:

Internet of Things (IoT) gadgets like wearable tech, smart home sensors, and mobile health apps can offer quick access to real-time information about a patient's health state that can be incorporated into their EHR. This can let medical professionals observe patients from a distance and decide on treatments with more knowledge. Improvements in patient engagement and self-management are also possible with IoT technology. IoT-enabled gadgets, for instance, can give patients real-time feedback on their health status, enabling them to make better decisions about their care.

IoT devices can be utilized to automatically gather data and communicate it to EHR systems, reducing the need for manual data entry and enhancing the accuracy of EHRs. IoT devices can generate a large amount of data that can be analyzed and used to spot patterns and trends. This can aid medical professionals in forecasting future health consequences and enhancing patient outcomes.

IoT devices can also be utilized to enhance care coordination in various situations. To quickly access and monitor a patient's health and keep track of their medical history, IoT devices can be used to communicate data with hospitals, clinics, and home care providers. Additionally, there are serious security issues that need to be resolved when IoT devices are integrated with EHRs. Data privacy, secrecy, and maintaining data integrity are a few of them. The security and reliability of the IoT devices, as well as the EHR system's ability to secure data originating from them, are critical [7].

5.6 EHR Encryption at Different Levels

Different levels of encryption can be used to protect Electronic Health Records (EHRs) as shown below

File-level encryption: It encrypts individual files or directories with the aid of a particular encryption algorithm. This is a quick and efficient solution for encrypting EHRs at rest since it makes accessing the data when necessary and decrypting the data straightforward.

Full-disk encryption: The entire hard disk or storage device where EHRs are kept is encrypted under this sort of encryption. This approach ensures that all data saved on the device is encrypted and secured, offering a better level of security than file-level encryption.

Database encryption: This method of encryption entails completely encrypting the database that houses the EHRs. Due to the fact that it guarantees that all information saved in the database is encrypted and safeguarded, this technique is especially helpful for EHR systems that employ database management systems.

Virtual disk encryption: Here it entails the creation of an encrypted virtual drive. This approach is advantageous for cloud-based EHR systems since it enables data encryption and cloud storage.

Tokenization: By using a non-sensitive equivalent known as a token instead of sensitive data, such as credit card numbers or Aadhar numbers, this type of encryption can protect sensitive information. Because the sensitive data is not saved on the device but rather a non-sensitive token is, this method offers a higher level of security than file-level encryption.

5.6.1 Encryption Methods

Electronic Health Records (EHRs) can be protected using a variety of encryption techniques while the data is being transmitted:

SSH or TLS: Secure Sockets Layer and Transport Layer Security Secure online communications are made possible by these methods. Between IoT devices and EHR systems, they can be utilized to secure data transmission.

VPN: A Virtual Private Network VPN establishes a safe, encrypted link between two devices, enabling communication as though the devices were both connected to the same network. This technique is effective for securing data sent over open networks like the Internet and can be used to encrypt data exchanged between IoT devices and EHR systems.

Secure MQTT: Mobile devices and small sensors can communicate using the lightweight Secure Message Queuing Telemetry Transport (MQTT) protocol. An addition to MQTT called Secure MQTT adds functionality for secure conversations. Data sent between IoT devices and EHR systems can be encrypted using this method.

Secure CoAP: Constrained Application Protocol (CoAP) is an Internet of Things (IoT)-specific web transfer protocol that is primarily utilized with limited nodes and networks. A CoAP extension that supports secure communications is called Secure CoAP. Data sent between IoT devices and EHR systems can be encrypted using this method.

Secure SHC: Secure Health Transport (SHC) is a protocol created expressly for the safe and dependable transmission of health data over the Internet. It can be used to encrypt data sent between IoT devices and EHR systems and is based on the CoAP and DTLS protocols.

5.7 Elliptic Curve Cryptography

5.7.1 Cryptography Basics

The study of encoding information into a code or cipher that may be sent safely via a communication channel is known as cryptography [8, 9]. It entails developing a safe method of information exchange utilizing mathematical ideas and algorithms.

Encryption: Ordinary text is changed into a coded format that can only be read by someone who has the right decryption key.
Decryption: A secret key is used during the decryption process to transform the encrypted message back into the original message.

5.7.1.1 Types of Cryptography

Symmetric Key Cryptography: Data is encrypted and decrypted using the same key in symmetric key cryptography, also known as private key cryptography. As both the sender and the receiver must have the same secret key, it is typically faster than asymmetric cryptography but necessitates secure key distribution. Because it is effective for bulk data encryption, symmetric encryption is frequently employed for protecting the real data while it is in transit.
Asymmetric Key Cryptography: A pair of keys—a public key and a private key—are used in asymmetric key cryptography, sometimes known as public key cryptography. While the private key needs to be kept a secret, the public key can be freely distributed. This method offers a technique to encrypt messages or securely exchange keys without requiring both parties to possess the same secret key. Insecure key exchange, digital signatures, and secure communication over untrusted networks all require the use of asymmetric cryptography, which is slower than symmetric encryption.
Hash Function: A mathematical function or technique known as a hash function takes an input (or "message") and outputs a fixed-length string of characters, usually a hexadecimal integer. The output is a distinct representation of the input data known as the hash value or hash code. In

computer science and cryptography, hash functions are frequently used for a variety of tasks, including data retrieval, data verification, data integrity, and password storage. A hash function must demonstrate a number of critical properties, including determinism, fixed output length, efficiency, pre-image resistance, collision resistance, and the avalanche effect.

Digital signature: A technique used to authenticate the integrity and authenticity of a digital document or message.

Authentication: The process of verifying the identity of a user or system. In cryptography, authentication is often used to ensure that the recipient of a message is who they claim to be.

The functions and properties of elliptic curves is studied for more than 100 years and their uses in the cryptographic algorithm were proposed in 1985 by Koblitz from the University of Washington and Victor Miller at IBM. It laid and mapped the road for Elliptic Curve Cryptography (ECC), first developed by a mobile electronic business security provider, Certicom. ECC is a public key cryptographic-based algorithm that depends on the algebraic structure of elliptic curves run over finite fields. It helps to perform critical computer security/Information security functionalities which include encryption, authentication, and digital signatures. In ECC, the elliptic curve is a plane curve over a finite field that is relaying on the finite points satisfies the equation,

$$y^2 = x^3+ax+b \tag{5.1}$$

for some constants 'a' and 'b'.

For example, consider any point on the curve in ECC, it is mirrored over the X-axis and the curve stays the same as earlier and any non-vertical line is intersecting the curve in three places or lower. ECC is given in the context of Riverst-Shamir-Adleman (RSA), the frequently used and powerful cryptographic algorithm used in the field of security enhancement. RSA is known for one-way encryption and is used in major applications like emails, data, information, etc. using Prime factorization techniques [12].

ECC allows smaller keys compared to non-EC cryptography algorithms without compromising the security perspectives. ECC is stronger than RSA for key sizes. For Example, the typical key size of 521 bits is equivalent to a 15360 bits RSA key and proves to achieve the same level of security. This clearly states ECC uses less memory when compared to RSA. Also, ECC key generation and signing are considerably quicker than RSA, both encryption and decryption speeds are faster. The core techniques that the

ECC algorithm uses are that private and public keys in ECC are not equally exchangeable like the RSA algorithm. In ECC, the public key is a point that lies on the curve and the private key is an integer value. Also, ECC features very strong protocols for authenticated key exchange, and technical support is most confident. So, the efficient benefits of ECC attract many enterprises to use it in their applications or products nowadays.

ECC has its own limitations, it is tricky and complicated to implement securely on some occasions, and public key operations are considerably slower [12]. The ECC is a little expensive to implement, it is debatable based on the application usage benefits and return values. In general, all newer algorithms might have unknown weaknesses as always.

5.7.2 Key Generation Steps

The encryption process where A is sending a message 'm' which is represented as a point 'M' on the elliptic curve 'Ec'.

1. A randomly selects a number 'k' within the range of [1 - (n-1)], where 'n' is the number of points on the elliptic curve.
2. A chooses a point 'P' on the curve to use in the encryption process.
3. A computes the first ciphertext 'Ct1' using the equation Ct1 = k * P. 'Ct1' is the point on the curve resulting from the multiplication of the random number 'k' and the point 'P'.
4. A computes the second ciphertext 'Ct2' using the equation Ct2 = M + k * Q, where 'Q' is B's public key. 'Ct2' is the point on the curve resulting from adding the point 'M' and the multiplication of the random number 'k' and B 's public key 'Q'.
5. A sends both ciphertexts 'Ct1' and 'Ct2' to B.

5.7.3 Message Encryption and Decryption

The steps involved in generating the public and private keys for B and using them to encrypt and decrypt a message sent by A:

1. B selects a random number 'd' within the range of 1 to n-1, where 'n' is the number of points on the elliptic curve being used for encryption.

2. B chooses a point 'P' on the curve to use in the key generation process.
3. B computes the public key 'Q' using the equation Q = d * P, where 'Q' is the point on the curve resulting from the multiplication of the random number 'd' and the point 'P'.
4. B keeps its private key 'd' secret and securely stores it while sharing his public key 'Q' with A.
5. A wants to send a message to B, so he encrypts the message using B's public key 'Q'.
6. B receives the encrypted message and decrypts it using its private key 'd', which only B knows. This allows B to read the original message sent by A.

B can then decrypt the message using his private key 'd' and the following steps:

- B then calculates the point 'k * Q' by using d which is his private key and the equation k * Q = d * Ct1.
- Next B subtracts 'k * Q' from 'Ct2' to get the point 'M', which is the original message sent by A.

5.7.3.1 *Math Involved in Decryption*

$$M = Ct2 - d * Ct1 \tag{5.2}$$

Substituting 'Ct2 – d * Ct1* for M from Equation (5.2)

$$Ct2 - d * Ct1 = (M + k * Q) - d * (k * P)\ (Ct2 = M + k * Q \text{ and } Ct1 = k * P)$$

$$= M + k * d * P - d * k * P$$

$$= M \text{ (original message)}$$

The above encryption process is called Elliptic Curve ElGamal encryption. It gives integrity and also confidentiality for the message that is being sent. A set of algorithms and procedures used for encryption and decryption is Cipher and the information used to encrypt or decrypt a message is called a key. The study of breaking codes and ciphers is called Cryptanalysis. The above is an example of how elliptic curve cryptography can be used to generate and use public and private keys. There are many different methods and variations of this process, depending on the specific cryptographic algorithm being used.

The usage of ECC in securing EHR is given/discussed by different researchers from different perspectives. Hema and Kesavan [6] portray the importance of e-healthcare current time period, bringing to ensure security through confidentiality and integrity, apparently the overhead time insider threats are convinced. The author Tsai *et al.* briefs out the ECC-based EMR system, ESEMR that could handle medical records in a cloud database, incorporates an integration unit, a smart card, and a portable device that ensures secured data transmission and maintaining critical data quality [11].

In today's market, IoT-based wearable devices are put into use to collect patient medical data and help to send alert messages to healthcare providers/relatives if the patient is at risk or any changes in the normal health situation. One such application is evidenced by Vijayakumar *et al.* in their research paper. Eshraq *et al.* discussed a method to enhance medical data security by combining ECC and Image Steganography. The consideration of ECC for the encryption of medical data provides higher security compared to the earlier methods [4].

The working functionality of ECC [12] for the encryption and decryption of Electronic Health Records (EHRs) is given in the Figure 5.1 below:

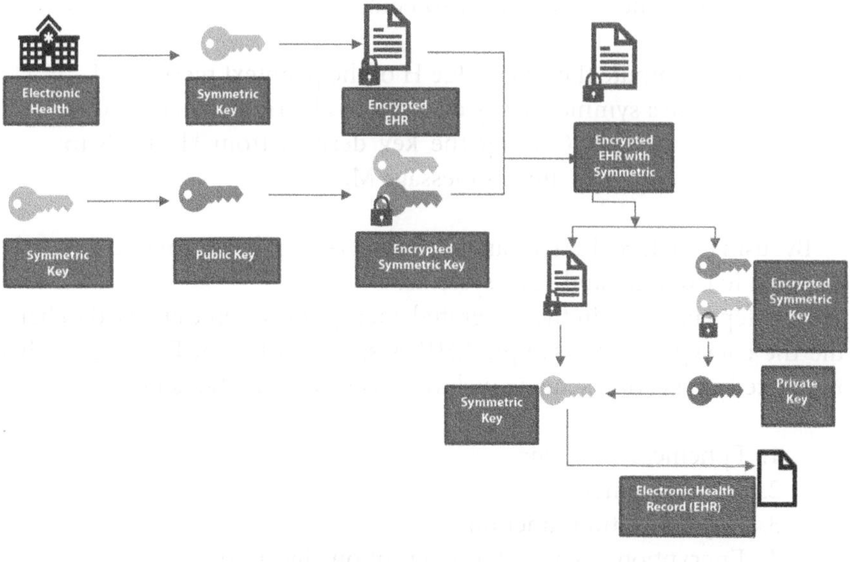

Figure 5.1 ECC encryption/decryption flowchart.

5.8 Elliptic Curve Integrated Encryption Scheme (ECIES)

ECIES combines the Elliptic Curve Diffie-Hellman (ECDH) key agreement protocol with symmetric key encryption to provide a secure and efficient encryption scheme.

The steps in ECIES are as follows:

1. **Key Generation:**
    - Choose an elliptic curve E over a finite field Fp, where p is a large prime number.
    - Choose a base point G on curve E.
    - Choose a random integer d as the private key.
    - Calculate the public key Q = dG.
2. **Encryption:**
    - Choose a random integer k as the ephemeral key.
    - Calculate the shared secret S = kQ.
    - Compute the hash value H of the plaintext message M.
    - Use a symmetric key encryption algorithm, such as AES, to encrypt M using the key derived from H and S.
    - Send the ciphertext C and the ephemeral key k to the receiver.
3. **Decryption:**
    - Use the private key d to compute the shared secret S = kQ.
    - Compute the hash value H of the plaintext message M.
    - Use a symmetric key decryption algorithm, such as AES, to decrypt C using the key derived from H and S to obtain the plaintext message M.

By using ECIES, EHRs can be encrypted and transmitted securely between IoT devices and EHR systems.

The steps involved in the integrated encryption scheme are used to handle the encryption of a sample EHR is shown below in Figure 5.2. This integrated encryption scheme includes the below functions [9].

1. Ephemeral Key Pair
2. Key Agreement
3. Key Derivation function
4. Encryption – Symmetric encryption algorithm

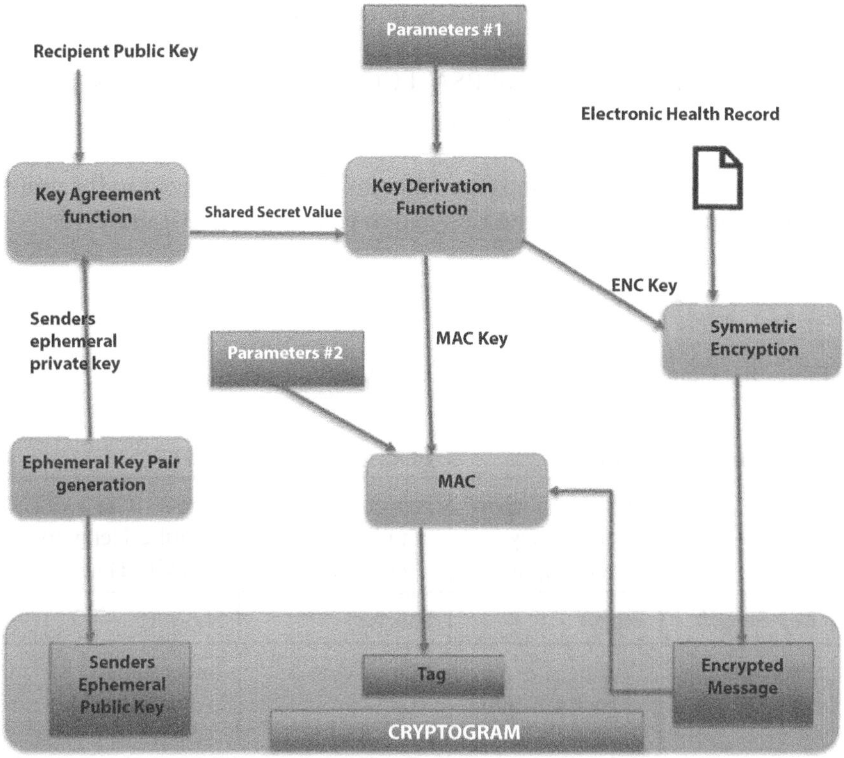

Figure 5.2 ECIES encryption flowchart for EHR.

5. Message Authentication Code (MAC)
6. Hash (HASH)

The main use is the Key Encapsulation Mechanism (KEM) which generates shared keys which are shared between two parties who have never communicated. Based on quantum physics, a model of computing constructed to handle the functionalities/tasks that traditional computers could not handle is called Quantum Computing. The most notable importance of quantum computing is that it could break RSA and ECC algorithms efficiently. In the world of computing, Quantum computing is known for breaking some cryptographic algorithms, mainly RSA, ECC, and ECDSA and so these cryptosystems based on these algorithms are considered quantum unsafe. Cryptographic algorithms like cryptographic hashes, MAC algorithms, and Symmetric key ciphers are quantum-safe [7, 10]. It is apparent that the integration of Quantum Cryptography and

ECC for encryption using ECIES is one of the recommended methods [9, 10].

The comparative analysis of RSA, ECC, and ECIES algorithms is given below in the table by considering the benefits and complexity of the algorithms.

The key length comparisons for different bits are visualized in the graph below, Figure 5.3 to justify the Key-length feature given in Table 5.1.

Table 5.1 Comparison of RSA, ECC, and ECIES.

Algorithm/ features	RSA	ECC	ECIES
Key	Well-established public-key cryptography	Newer public key cryptography	Elliptic -Curve Diffie-Hellman (ECDH) key
Key-Length	Bigger	Shorter	Shorter
Principle	Prime Factorization	Elliptic curves	Integrated Encryption Scheme
Speed	Faster	More time	Differ with clients
Security	Less	Highly Secure	High

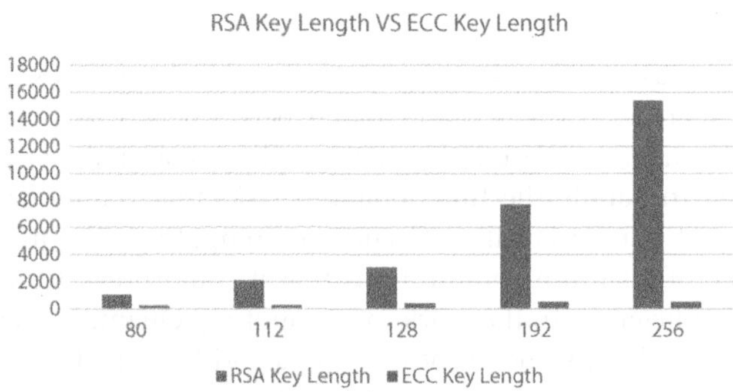

Figure 5.3 RSA vs ECC key length.

5.9 Conclusion

Maintaining Electronic Health Records of patients in the IoT-based cloud environment is highly challenging in terms of the security and privacy of sensitive information. To handle these security and privacy concerns, typical encryption and decryption algorithms are used. This chapter details the encryption methods, cryptography methods, ECC, and its advantages over RSA and ECIES. The different levels of EHR storage and processing and various steps involved in the ECIES algorithm are detailed in this chapter which evidences and gives confidence to the readers that ECC with ECIES algorithm gives recommended security features in EHR in an IoT environment.

References

1. Murala, D.K., Panda, S.K., Sahoo, S.K., Securing Electronic Health Record System using Cloud Environment Using Blockchain Technology, in: *Recent Advances in Blockchain Technology, Intelligent Systems*, 2023.
2. Koran, A. and Prasad, R., IoT Health Data in Electronic Health Records (EHR): Security and Privacy Issues in Era of 6G. *J. ICT Stand.*, 10, 1, 63–84, 2022.
3. Sarath, S., Ramalingam, H.M., Vishaka, M., Swapna, H.R., Swaraj, H., Implementation of a secure and privacy-aware E-Health record and IoT data sharing using Blockchain. *Global Transitions Proc.*, 2, 429–433, 2021.
4. Eshraq, H. and Adnan, G., Enhancing Medical Data Security via Combining Elliptic Curve Cryptography and Image Steganography. *Int. J. Comput. Netw. Secur.*, 20, 8, 2020.
5. Chen., C.-L., Huang., P.-T., Deng., Y.-Y., Chen., H.-C., Wang., Y.-C., A Secure electronic medical record authorization system for smart device applications in cloud computing environments, in: *Human-Centric Computing and Information Sciences*, 2020.
6. Hema, V.S.V. and Kesavan, R., ECC-based secure sharing of healthcare data in the health cloud environment. *Wirel. Pers. Commun.*, 108, 1021–1035, 2019.
7. Badr., S., Gomaa., I., Abd-Elrahman., E., Multi-tier Blockchain Framework for IoT-EHRs Systems. ScienceDirect. *Proc. Comput. Sci.*, 141, 159–166, 2018.
8. Khan., N., Quantum-Elliptic Curve Cryptography for Multihop Communication in 5G Networks. *Int. J. Comput. Netw. Secur.*, 17, 5, 2017.

9. Ahmed, D.E. and Khalifa, O.O., Robust and Secure Image Steganography Based on Elliptic Curve Cryptography. *International Conference on Computer and Communication Engineering*, 2014.
10. Gayoso Martínez, V., Hernández Encinas, L., Sánchez Ávila, C., A Survey of the Elliptic Curve Integrated Encryption Scheme. *Indian J. Comput. Sci. Eng.*, 2, 2, 2010.
11. Bennet, C.H. and Brassard, G., Quantum cryptography: Public key distribution and coin tossing. *Proceedings of the International Conference on Computers, Systems and Signal Processing*, 1984.
12. Tsai., K.-L., Lue., F.-Y., Wu., T.-H., Chiou., S.-S., Liu., Y.-W., Liu., H.-Y., A Secure ECC based Electronic Medical Record System. *J. Internet Serv. Inf. Secur.*, 4, 1, 47–57, 2014.
13. Gobi, M. and Vivekanandan, K., A New Digital Envelope Approach for Secure Electronic Medical Records. *Int. J. Comput. Sci. Netw. Secur.*, 9, 1, 1–6, 2009.

6

2D Photonic Crystal Nano Biosensor with IoT Intelligence

Balaji V. R.[1], Jesuwanth Sugesh R. G.[2*], Sreevani N.R.G.[3], Shanmuga Sundar Dhanabalan[4], T. Sridarshini[5] and Gopalkrishna Hegde[6]

[1]Centre for Healthcare Advancement, Innovation and Research, Vellore Institute of Technology, Chennai, Tamil Nadu, India
[2]Department of Electronics and Communication Engineering, CHRIST University, Bangalore, Karnataka, India
[3]Department of Computer Science and Engineering, S.A. Engineering College Tamil Nadu, India
[4]Functional Materials and Microsystems Research Group, School of Engineering, RMIT University Melbourne, Victoria, Australia
[5]Department of Electronics and Communication Engineering, College of Engineering Guindy Campus, Anna University, Chennai, Tamil Nadu, India
[6]Centre for Nanoscience and Engineering, Indian Institute of Science, Bengaluru, Karnataka, India

Abstract
Optical biosensors based on photonic crystals (PCs) offer interesting possibilities for the analysis and identification of bioanalytes. PC is a periodically varying artificial dielectric material that determines the propagation of modes present in the structure. Within dielectric media, there are modes that are selected based on structural perturbations. Changes in the refractive index of biological analytes are used to identify biological samples and are therefore used as sensing media in many applications. Because these PC sensors are designed in the nano range, they have excellent selectivity and sensitivity. The PC is ultra-compact and only small amounts of analyte are required for bioanalyte detection. Quantification of bioanalytes and biochemicals is one of the greatest challenges in the medical and diagnostic fields. However, these electronic devices cannot be directly connected

**Corresponding author*: jesuwanth.sugesh@christuniversity.in; ORCID: 0000-0002-2228-8020
Balaji V. R.: ORCID: 0000-0002-9239-7724

Hari Murthy, Marta Zurek-Mortka, Vinay Jha Pillai and Kukatlapalli Pradeep Kumar (eds.)
Internet of Things in Bioelectronics: Emerging Technologies and Applications, (107–124) © 2024 Scrivener Publishing LLC

to biological analytes, so the most difficult task is to extract the analyte information and convert it into electronic signals. Optical biosensors offer an attractive way to interrogate the content of bioanalytes because they directly convert biological events into electrical signals. It is also called a self-contained integrated physical medium because of its many applications such as food industry, drug delivery, point-of-care diagnostic sensing devices, and environmental monitoring. Based on the analyte placed on the PC sensor, resonant wavelengths are observed and the measurements are stored in a database. Diseases are identified based on the current user's cognitive value, and data is transmitted and monitored over the Internet of Things.

***Keywords*:** Photonic crystal, internet of things, bio-analyte, nano biosensor, photonic sensor

6.1 Introduction

In photonic crystals (PCs), the refractive index is periodically modulated, usually by creating periodic arrays of dielectric or metallic materials. This periodicity causes constructive and destructive interference of light waves at specific frequencies, leading to the formation of energy bands. Similar to the electronic band structure in solid-state physics, PCs have allowed and forbidden frequency ranges known as the photonic band and photonic band gap (PBG), respectively. Within the photonic bandgap, the crystal behaves as a perfect photonic isolator, reflecting or trapping light of specific frequencies or wavelengths. This property of the photonic bandgap allows precise control of the luminous flux, enabling a variety of applications [1]. The width and position of the PBG depend on parameters such as PC geometry, refractive index contrast and lattice symmetry. By tuning these parameters, engineers and researchers can tune the properties of PCs to produce specific bandgaps, optical filters [2], waveguides [3], lasers [4], It enables the control and manipulation of light in numerous applications such as sensors [5] and demultiplexer [6]. There are many types of PCs, each with its own structure and characteristics. Here are some well-studied and used types. One-dimensional (1D) photonic crystals: These PCs have periodicity in one dimension. They consist of alternating layers or regions of different refractive materials. Examples include distributed Bragg reflectors (DBRs) and multilayer dielectric stacks. 1D-PC is widely used in optical coatings, mirrors and filters. 2D photonic crystals: These PCs exhibit periodicity in two dimensions. These typically consist of a square or hexagonal grid of holes or rods in high index material. The arrangement of these holes or bars creates a 2D periodic pattern. 2D PC can be used to control the propagation of light in planar waveguides, microcavities, and PC fibers. 3D Photonic Crystals: These PCs are periodic in three dimensions. They consist of periodic arrangements of materials in all three dimensions. 3D PC offers the most comprehensive control over light, including full PBG formation.

Researchers continue to explore new structures and materials to develop PCs with properties tailored for specific applications in fields such as telecommunications, optical computing and sensing. The advantages of 2D PCs over 3D PCs depend on specific applications and requirements. Both types have their advantages and limitations, but the advantages of 2D PCs are that they are easy to manufacture, can be integrated into planar devices, simulate time, and are easy to reason theoretically.

Square or hexagonal grids of holes or bars are common geometries used in the manufacture of 2D PCs. These structures are designed to be periodic in his two dimensions, allowing the manipulation and control of light propagation. A square grid has holes or bars arranged in a repeating pattern of squares. Each hole or bar is surrounded by four adjacent holes or bars to form a square grid. This arrangement results in a simple and regular structure that is relatively easy to fabricate and analyze. Hexagonal grids, on the other hand, consist of holes or bars arranged in a repeating hexagonal pattern. Each hole or bar is surrounded by 6 adjacent holes or bars to create a honeycomb structure. A hexagonal grid has its own advantages: B. Higher packing density and more efficient use of space compared to a square grid. The hexagonal symmetry also enables the formation of circularly symmetric band structures. Both square and hexagonal lattice arrangements have been extensively studied and used in the design of 2D PCs.

6.1.1 Structural Parameter

The two basic topologies of PC slabs are a cubic lattice of silicon (dielectric) rods in air and a triangular lattice of air holes in a solid (silicon) dielectric slab.

1. Square lattice of rods
2. Square lattice of holes
3. Hexagonal lattice consists of holes or rods

A. Cubic Lattice (2D XZ) (Rods in air)
Lattice Constant (a) of lattice: 500 nm
Radius of Silicon (dielectric) rods: 120 nm

Dielectric constant of d rod: 11.56
Height of silicon (dielectric) rods: 5000 nm
Refractive Index (RI) of Rod (n): 3.476
Refractive Index difference (Δn): 2.476
Lattice Size (2D XZ):10×10

To design the PC biosensor, we need to study the band gap analysis of a PC with a cubic lattice of periodic dielectric rods. The lattice size is 10x10 in the X and Z directions, with the above structural parameter shown in Figure 6.1 (a). The 3D view of PC is shown in Figure 6.1 (b).

Figure 6.1 (c) shows the PBG for cubic lattice before introducing the defects complete bandgap exists in TM mode. According to the structure shown in Figure 6.1 (c), the structure has two TE modes. The TE1 mode exits in between 0.258 ≤ a/λ ≤0.362, in the λ range of 1381 nm ≤ λ ≤ 1937 nm. This is a suitable range for optical systems applications. The TE2 exits between the λ range of 929 nm ≤ λ ≤ 1028 nm which is not suitable for optical communication systems.

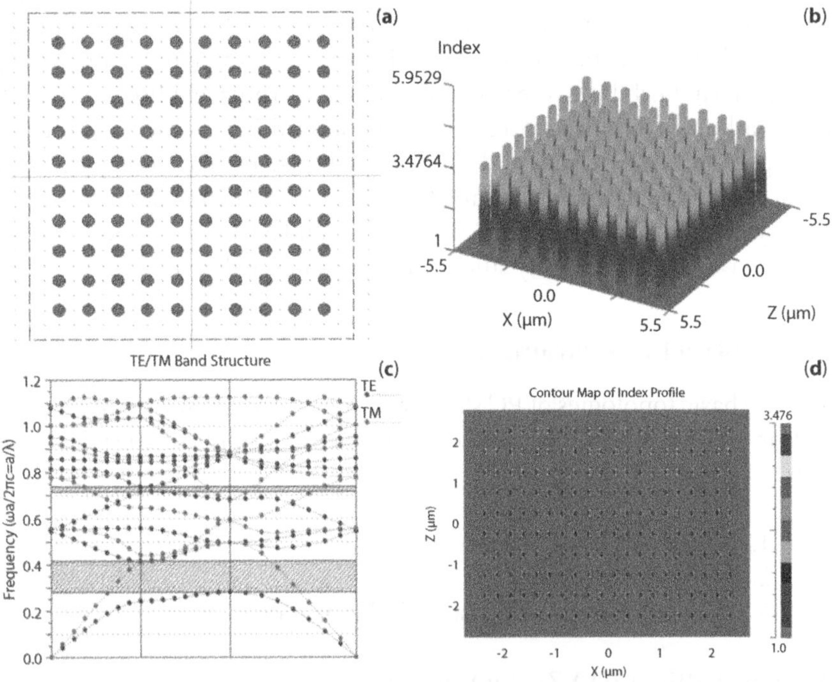

Figure 6.1 (a) A 3D view of 2D PC slab on a square lattice (b) 2D view of slab (c) TE PBG before introducing the defects (d) Contour map profile.

Figure 6.1 (d) shows the contour map profile illustrating a cubic lattice structure. In this map, different colors are used to represent different materials and their refractive indices. In particular, the violet color represents the air medium, which has a refractive index of 1. This means that light passing through the air will not undergo significant bending or refraction. On the other hand, the red color circle represents silicon rods. Silicon is known to have a relatively high refractive index of 3.476. When light passes through silicon, its speed decreases and it undergoes refraction, resulting in a change in direction. By using different colors to differentiate between air and silicon, the contour map profile provides a visual representation of the refractive index distribution within the cubic lattice structure.

B. Hexagonal Lattice (2D XZ) (Holes in Slab)
Lattice Constant (a) of lattice: 400 nm
Radius of Silicon dielectric rods: 120 nm
Dielectric constant of dielectric rod: 11.56
Height of Si slab: 220 nm
Effective Refractive Index of slab (N_{eff}): 3.399523
Mode: 0
Refractive Index difference (Δn): 2.476
Lattice Size (2D XZ): 10×10

To design an optical biosensor with a 10 × 10 lattice type of hexagonal and etched holes in the dielectric slab as shown in Figure 6.2 (a) (indicating that there are 10 holes in both the x and z directions.), the refractive index of the dielectric slab should be 3.476. The slab represents the material in which the etched holes are present. The etched holes have a refractive index of n = 1. The 3D view of the 2D PC is shown in Figure 6.2 (b). Figure 6.2 (c) shows the PBG for hexoganal lattice before introducing the defects complete bandgap exists in TM mode. According to the structure shown in Figure 6.2 (c), the structure has two TM modes. The TM1 mode exits in between $0.212 \leq a/\lambda \leq 0.28$, includes in the wavelength range of 1428 nm $\leq \lambda \leq$1886 nm., which is a suitable range for optical systems applications. The TM2 exits between the wavelength range of 673 nm $\leq \lambda \leq$ 643 nm which is not suitable for optical communication systems.

Figure 6.2 (d) shows the contour map profile illustrating a hexagonal lattice structure. The red color represents the silicon medium with a refractive index of 3.467. When light encounters the boundary between air and silicon, it will bend or refract due to the refractive index mismatch. The etched holes represented by the red circles in the contour map indicate regions where the silicon material has been modified or removed. Light

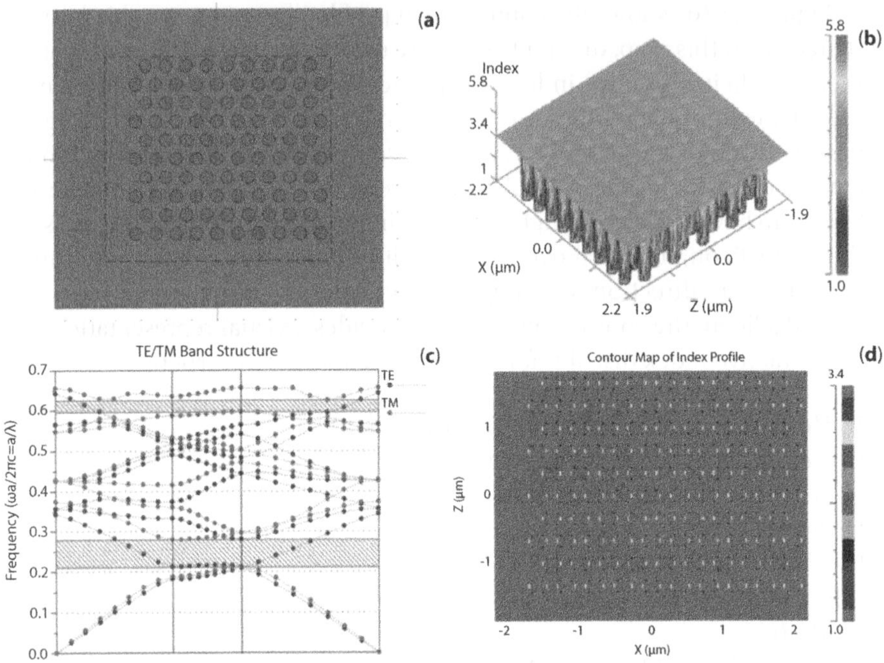

Figure 6.2 (a) A 3D view of 2D PC slab on a Hexagonal lattice consisting of holes (b) 2D view of slab (c) Photonic band gap before introducing the defects (d) Contour map profile.

passing through these regions will interact differently compared to the surrounding silicon material. The change in refractive index due to the presence of these holes will affect the path of light and result in variations in the contour map.

2D PC sensors are optical sensors that utilize the properties of 2D PCs to detect and measure changes in the surrounding environment. These sensors are designed with a periodic arrangement of holes or rods in a high refractive index material, forming a 2D lattice structure. The interaction of light with the PC structure enables the sensing of various parameters, such as refractive index, temperature, pressure, humidity, and chemical composition.

The most important parameters of 2D PC sensors

Detection mechanism: The sensing mechanism of sensors works based on photonic or resonant band structure modulation, changing the refractive index or binding events to specific molecules and changing the resonant frequency band or wavelength, causing measurable observation in the resonant wavelengths.

Sensitivity and selectivity: The 2D PC sensors provide the high sensitivity and selectivity for specific analytes or parameters. Through proper optimization of the photonic crystal structure the sensor can be tuned to a specific wavelength or frequency range, thereby increasing the selectivity of the detection process.

Labeless sensor: 2D PC sensors work on the principle of labeless sensing. This means no labels are essential for analyte detection. This makes simpler the detection process, reduces costs and enables direct detection of the target analytes.

Miniaturization and integration: 2D PC sensors can be fabricated on a Nano scale, allowing miniaturization and integration into compact sensing devices. These sensors can be easily integrated into light sources, optical detectors and microfluidic systems, allowing and on-chip sensing applications.

Real-time monitoring: 2D PC sensors are suitable for real-time monitoring of effective and dynamic processes to provide the high sensitivity and fast response. The sensor ability to detect environmental and pattern changes in near real time enables uninterrupted monitoring and provides valuable information for process feedback and control.

2D photonic crystal sensors have applications in various fields such as mechanics, electricity, chemical analysis, biosensors, radiation, magnetism and heat, as shown in Figure 6.3.

Electrical domain: PC sensors used to sense and detect the parameters in the electrical domain applications such as electric field sensing and load sensing. Through combining electrodes and manipulating the interaction among light and electric fields. PCs can measure electrical parameters and phenomena.

Mechanical field: In the domain of mechanics, photonic crystal sensors can detect and measure the mechanical stress, strain or vibration, through the changes in the mechanical properties of the photonic crystal structure can affect light transmission, allowing sensitive detection of mechanical phenomena.

Chemical domain: PC sensors are used in chemical and Biological detection and analysis. By functionalizing the PC structure with specific receptors or wastes, changes in chemical composition, concentration or reactivity can be sensed and measured.

Radiation domain: PC sensors can be used to sense, detect and measure radiation such as visible light, ultraviolet, and infrared. PC structures exhibit changes in optical properties, allowing detection and characterization of radiation sources and levels.

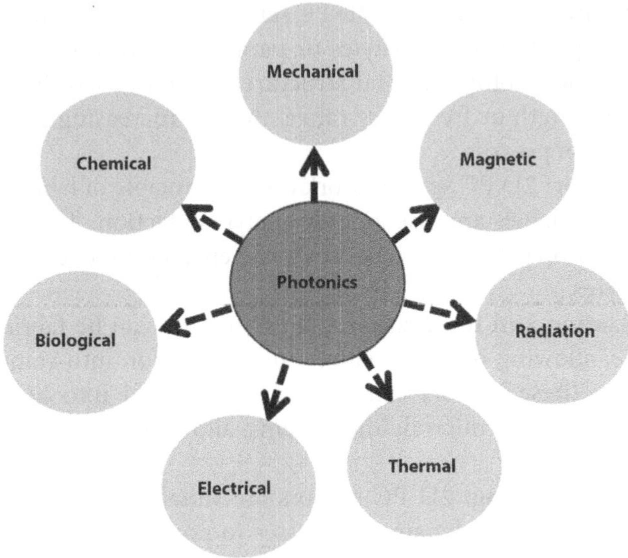

Figure 6.3 Different domain of 2D Photonic sensor.

Magnetic domain: Magnetic Domain able to detect magnetic fields using PC sensors. Photonic crystals can be used to observe the magnetic fields and the presence of magnetic materials, either by integrating magnetic materials or by using the magneto-optic effect.
Thermal domain: PC sensors used for temperature measurement and thermal analysis temperature ranges. Temperature changes modulate the optical properties of PCs, so temperature changes can be measured and detect with high sensitivity and accuracy.

6.1.2 Performance Parameters of Sensor

Quality factor: The quality factor (Q), is a parameter used to characterize the quality or performance of a resonant system The quality factor describes the sharpness or narrowness of a resonance, indicating how well a system can store and release energy at a specific frequency [7]. Mathematically, the quality factor can be expressed as,

$$Q = \omega_0/\Delta\omega \tag{6.1}$$

where ω_0 represents the resonant frequency of the system, and $\Delta\omega$ represents the FWHM of the resonance curve, which is a measure of the bandwidth around the resonant frequency.

Sensitivity: The sensitivity (S) [7], as expressed by the equation, quantifies the relationship between the change in wavelength ($\Delta\lambda$) and the corresponding change in the measured quantity (ΔN). It indicates how sensitive the sensor is to variations in the parameter being measured. A higher sensitivity value suggests that small changes in the measured quantity will result in larger changes in the detected wavelength.

$$S = \Delta\lambda / \Delta N \tag{6.2}$$

$\Delta\lambda$: Change in wavelength. This refers to the difference or variation in the wavelength of the incident light or the detected light signal.
ΔN: Change in the measured quantity. This represents the variation in the physical or chemical parameter being measured by the sensor. It could be a change in refractive index, concentration, temperature, pressure, or any other relevant parameter.

Spectral response: Spectral response (R) [7] or spectral shift of the sensor. It indicates the displacement or change in the wavelength of the detected light compared to a reference wavelength.

$$R = \Delta\lambda = \lambda r - \lambda s \tag{6.3}$$

λr: Reference wavelength. It represents the known or predefined wavelength used as a reference point for comparison.

λs: Sensed or detected wavelength. This is the wavelength of the light signal that is captured or measured by the sensor.

Detection limit or limit of detection (D): It represents the less detectable change or concentration of the measured parameter that the sensor can reliably differentiate from the background noise [7].

$$D = R/S \tag{6.4}$$

Figure of Merit (FOM): FOM represents a metric used to assess the quality of a photonic sensor [7].

$$FOM = S \times Q / \lambda r \tag{6.5}$$

Transmission Efficiency: It represents the percentage of the incident power that is transmitted through the sensor. It indicates how effectively the sensor allows the passage of light or signals [7].

$$T.E = (\text{Transmitted Power} / \text{Incident Power}) * 100\% \quad (6.6)$$

Transmitted Power refers to the power of the light transmitted over the sensor.

Incident Power refers to the power of the incident light launched to the sensor.

6.1.3 Sensing and Detection Mechanism

Photonic biosensors operate on two main detection mechanisms: resonant wavelength shift and intensity Variation. These mechanisms can be used for sensor calibration and characterization [8].

Resonance wavelength shift: In this mechanism, the biosensor is designed to have a resonance peak that is sensitive to refractive index changes. If the refractive index of the sample being observed (such as blood composition) changes, the resonant wavelength will change. This change can be detected and correlated with the concentration of the analyte or with a specific property of material. A reference sample of recognized refractive index can be used to adjust the sensor and determine the baseline resonant wavelength. Accurate measurements and calibrations can be made by comparing the variations in resonance wavelength induced by the target analyte to a reference.

Intensity shift: This system detects biosensors by varying the intensity of light emitted. The interaction of light inside the biosensor structure is affected by changes in the refractive index of the sample, causing the intensity of the recorded signal to vary. This shift in intensity can be attributed to a variety of phenomena, including scattering, absorption, and variations in optical path length. To calibrate the sensor and generate a calibration curve that links changes in observed intensity to characteristics of interest such as analyte concentration, a number of known samples or standards with varying attributes can be utilized.

6.2 Photonic Crystal Biosensor

A PC-based biosensor is an optical sensor that detects and analyses biological biomarkers or analytes using a PC. PC is a man-made periodic Nanomaterial with unique optical features, such as the capacity to regulate and change light transmission via its band structure. PC structures are created with the intention of interacting with biological substances or cells. The interaction between the target analyte and the PC creates variations in the structure's optical characteristics, which can be viewed, detected, and measured.

The principle of a PC-based biosensor typically includes the following steps:

Detection surface preparation: The PC surface is modified using definite captured molecules that can selectively bind to the target analyte of interest, such as proteins, DNA, or cells.
Analyte binding: When the sample containing the target analyte is taken to the sensor position, the analyte molecules bind to immobilized receptors, creating a specific molecular interaction.
Optical signal sensor: The PC structure is designed to have a resonant mode or frequency band that is sensitive to variations in the refractive index. The position of the analyte molecules induces changes in the local refractive index or thickness, causing a change in the resonant frequency or wavelength in the band gap of the PC.
Signal analysis: The change in resonant frequency or wavelength is detected and measured using various optical techniques, such as spectroscopy, and interferometer. The degree of change compares with the properties of the target analyte.

6.2.1 Highlights of PC Biosensors

PC-based biosensors have several advantages such as high sensitivity, label-free detection, and the possibility of multiplex analysis. Accurate design and optimization of the PC structure is essential to achieve high-performance biosensing capabilities.

6.2.2 IoT-Enabled 2D PC Biosensor

2D PC biosensors with Internet of Things (IoT) intelligence integrate PC principles with IoT technological capabilities to form an intelligent biosensor system [9]. This connectivity enables biosensors to be monitored in real time, analyzed, and controlled remotely. 2D PC biosensors are made up of PC structures that are designed to interact with biomolecules such as DNA and proteins in order to detect and analyze them. The PC structure increased environmental change detection sensitivity and selectivity.

Integration via IoT intelligence provides several benefits to biosensing devices. For starters, it enables continuous monitoring of biosensor functioning as well as ambient variables. Sensor data, including photon responses from biosensors, can be collected in real time and wirelessly transferred to a central server or cloud platform. Advanced data analysis and processing are also possible with IoT intelligence. Machine learning algorithms can be applied to acquired data to provide important insights, recognize trends, and improve biosensor measurement accuracy. It enables the automatic detection of specific biological targets or aberrant circumstances, which improves the reliability and efficiency of biosensing systems. Furthermore, IoT intelligence allows for remote control and management of biosensors. Users can remotely configure biosensors, establish detection thresholds, and receive messages and alerts when certain events and circumstances are detected via a dedicated app or user interface. This capability is very beneficial in circumstances requiring constant monitoring, such as environmental or medical applications. Overall, incorporating IoT intelligence into a 2D PC biosensor improves its capabilities by allowing for real-time monitoring, enhanced data analysis, and remote control. With this combination, smart and efficient biosensing applications with better accuracy, convenience, and accessibility are possible.

6.2.3 PC Block Diagram

Figure 6.4 depicts the schematic diagram of a PC-based biosensor.

The light beam or signal that interacts with the photonic crystal structure and the analyte is provided by the light source.

Photonic Crystal Structure: A nanostructured manufactured material with a photonic bandgap or resonant mode. It interacts with the analyte and modifies its optical characteristics as a result of the binding events.
Sensing Surface: The surface of the photonic crystal structure where specific receptors or capture molecules are immobilized. It allows for selective binding of the target analyte.
Analyte Solution: The sample or solution containing the target analyte. It is introduced onto the sensing surface for the binding interaction with the immobilized receptors.

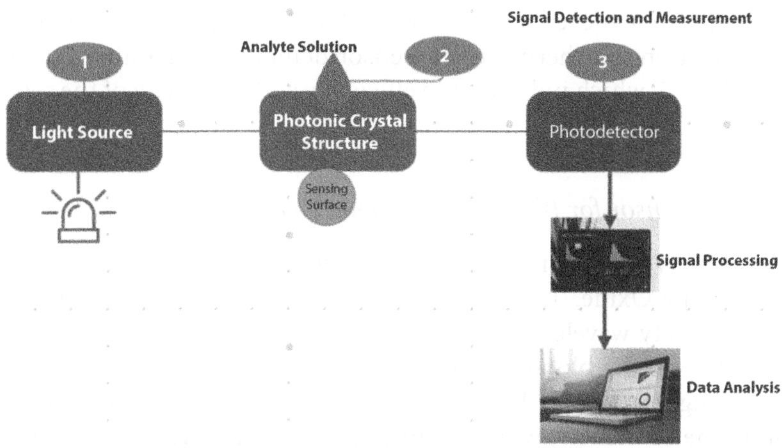

Figure 6.4 Schematic diagram of PC based biosensor.

Signal Detection and Measurement

a. Photodetector: Receives and converts the optical signal from the photonic crystal structure into an electrical signal.
b. Signal Processing: Amplifies, filters, and conditions the electrical signal from the photodetector for further processing.
c. Data Analysis: Analyzes the processed signal to extract information about the presence, concentration, or properties of the target analyte.
d. Output/Display: Presents the results of the analysis, such as the concentration of the analyte or a visual indication of the detection.

6.2.3.1 *Biosensor for Cancerous Cell Detection*

Abinash Panda *et al.* [10] reported the 2D PC waveguide to sense and detect the normal and cancerous cells. The structure consists of a 5x5 array of silicon rods etched on a cubic lattice, with a central line defect and air as the background material. The simulation results demonstrated that for normal cells (INOK), the resonant wavelengths dropped into the orange color range, while for cancerous cells (YD-10B), the resonant wavelengths dropped into the yellow color wavelength. The sensor exhibited high sensitivity, with a value of 2360.12 nm/RIU (refractive index unit), indicating its ability to detect small changes in the surrounding medium. It also achieved a very low resolution of 1.78×10^{-6}, enabling precise detection. Furthermore, the sensor demonstrated a high-quality factor of 99.765, which indicates the efficiency and selectivity of the sensing mechanism.

6.2.3.2 Biosensor for Blood Components Detection

Fatemeh Baraty [11] devised a two-dimensional PC biosensor designed with Graphene Oxide. The biosensor is designed based on the mechanism of intensity wavelength shift based on the different blood components present in the blood. The design uses the X-shape ring resonator on the triangular lattice. The overall size of the biosensor is 21mm × 16.5mm. The sensitivity, which denotes the change in resonance wavelength per refractive index unit (RIU), is calculated to be 375 nm/RIU. The Q of the biosensor is determined to be 14665.8. The full-width half maximum (FWHM) is reported as 0.14nm, indicating the spectral width of the resonance peak. A narrower FWHM implies better spectral resolution, enabling the biosensor to differentiate between closely spaced resonance wavelengths. The FOM is calculated to be 2500 RIU^{-1}, which is a measure of the sensor's overall performance and the transmission efficiency of the biosensor is reported to be 99.8%. This signifies the percentage of incident light that is transmitted through the device, highlighting its capability to efficiently interact with the sample and detect changes in the refractive index.

6.2.3.3 Biosensor for Chikungunya Virus Detection

Sanjeev Sharma *et al.* [12] reported a 2D PC double ring resonator-based biosensor for detecting the chikungunya virus using the resonant wavelength shift method. The biosensor is designed to sense and detect normal and infected uric acid, red blood cells, platelets, and plasma in the blood. The transmission characteristics, quality factor, and power efficiency of the biosensor are studied based on the refractive index variations of these blood components. The sensor detects the shift in the resonant peak exposed to different refractive indices of the blood components. Based on the changes in the resonant wavelength, the sensitivity of the sensor is calculated as 3.43×10^3nm/RIU. Transmission efficiency is 98%, and the quality factor is 60.12. The sensor reported a low-quality factor and high sensitivity.

6.2.3.4 *Biosensor for Glucose Monitoring*

S. Mohamed *et al.* [13] reported the biosensor for the detection of glucose monitoring. The performance of the biosensor design is evaluated by calculating the transmission spectrum through the structure. This investigation aimed to enhance the detection capability of the biosensor for small variations in the physical properties of the analyte, specifically glucose. The sensor reported a high sensitivity of 422 nm/RIU. The design is simple for implementation and potential integration into practical glucose monitoring devices.

6.2.3.5 *Biosensor for Glucose Concentration in Urine*

P. Sharma *et al.* [14] devised the simple line defect based 2D PC Biosensor for detecting glucose concentration in urine. The finite-difference time-domain method has been employed for the analysis, which is a computational technique used to solve electromagnetic wave propagation problems. The reported structure and structural parameters revealed that even a small change in the refractive index leads to a good shift in higher wavelength and normalized transmitted output power. This indicates that the designed biosensor is highly sensitive to changes in the refractive index. By measuring the shift in the transmitted output power or frequency, the biosensor can detect variations in the glucose concentration in urine samples.

6.2.3.6 *Biosensor for Abnormal Tissues Analysis Detection*

A. Asuvaran *et al.* [15] reported the 2D PC optical sensor presents a promising option for real-time detection of distinct brain tissue categories during robot-assisted minimally invasive surgery. The sensor has been designed to detect and respond to changes in the refractive index of certain brain tissues. Notably, aberrant tissues, such as tumors or cancer-infected brain tissues, have different refractive indices than normal brain tissues. This biosensor has a high sensitivity, with a value of 4615.38nm/RIU (refractive index unit). The quality factor, which represents the sharpness of the sensor's response, is 573. Furthermore, the sensor's detection limit is reported to be 0.0013 RIU, suggesting its capacity to detect even minor changes in the refractive index's value.

6.2.3.7 *Biosensor for DNA Detection*

Benmerkhi *et al.* [16] reported a 2D PC biosensor for DNA detection. The design includes an L2 resonant cavity formed by removing two air holes in the middle, input waveguide 1, and output waveguide 2 formed by removing three air holes on the PC. To improve sensing, four slots are inserted into the resonant cavity's center, and the functionalized holes near the cavities are filled with DNA. These changes improve the sensitivity and detection of biological substances. The biosensor's sensitivity is a critical parameter in biosensing applications because it determines the ability to detect minor changes in the refractive index of the surrounding medium.

6.3 Inference and Future Enhancements

1. When designing a 2D PC biosensor through a rod or hole structure, certain dimensions, refractive indices, cavity design, sensing region must be optimized to achieve the desired sensing performance parameters. Computational techniques such as FDTD and PWE are commonly used to simulate and analyze the band structure and design parameters of PCs.
2. Hexagonal air holes are used in most designs. By optimizing the parameters and considering the refractive index of the material involved, it is possible to obtain a larger PBG in the desired spectral range than a cubic lattice. This is beneficial for applications such as integrated optics, biosensors and photonic filters.
3. PC sensors can be designed using both resonant intensity and wavelength based methods, and the two can be combined to improve the sensitivity and selectivity of the sensing platform.
4. It is important to note that increasing the sensitivity can decrease the Q-factor.
5. PC sensors integrated with IoT intelligence can be used for advanced applications such as real-time monitoring, wireless connectivity, data analysis and machine learning, cloud integration of autonomous and adaptive systems, remote configuration and management, and integration with other IoT devices. It offers multiple benefits for sensor applications.

6. PC sensors are particularly advantageous for biosensing applications where specific biomolecular interactions need to be detected. B. Antibody-antigen binding, DNA hybridization, or enzyme-substrate interaction. It offers label-free detection, high sensitivity, and multiplex analysis options. However, for analytes that do not involve specific biomolecular interactions or induce refractive index changes, alternative sensing platforms may need to be considered.

Conclusion

2D Photonic crystal biosensors offer high sensitivity, label-free detection, multiplexing capabilities, and real-time monitoring, making them powerful tools for various bio sensing applications. .Integration through other technologies opens up even further possibilities, paving the way for advanced detection systems with improved performance and capabilities. Biosensor performance is monitored using the resonant wavelength. With the right database, you can connect to IoT and enable smart detection. Photonic crystal sensors integrated with IoT intelligence can improve performance through real-time monitoring, data analysis, remote management, and integration with IoT devices. This integration enables intelligent, data-driven decision making and improves the overall performance and functionality of sensor systems.

References

1. Joannopoulos, J.D., Johnson, S.G., Winn, J.N., Meade, R.D., *Molding the flow of light*, Princet. Univ. Press, Princeton, NJ [ua], 2008.
2. Qiu, M., Mulot, M., Swillo, M., Anand, S., Jaskorzynska, B., Karlsson, A., Forchel, A., Photonic crystal optical filter based on contra-directional waveguide coupling. *Appl. Phys. Lett.*, 83, 25, 5121–5123, 2003.
3. Krauss, T.F., Slow light in photonic crystal waveguides. *J. Phys. D: Appl. Phys.*, 40, 9, 2666, 2007.
4. Altug, H., Englund, D., Vučković, J., Ultrafast photonic crystal nanocavity laser. *Nat. Phys.*, 2, 7, 484–488, 2006.
5. Nair, R.V. and Vijaya, R., Photonic crystal sensors: An overview. *Prog. Quantum Electron.*, 34, 3, 89–134, 2010.
6. Balaji, V.R., Murugan, M., Robinson, S., Hegde, G., A novel hybrid channel DWDM demultiplexer using two dimensional photonic crystals meeting ITU standards. *Silicon*, 14, 1–12, 2021.

7. Fan, X., White, I.M., Shopova, S., II, Zhu, H., Suter, J.D., Sun, Y., Sensitive optical biosensors for unlabeled targets: A review. *Anal. Chim. Acta*, 620, 1–2, 8–26, 2008.
8. De Vos, K., Bartolozzi, I., Schacht, E., Bienstman, P., Baets, R., Silicon-on-Insulator microring resonator for sensitive and label-free biosensing. *Opt. Express*, 15, 12, 7610–7615, 2007.
9. Jain, S., Nehra, M., Kumar, R., Dilbaghi, N., Hu, T., Kumar, S., Li, C.Z., Internet of medical things (IoMT)-integrated biosensors for point-of-care testing of infectious diseases. *Biosens. Bioelectron.*, 179, 113074, 2021.
10. Panda, A. and Devi, P.P., Photonic crystal biosensor for refractive index based cancerous cell detection. *Opt. Fiber Technol.*, 54, 102123, 2020.
11. Baraty, F. and Hamedi, S., Design of a 2D photonic crystal biosensor using X-shape ring resonator based on Graphene Oxide (GO) for detection of blood components. *J. Electromagn. Waves Appl.*, 36, 17, 2401–2418, 2022.
12. Sharma, S., Kumar, A., Singh, K.S., Tyagi, H.K., 2D photonic crystal based biosensor for the detection of chikungunya virus. *Optik*, 237, 166575, 2021.
13. Mohamed, M.S., Hameed, M.F.O., Areed, N.F., El-Okr, M.M., Obayya, S.S.A., Analysis of highly sensitive photonic crystal biosensor for glucose monitoring. *Appl. Comput. Electromagn. Soc. J.*, 31, 836–842, 2016.
14. Sharma, P. and Sharan, P., Design of photonic crystal-based biosensor for detection of glucose concentration in urine. *IEEE Sens. J.*, 15, 2, 1035–1042, 2014.
15. Asuvaran, A. and Elatharasan, G., Design of two-dimensional photonic crystal-based biosensor for abnormal tissue analysis. *Silicon*, 14, 12, 7203–7210, 2022.
16. Benmerkhi, A., Bouchemat, M., Bouchemat, T., Design of two-dimensional photonic crystal biosensor using DNA detection. *Phosphorus Sulfur Rel. Elem.*, 195, 11, 960–964, 2020.

7

Portable IoT Smart Devices in Healthcare and Remote Health Monitoring

Boopathi Raja G.[1], Parimala Devi M.[1*], Deepa R.[2], Sathya T.[1] and Nithya S.[3]

[1]Department of ECE, Velalar College of Engineering and Technology, Erode, Tamil Nadu, India
[2]Department of ECE, CMR Institute of Technology, Bangalore, Karnataka, India
[3]Department of EEE, SRM Institute of Science and Technology, Chennai, Tamil Nadu, India

Abstract

Most of the people in the country reside in rural regions need good medical care. The significance of telemedicine and the application of the Internet of Things (IoT) are emphasized in this chapter. The significant developments in healthcare technology that have occurred recently are the result of the Internet of Things due to pervasive use of computers. By deploying IoT based devices, healthcare professionals are provide better service to the general public. This chapter explains how the recent issues in the healthcare system may be fixed by designing a remote health and environment monitoring system, with a focus on patients who are at a greater risk of complications. Since timely treatment is of the utmost importance, this system will enable physicians and other medical professionals to get information about a patient in real-time which provide the services instantly to the patients in different locations. The system is made up of several sensors that gather data on a variety of factors, including heart rate, body temperature, blood pressure, and air quality. It will analyze that data using a microcontroller and is connected to a mobile application seamlessly. All data are transmitted to the mobile application via a communication module. Since it is upgraded every few seconds, the medical staffs promptly monitor the condition of their patients and react accordingly to any circumstances. The proposed model assists medical experts and also the patient's family in the process of monitoring the patient's

Corresponding author: parimaladevi.vlsi@gmail.com

Hari Murthy, Marta Zurek-Mortka, Vinay Jha Pillai and Kukatlapalli Pradeep Kumar (eds.)
Internet of Things in Bioelectronics: Emerging Technologies and Applications, (125–144) © 2024 Scrivener Publishing LLC

physiological data from a distant place. The physiological state of the patient is uploaded to the cloud. Both analog and digital representations of the patient's data are sent via the mobile application that the doctor uses to treat patients. Also, the physician adjusts the rate of medicine infusion from a distant place. Patients who are admitted in hospital or traveling in an ambulance may successfully use the proposed model. This system is portable and is simple enough for anybody to use it. The error rates for the oxygen saturation in the blood, and heart rate measured are correspondingly 2.02%, and 2.63%. Measured values are uploaded to cloud after the data is processed at the fog and edge node in order to reduce the traffic to cloud. After receiving all the data, medical professionals were able to monitor the health of individuals in emergency care.

***Keywords*:** Data security, healthcare, IoMT, privacy issues, implant devices

7.1 Introduction

In the past decade, the Internet of Things (IoT) has facilitated the rapid growth of remote healthcare and telemedicine technology, where different kinds of medical sensors are combined to monitor medical parameters and transmit them to any location. Currently, intelligent portable devices are utilized to track human health by monitoring various medical aspects [1]. They may also pre-diagnose illnesses and identify organ dysfunction. This chapter describes the design as well as the creation of small, flexible health monitoring devices for everyday medical checks [2]. The developed system monitors a variety of medical parameters, including electrocardiography (ECG) signal, heart rate (HR), photoplethysmography (PPG) signal, blood oxygen saturation (SpO2), the temperature of the body, the temperature of the environment, and room humidity [3]. In local mode, measurements are observed on the device's panel or wirelessly transmitted to an application on the smartphone or cloud storage for observation from afar [4]. The framework that has been created is employed to track the people they are responsible for while allowing them to live their normal lives. In addition, statistical examinations revealed a strong relationship between the measured and standard measurements. The results indicate that the proposed system is extremely precise and suitable for implementation in routine medical applications.

7.2 Related Works

According to recently released statistics, between 7 and 12 percent of patients in the European Union have issues with their extant healthcare systems [5]. They are subjected to unsuitable service and the absence of case follow-up [6]. In addition, it has been reported that 5% of those admitted to hospitals without preventative measures have infectious diseases [7]. In addition, 60 percent of American adults older than 18 have a minimum of one chronic illness, and more than four often suffer from multiple chronic illnesses [8].

Researchers and commercial partners have competed to assist individuals in adjusting to a novel lifestyle [9]. This is due to the explosive growth of information and communication technology, and related industries, in addition to the rapid evolution of daily life [10]. Businesses and governments are promoting the use of electronic principles and information and communication technology in health sectors [11]. This contributes to the development of computerized healthcare systems [12]. Individuals should be able to monitor their health status without having any contact with or time commitment from medical professionals [13]. Intelligent health monitoring systems are required to prevent epidemics of infectious diseases from spreading in a wider sense [14]. In addition, personal health devices have been trustworthy options for the majority of people who are unable to have frequent hospital visits to track and trace their health conditions [15]. Consequently, small personal healthcare gadgets are attaining popularity and being a necessity in the marketplace [16].

The Internet of Medical Things (IoMT) and recent technological developments have made distant medical data transmission possible [17]. If these kinds of signals are transmitted and examined within a dependable framework, they provide crucial information about the different situations of individuals [18]. These applications utilize multiple communication protocols, including GSM, Wi-Fi, and Bluetooth [19]. In addition, the Internet of Things (IoT) has been integrated into this field to leverage its apparent advantages, including small-sized sensors, communication, and a vast array of additional features [20].

Numerous researchers have modeled IoT-based healthcare systems. Following are some of such investigations. Siam *et al.* [21] made a safe health tracking system for keeping an eye on the most important vital signs of a patient: Pulse Rate, SpO2, and temperature of the body. Before transmitting medical observations to the cloud, researchers encrypt them to safeguard the confidentiality of medical data records. There was a lot of agreement between the readings of the device and the results of the comparisons with widely available devices. Dagtas *et al.* [22] proposed a ZigBee-based wireless real-time health monitoring system. The proposed system has three-tier architecture, with the first level consisting of a mobile device that captures important data and offers local archive and transfer capabilities. The local server then processes and saves the incoming data. The diagnostic and storage facility receives processed data and outcomes. Using symmetric encryption algorithms to encrypt sensitive data has ensured their safety. Khan *et al.* [23] developed an organic PPG monitor that measures heart rate and SpO2 and worn on the inner wrist. One channel receives its data directly through the ulnar artery, whereas the other device receives its data through the radial artery. The unique sensor establishes improved PPG signal amplification and power consumption. It also performed well when compared to real-world data, meaning it might be employed in portable oximetry. Over the past few years, industrial and academic research on healthcare monitoring has been growing.

Majumder and Deen [24] conducted an in-depth investigation of how smartphone devices are used for health monitoring. They explained how the advanced computing and communication technology that is included in modern cell phones work. It includes a large number of built-in sensors, which have led to significant advancements in the health monitoring capabilities of smartphones. The sensors of the smartphone monitors blood pressure, cardiac activity, respiration rate, ocular problems, skin conditions, sleep quality, and accidents.

Philip *et al.* [25] conducted an in-depth examination of the IoT trend for in-home monitoring of health. They presented numerous applications, obstacles, and potential paths for home-based health monitoring systems. It portrays the significance of the Internet of Things, which enabled remote health applications to enhance diagnostics, staff-patient communication, prescribing of drugs, and preventative advice. They also raised concerns regarding the adoption of remote healthcare systems, including issues of dependability, stability, security, legality, and privacy, among others.

Ali *et al.* [26] gathered data on three physiological indicators, which included temperature of the body, saturation of oxygen, and heartbeat. The readings measured are then sent via Bluetooth to an application running on smartphone. Ghosh *et al.* [18] monitored multiple vital signs (ECG, temperature of the body, and patient position) using an IoT sensor module. This module may transmit measurements for remote monitoring to cloud storage. Swaroop *et al.* [27] developed a real-time heart rate, arterial pressure, and body temperature monitoring system. Sensors process and link a Raspberry Pi system. Specialists get medical data through GSM, BLE, and Wi-Fi.

Siam *et al.* [28] used IoT and cloud computing to monitor HR, SpO2, and body temperature. The ESP8266 microcontroller processes data and sends it through Wi-Fi to the Internet for remote monitoring. The device may email the caregiver if measurements surpass threshold levels. The PCB has a web server enabling remote data transfer but no data visualization interfaces. IOMT technology has evolved due to the growth of efficient, remarkable, and cost-effective methods as well as pervasive sensors.

7.3 Proposed Framework Design

In the local mode, the patient or a portion of the patient's relatives monitor the patient's vital signs and the measures that are linked to them locally. It has a remote mode that allows a medical professional to remotely monitor a patient's readings. It contacts a physician if certain parameters exceed normal ranges. This speeds up the health organization's ability to respond to emergencies and communicate with patients.

Figure 7.1 depicts the typical framework of an IoT-based healthcare tracking system. Medical sensors capture multiple health parameters, such as cardiovascular signs, blood pressure, body temperature, blood sugar level, and consciousness level. A local processing unit collects and processes these health-related data before transmitting them to a data center employing either short-range or distant communication protocols to be

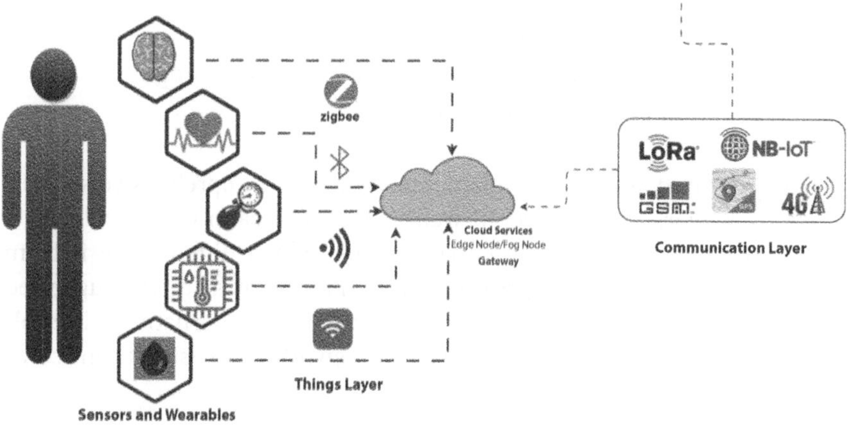

Figure 7.1 The framework of an IoT-based healthcare tracking system.

used for visualization, diagnosis, or storage. Data uploaded to the cloud is reduced by the data processing carried out at the fog and edge node.

Remote health monitoring technique allows patients to self-monitor or send data to a doctor to determine the next steps. However, such healthcare systems must capture a variety of signals for in-depth knowledge of human health, develop an efficient monitoring algorithm alongside a limited amount of complexity, transfer the signals to a centralized location to analyze and store them while maintaining them not affected by the channel, and ensure that the signals remain unaffected by the communication channel.

This chapter discusses a dependable, lightweight, and independent healthcare monitoring system that offers both remote and in-person health monitoring modes and operates in real-time. Consequently, medical personnel remotely manage patient cases, leading to an excellent degree of medical productivity. Multiple biomedical aspects are reliably monitored and tracked using the proposed system. This may facilitate the early prediction as well as examination of diseases related to these abnormalities. The following parameters are measured by this system: Heart Rate (HR), Electrocardiogram (ECG), body temperature (T), the temperature of the surrounding air, Photoplethysmograph (PPG), blood oxygen saturation (SpO2), and ambient humidity. Furthermore, it sends immediate alerts (messages) to caretakers if certain values reach predefined thresholds. The normal and aberrant ranges for different measurements are defined by medical sources and authorities.

In the method that is being suggested,

The following ranges to be abnormal are considered; whenever one of these ranges is achieved, the appropriate caregiver will be contacted.

1. SpO2: Less than 93%.
2. Heart Rate: More than 140 BPM or less than 45 BPM.
3. Body Temperature (T): More than 36.

The proposed system is implemented within a comprehensive surveillance framework for the overall well-being and health of individuals. It offers various novel strategic enhancements which differentiate it from existing rival products and prior research in a similar field. The suggested approach provides numerous benefits over existing alternatives. The following is a summary of the proposed framework's most significant competitive features.

1. The suggested system assessed a variety of vital data including heart rate, SpO_2, temperature of the body, ambient temperature, PPG, ECG, and humidity. Consequently, it is adequate to use this system solely for measuring and monitoring all kinds of physiological processes and external influences.
2. In contrast to certain commercial devices, such as smartwatches, which measure physiological functions in non-standard locations, the system measures a wide range of physiological processes in standard positions.
3. The measurements of the system may be interpreted in a variety of ways. Measurements are displayed using an integrated Organic Light Emitting Diode (OLED) display, a smartphone program, or a web application.
4. The system may send warnings to rescue centers or caretakers if bodily processes are disrupted or if the observed bio-signals deviate from the set parameters.
5. The coordinating expert may have virtual access to the patient side to monitor observations and react immediately to issues.
6. A 160 MHz microprocessor ensures the system's measurement speed and precision.
7. The system is lightweight and portable.
8. Since the environment affects most biological activities, the system monitors temperature and humidity. If the patient has to be maintained in a controlled environment, it may also be used.

The suggested system uses hardware and software to provide reliable, real-time, multifunctional health monitoring in an overall healthcare framework. The output channels for both nearby and remote monitoring are depicted in Figure 7.2. Sensors at the input side of Node MCU microcontroller is used to collect the data heart rate, oxygen saturation level, temperature and humidity level of the patients. Output values from the Node MCU are uploaded to the cloud. Output is also displayed through mobile App and OLED display.

Figure 7.3 shows the remote health monitoring system's layout. Medical sensors provide data to the ESP8266 microcontroller. ESP8266 sends data to Firebase cloud storage over Wi-Fi. The hospital server processes and displays these measurements for medical professionals on the monitoring interface.

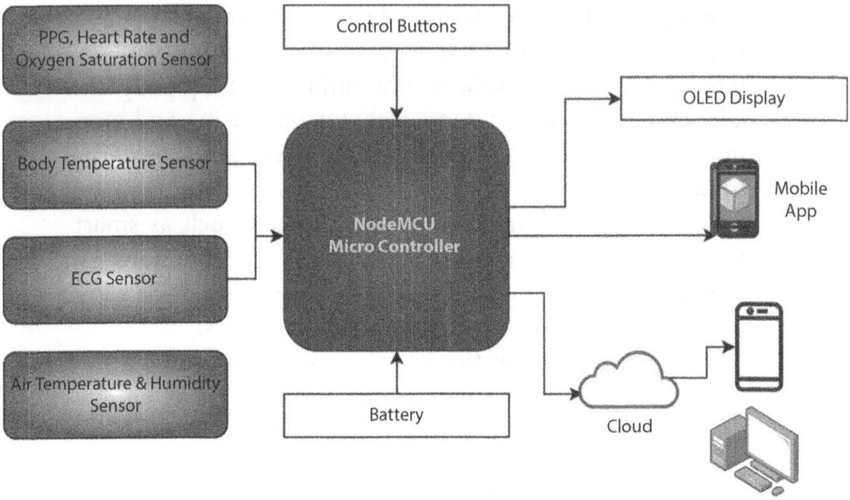

Figure 7.2 Architecture of portable health monitoring system.

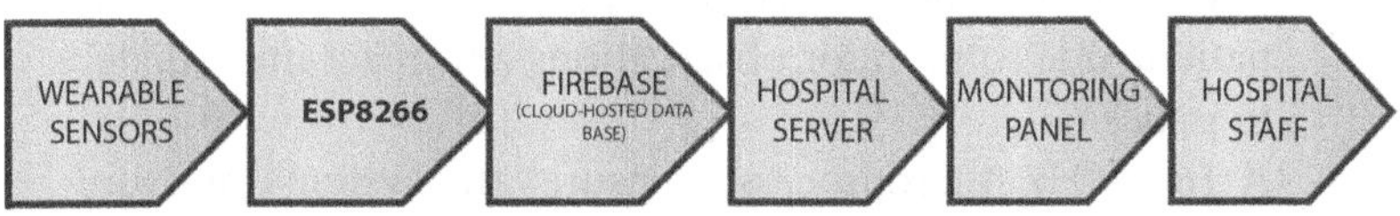

Figure 7.3 The layout of remote health monitoring system.

7.4 Implementation of Hardware Module

7.4.1 Required Hardware Components

The hardware devices and components deployed in the implementation of this system are outlined below.

1) **HR Sensor:** The MAX30102 is a reflecting pulse oximeter that is used to detect the saturation of oxygen in the blood (SpO2) in addition to the heart rate (HR).
2) **ESP8266 Node MCU:** ESP8266 Node MCU is a novel Internet of Things device with a compact form factor. It has a low cost, an integrated Wi-Fi module, and a speedy processor. Figure 7.4(a) depicts the ESP8266 NodeMCU Wi-Fi Devkit from the top perspective.

   Moreover, it is employed in the PPG signal acquisition procedure. The MAX30102 is equipped with a photodiode,

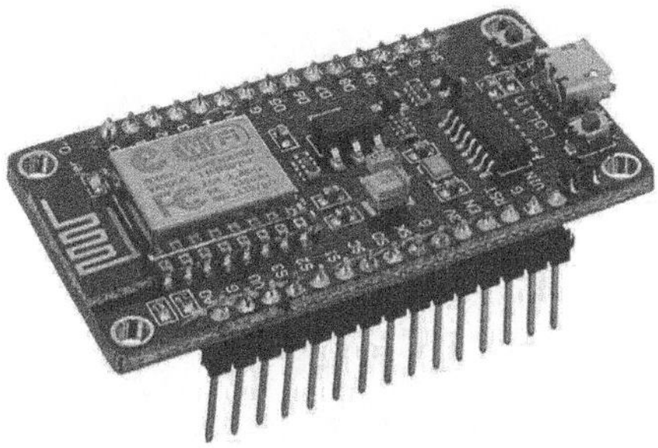

(a)

Figure 7.4 (a) ESP8266 NodeMCU Wi-Fi Devkit.

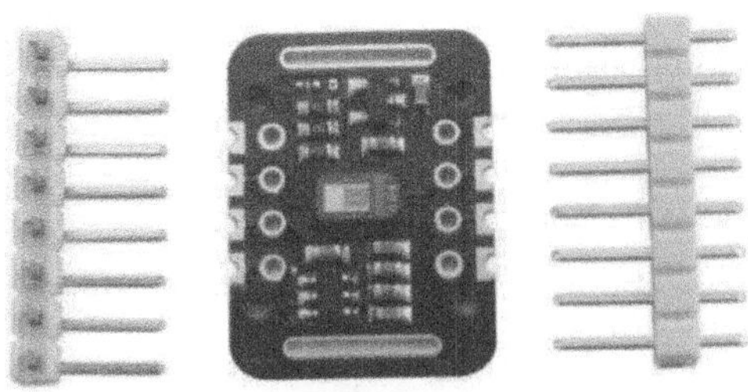

(b)

Figure 7.4 (b) MAX30102 sensor's upper view.

a filter, an amplifier, and two light sources (red and infrared LEDs). The quantity of light reflected after colliding with a liquid (particularly blood) is measured to generate the PPG signal. Consequently, the HR is computed by counting the number of pulses in the generated signal. In addition, a correlation exists between the amount of light reflected and the amount of oxygen in the blood, allowing for the estimation of blood oxygen levels. Figure 7.4(b) depicts the MAX30102 sensor's upper view. Figure 7.4(c) illustrates the MAX30102 board after cabling and before measurement.

3) **ECG Sensor (AD8232):** The AD8232 board is utilized for ECG signal detection and plotting. Figure 7.4(d) depicts the upper perspective of the AD8232 sensor.
4) **Temperature and Humidity Sensor (DHT22):** It is employed for determining a room's temperature and humidity because the majority of biological processes are weather-dependent. This is also beneficial when the patient has to be

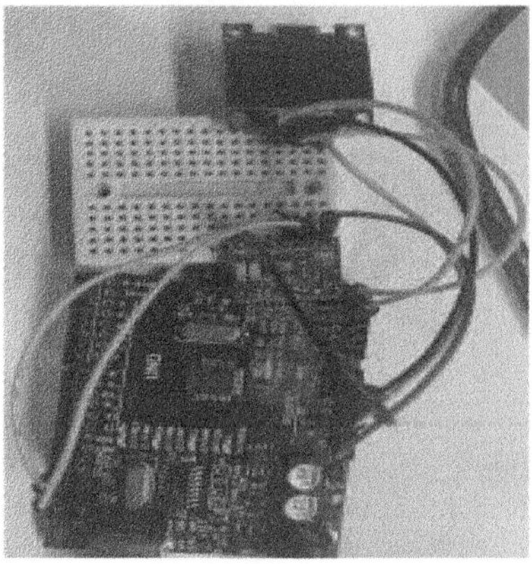

(c)

Figure 7.4 **(c)** MAX30102 board after cabling.

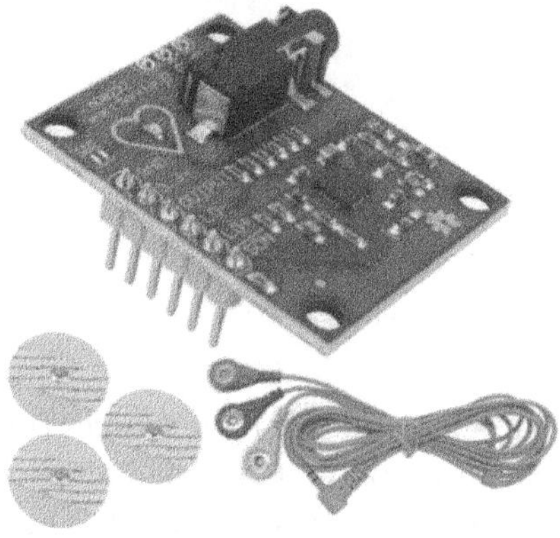

(d)

Figure 7.4 **(d)** AD8232 sensor.

endured adverse conditions. The DHT22 sensor is shown in Figure 7.4(e), which illustrates it from the top down.

5) **Body Temperate Sensor (DS18b20):** This sensor measures the body temperature of the epidermis of the patient. Figure 7.4(f) depicts the DS18b20 sensor. It is distinguished through its high-precision (9- to 12-bit) readings.
6) **OLED Display:** The proposed device may include a 1.3-inch OLED display for accurate medical measurement observations. Figure 7.4(g) depicts a perspective of the OLED display from the top.

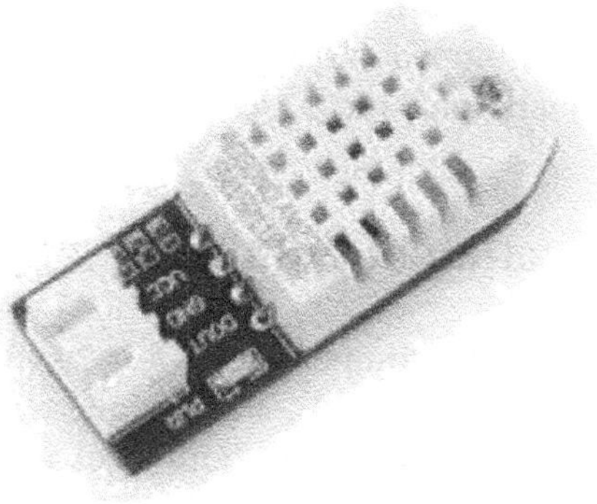

(e)

Figure 7.4 **(e)** The DHT22 sensor.

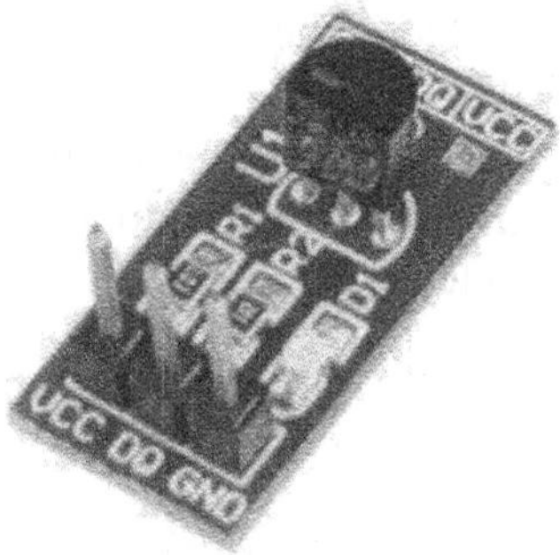

(f)

Figure 7.4 **(f)** DS18b20 sensor.

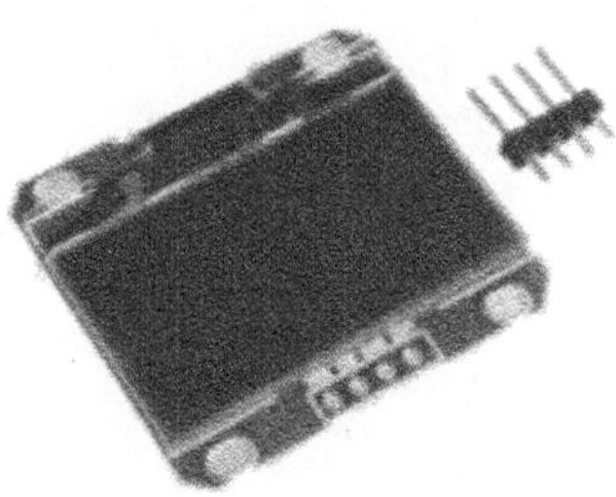

(g)

Figure 7.4 **(g)** Perspective of the OLED.

7) **Battery:** The proposed system is going to be outfitted with a rechargeable lithium-ion battery with a rating of 3.7 volts to extend its operational life.

7.5 Implementation of Prototype

During this stage, all of the components will be assembled onto an individual Printed Circuit Board (PCB), and the microcontroller's programming code will be developed to enable both local and remote continuous health monitoring capabilities. The proposed health monitoring system is depicted in its totality in Figure 7.5, which depicts the system's prototype. Implementation results are shown in Figures 7.6, 7.7, and 7.8.

Our information is stored on a Firebase cloud platform. Figure 7.6 shows the heartbeat sweat and temperature measurements from the prototype constructed using ESP8266. The measured values are sent to mobile app and also it is uploaded to cloud.

Figure 7.7 shows the data stored in the database in the Firebase cloud platform. Data uploading to the cloud is done only after processing the data in the fog and edge node.

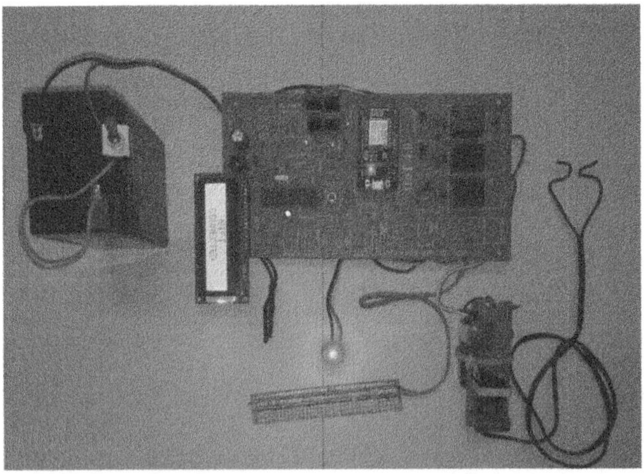

Figure 7.5 The system's prototype.

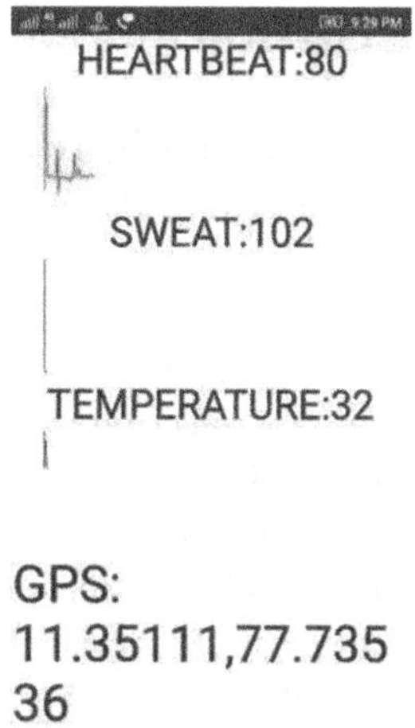

Figure 7.6 Heart beat sweat and temperature measurements from prototype.

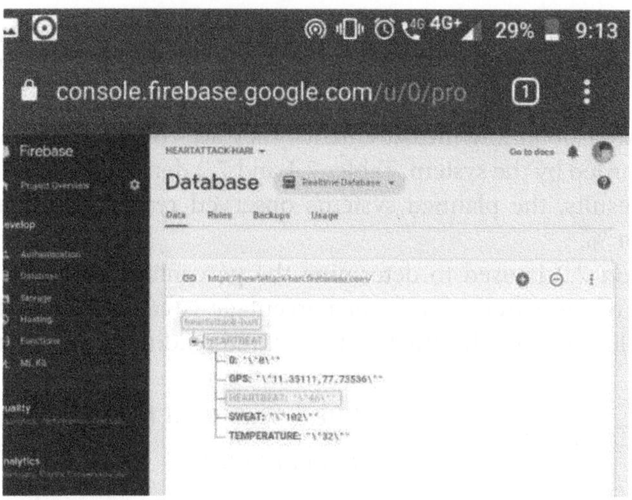

Figure 7.7 Data Stored in the database in the Firebase Cloud Platform.

The Arduino IDE package is used for creating the programming code required for the microcontroller to operate as specified. The hardware cannot execute its functions without these sensor libraries (e.g., DHT22, DS18b20, MAX30102).

7.6 Results and Discussion

When it comes to ensuring the dependability of the system that has been suggested, one of the most important players and goals is ensuring the accuracy of the measurements. As a result, to guarantee a high level of dependability and trust, we will give careful consideration to the precision of the measurements produced by the proposed system in comparison to other measures. To determine how accurately the proposed system measures, the measurements obtained from several people of different ages and genders were analyzed and compared to those obtained from commercially available medical equipment. Tests have been performed on the measures of heart rate and SpO_2 as well as the temperature of the body.

The following formula estimates the number of cardiac cycles the heart completes each minute to calculate Heart Rate (HR). Equation to calculate heart rate is given by Equation 7.1

$$\text{Heart Rate} = 60\text{T (bpm)} \tag{7.1}$$

where T is the time required to complete one cardiac cycle and bpm is beats per minute. The assessment of HR and SpO_2 is carried out with the use of an IMDK pulse oximeter. It is utilized frequently by medical professionals. After obtaining measurements, they are compared to those previously recorded by the system. Tables 7.1 and 7.2 demonstrate the proposed device's results, the planned system's observed results, and the HR and SpO_2 error %.

Equation 7.2 is used to determine the percentage inaccuracy for any given set of measurements. Error percentage is calculated for heart rate and SpO_2 levels through actual and measured readings using Equation 7.2.

$$Error(\%) = \frac{actual\ reading - measured\ reading}{actual\ reading} \times 100 \tag{7.2}$$

The measurements of the system's body temperature that were obtained using a medical thermometer were analyzed. The values of oxygen saturation (SpO2), and heart rate are compared and contrasted in the graphs that may be seen in Figures 7.8 and 7.9. The values that were measured and those that were used as references varied from one another, although only slightly. 10 samples are considered for analysis of heart rate. Measured

Table 7.1 Heart rate readings (reference) and proposed system (measured).

Sample	Reference value (bpm)	Measured value (bpm)	Error (%)
1	110	108	1.82
2	118	116	1.69
3	99	100	1.01
4	105	104	0.95
5	89	89	0.00
6	113	112	0.88
7	90	92	2.22
8	115	116	0.87
9	106	106	0.00
10	98	97	1.02

Table 7.2 SPO_2 readings (reference) and proposed system (measured).

Sample	Reference value (%)	Measured value (%)	Error (%)
1	98	97	1.02
2	97	98	1.03
3	98	99	1.02
4	96	96	0.00
5	97	98	1.03
6	98	99	1.02
7	99	98	1.01
8	97	97	0.00
9	99	98	1.01
10	99	98	1.01

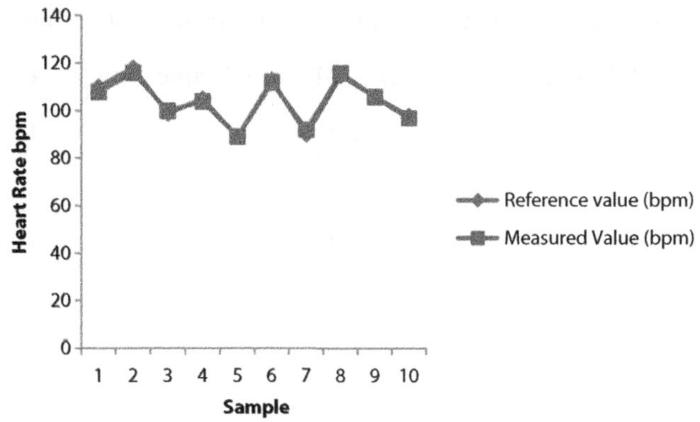

Figure 7.8 Heart rate level comparison between the reference and measured values.

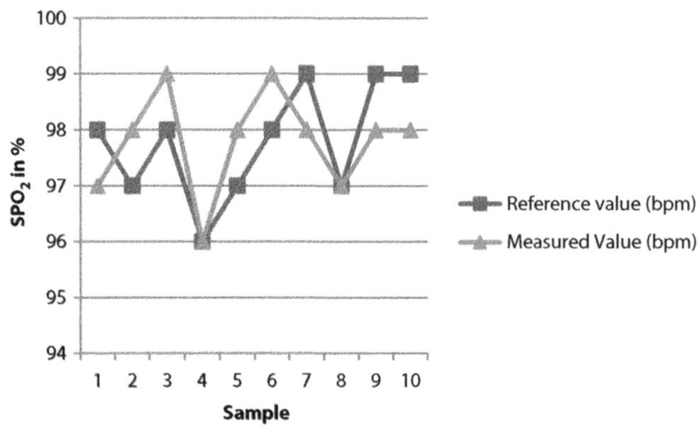

Figure 7.9 Oxygen saturation (SpO2) level comparison between the reference and measured values.

heart rate values are matching with the reference value with little deviation. For the oxygen saturation levels, deviation is noted from the reference values.

The highest error percentages for measurements of heart rate (HR), oxygen saturation (SpO2), and body temperature are respectively 2.63% and 2.02%. These values fall outside the permissible error range for these measures. These findings provide evidence that the suggested medical system may be implemented successfully. The suggested system's measurements match the conventional observations well.

7.7 Conclusion

A gadget that is both portable and capable of real-time operation has been developed. It is suitable for generally accepted medical purposes. Using a variety of sensors, the system logs the patient's vital signs and accompanying biomarkers. It additionally makes it possible to obtain this information both locally and remotely. To simplify the transmission of medical data, a microcontroller is used for data analysis and to establish connectivity with the Firebase server. Readings and diagrams might be shown on the device's display or transferred to a local mobile app for local monitoring. Alternatively, readings and diagrams are displayed on the device's external display. Sending measurements to a cloud server hosted by Firebase enables remote monitoring. In the final arrangement, the interface for remote monitoring is located within a reputable medical institution. The suggested system's readings were compared to standard medical equipment to confirm accuracy. Both devices provide results that are shown to have a high degree of consistency with one another. The error rates for the oxygen saturation in the blood, and heart rate are correspondingly 2.02%, and 2.63%, as stated in the reports. This demonstrates that the suggested method is successful and easily accessed by patients and elderly people in the hospital facilities in which they are located as well as in their homes.

References

1. Siam, A., II, El-Affendi, M.A., Abou Elazm, A., El-Banby, G.M., El-Bahnasawy, N.A., Abd El-Samie, F.E., Abd El-Latif, A.A., Portable and real-time IoT-based healthcare monitoring system for daily medical applications. *IEEE Trans. Comput. Soc. Syst.*, 2022.
2. Simerka, P., Council Recommendation of 9 June 2009 on patient safety, including the prevention and control of healthcare associated infections. pp. 1–6, Official journal of the European Union, Luxembourg, 2009.
3. Centers for Disease Control and Prevention. About Chronic Diseases, Accessed: Jul. 30, 2023. https://www.cdc.gov/chronicdisease/about/index.htm.
4. Majumder, S., Mondal, T., Deen, M.J., Wearable sensors for remote health monitoring. *Sensors*, 17, 1, 130, 2017.
5. Pantelopoulos, A. and Bourbakis, N.G., A survey on wearable sensor-based systems for health monitoring and prognosis. *IEEE Trans. Syst. Man Cybern. Part C Appl. Rev.*, 40, 1, 1–12, 2009.

6. Kharel, J., Reda, H.T., Shin, S.Y., Fog computing-based smart health monitoring system deploying LoRa wireless communication. *IETE Tech. Rev.*, 36, 1, 69–82, 2019.
7. Siam, A., II, El-Bahnasawy, N.A., El Banby, G.M., Abou Elazm, A., Abd El-Samie, F.E., Efficient video-based breathing pattern and respiration rate monitoring for remote health monitoring. *JOSA A*, 37, 11, C118–C124, 2020.
8. Taiwo, O. and Ezugwu, A.E., Smart healthcare support for remote patient monitoring during covid-19 quarantine. *Inf. Med. Unlocked*, 20, 100428, 2020.
9. Siam, A., II, Almaiah, M.A., Al Zahrani, A., Elazm, A.A., El Banby, G.M., El-Shafai, W., El-Bahnasawy, N.A., Secure health monitoring communication systems based on IoT and cloud computing for medical emergency applications. *Comput. Intell. Neurosci.*, 20212021.
10. Alharbey, R., Dessouky, M.M., Sedik, A., Siam, A., II, Elaskily, M.A., Fatigue state detection for tired persons in the presence of driving periods. *IEEE Access*, 10, 79403–79418, 2022.
11. Soufiene, B.O., Bahattab, A.A., Trad, A., Youssef, H., LSDA: lightweight secure data aggregation scheme in healthcare using IoT, in: *Proceedings of the 10th International Conference on Information Systems and Technologies*, 2020, June, pp. 1–4.
12. Ghosh, A.M., Halder, D., Hossain, S.A., Remote health monitoring system through IoT, in: *2016 5th International Conference on Informatics, Electronics and Vision (ICIEV)*, 2016, May, IEEE, pp. 921–926.
13. Khoi, N.M., Saguna, S., Mitra, K., Åhlund, C., IReHMo: An efficient IoT-based remote health monitoring system for smart regions, in: *2015 17th International Conference on e-health Networking, Application & Services (HealthCom)*, 2015, October, IEEE, pp. 563–568.
14. Al-Khafajiy, M., Baker, T., Chalmers, C., Asim, M., Kolivand, H., Fahim, M., Waraich, A., Remote health monitoring of elderly through wearable sensors. *Multimed. Tools Appl.*, 78, 17, 24681–24706, 2019.
15. Baig, M.M. and Gholamhosseini, H., Smart health monitoring systems: an overview of design and modeling. *J. Med. Syst.*, 37, 1–14, 2013.
16. Devi, M.P., Choudhry, M.D., Sundarrajan, M., Sivapriyanga, P., An efficient 24× 7 patient's vital parameter monitoring framework using machine learning based Internet of Biomedical Things: a comprehensive approach, in: *Advances in Image and Data Processing using VLSI Design Biomedical Applications*, vol. 2, IOP Publishing, Bristol, UK, 2022.
17. Parimala Devi, M., Raja, G.B., Gowrishankar, V., Sathya, T., IoMT-based smart diagnostic/therapeutic kit for pandemic patients, in: *Internet of Medical Things for Smart Healthcare: Covid-19 Pandemic*, pp. 141–165, 2020.
18. Devi, M.P., Sathya, T., Raja, G.B., Remote Human's Health and Activities Monitoring Using Wearable Sensor-Based System—A Review, in: *Efficient Data Handling for Massive Internet of Medical Things: Healthcare Data Analytics*, pp. 203–228, 2021.

19. Parimala Devi, M., Boopathi Raja, G., Sathya, T., Gowrishankar, V., Post-analysis of COVID-19 pneumonia based on chest CT images using AI algorithms: a clinical point of view, in: *Artificial Intelligence Strategies for Analyzing COVID-19 Pneumonia Lung Imaging Characterization Approaches*, vol. 1, pp. 9–1, IOP Publishing, Bristol, UK, 2022.
20. Chakraborty, C., Banerjee, A., Garg, L., Rodrigues, J.J., Internet of medical things for smart healthcare, in: *Studies in big data*, vol. 80, Springer, Cham, Switzerland, 2020.
21. Siam, A., II, Soliman, N.F., Algarni, A.D., El-Samie, A., Fathi, E., Sedik, A., Deploying machine learning techniques for human emotion detection. *Comput. Intell. Neurosci.*, 2022.
22. Dağtaş, S., Pekhteryev, G., Şahinoğlu, Z., Cam, H., Challa, N., Real-time and secure wireless health monitoring. *Int. J. Telemed. Appl.*, 2008.
23. Khan, Y., Han, D., Ting, J., Ahmed, M., Nagisetty, R., Arias, A.C., Organic multi-channel optoelectronic sensors for wearable health monitoring. *IEEE Access*, 7, 128114–128124, 2019.
24. Majumder, S. and Deen, M.J., Smartphone sensors for health monitoring and diagnosis. *Sensors*, 19, 9, 2164, 2019.
25. Philip, N.Y., Rodrigues, J.J., Wang, H., Fong, S.J., Chen, J., Internet of Things for in-home health monitoring systems: Current advances, challenges and future directions. *IEEE J. Sel. Areas Commun.*, 39, 2, 300–310, 2021.
26. Ali, M.M., Haxha, S., Alam, M.M., Nwibor, C., Sakel, M., Design of Internet of Things (IoT) and Android Based Low-Cost Health Monitoring Embedded System Wearable Sensor for Measuring SpO2, Heart Rate and Body Temperature Simultaneously. *Wirel. Pers. Commun.*, 111, 2449–2463, 2020.
27. Swaroop, K.N., Chandu, K., Gorrepotu, R., Deb, S., A health monitoring system for vital signs using IoT. *Internet Things*, 5, 116–129, 2019.
28. Siam, A., II, Abou Elazm, A., El-Bahnasawy, N.A., El Banby, G., Abd El-Samie, F.E., Abd El-Samie, F.E., Smart health monitoring system based on IoT and cloud computing. *Menoufia J. Electron. Eng. Res.*, 28, 1, 37–42, 2019.

8

Pioneering Implantable IoT: A New Era of Precision Medicine for Humans and Animals Unveiling the Future of Medicine Through Implantable Technology

Md. Afroz[1]*, Emmanuel Nyakwende[1] and Birendra Goswami[2]

[1]Department of IT, Al Faisal University, Prince Sultan College of Business, Jeddah, Saudi Arabia
[2]Department of Computer Science & IT, Sai Nath University, Ranchi, Jharkhand, India

Abstract

The emergence of implantable Internet of Things (IoT) technology represents a momentous milestone in the evolution of precision medicine, encompassing both human and veterinary healthcare domains. Implantable IoT devices, comprising sensors and microchips, possess the capability to continuously monitor vital signs, organ function, and other pivotal health parameters in real-time. This transformative technology has the potential to revolutionize medical diagnostics and treatment modalities, facilitating personalized therapies that can be dynamically adjusted to individual patient needs. In the context of diabetic patients, for instance, implanted IoT devices can monitor blood glucose levels and administer insulin as necessitated. Furthermore, these devices offer the promise of remote patient monitoring, reducing hospitalizations and enhancing recovery periods. This paper delves into the far-reaching implications and prospects of implantable IoT technology in the realm of precision medicine, highlighting its potential to reshape the healthcare landscape. Notably, this innovation stands poised to improve patient outcomes while simultaneously mitigating healthcare costs, with similar benefits extending to veterinary care through real-time monitoring of animal patients' vital signs.

**Corresponding author*: afrozhasnain@gmail.com

Hari Murthy, Marta Zurek-Mortka, Vinay Jha Pillai and Kukatlapalli Pradeep Kumar (eds.)
Internet of Things in Bioelectronics: Emerging Technologies and Applications, (145–170) © 2024 Scrivener Publishing LLC

Keywords: Implantable devices, Internet of Things (IoT), IoMT (internet of medical things), precision medicine, pioneering technology, human health, animal health, implantable IoT

8.1 Introduction

The Internet of Things (IoT) has brought about a paradigm shift across various sectors, fundamentally altering our engagement with the environment that surrounds us. One of the most noteworthy progressions in this domain is the utilization of IoT implant devices for therapeutic objectives in both humans and animals [1]. IoT implant devices, diminutive biocompatible electronic constituents engineered to be integrated within the organisms of humans or animals, pave the way for a plethora of functions. These range from monitoring critical signs, dispensing medication, or delivering real-time feedback on the body's condition, all while connecting to the internet or local networks for communication and data exchange with external apparatus or systems.

The purpose of this chapter is to provide a thorough introduction to IoT implant devices, analyze their many therapeutic uses, highlight the relevance of these devices in healthcare and veterinary medicine, and define the scope of this book chapter. These gadgets process and send data and have a sensor, an actuator, a power supply, and a communication module [2]. IoT implant devices have sensors that can assess parameters like body temperature, blood pressure, and glucose levels, and actuators that may initiate actions like medicine administration or electrical stimulation. With the help of the communication module, these gadgets may share information with other devices like computers and mobile phones.

Medical implant devices that use the IoT are a promising new area of research that might significantly improve patient care. These gadgets have several potential uses, including but not limited to the tracking of chronic illness progression, the monitoring of medication adherence, and the facilitation of remote patient monitoring. The potential for hacks and illegal access to these devices raises privacy and security issues, however. IoT implant devices have showed promise in improving patient outcomes and lowering healthcare expenditures, according to a recent research published in [3]. The research looked at the effectiveness of monitoring heart failure patients using IoT implant devices, and it revealed that the number of patients requiring hospitalization or emergency department visits dropped significantly. The authors suggest that IoT implant devices have

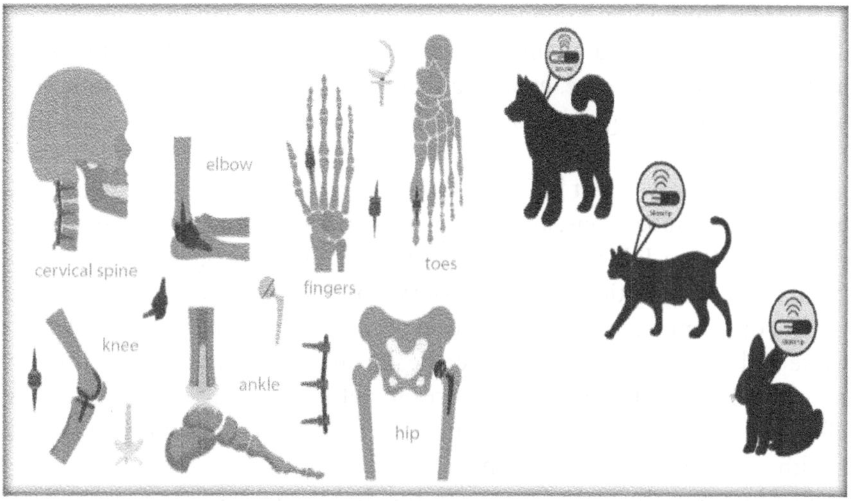

Figure 8.1 A schematic representation of implantable technology in human and animals. Adapted with permission from www.istockphoto.com.

the potential to transform healthcare by enabling more personalized and proactive care.

IoT implant devices as shown in Figure 8.1, [33] boast an array of therapeutic applications in human and veterinary medicine. One prominent application is pain management, where devices can mitigate chronic pain through targeted electrical stimulation to the nervous system or dispensing precise medication dosages. This method can decrease the necessity for systemic opioids and minimize adverse effects. In the realm of diabetes management, IoT implant devices can incessantly monitor glucose levels and autonomously release insulin as needed, offering superior glycemic control for diabetic patients. These devices can also be employed in neurostimulation, targeting specific brain or nervous system regions in patients with neurological disorders, such as epilepsy or Parkinson's disease, to alleviate symptoms and enhance their quality of life. Monitoring cardiac activity in real time with implanted IoT devices enables for early diagnosis of possible problems and rapid intervention if needed [4]. With the use of the IoT, prosthetic limbs and orthotic devices may provide real-time feedback to patients and healthcare professionals, allowing for more precise modifications and better patient outcomes. Health monitoring, drug administration, and even reproductive control in cattle are just some of the therapeutic uses for IoT implant devices in veterinary medicine [5].

There is substantial hope that IoT implant devices will improve human and animal health and quality of life. These tools enable for individualized and precise medical care, ensuring that each patient receives an intervention specifically designed to address their condition. A patient's vitals may be monitored in real time, allowing doctors to make better judgments and give prompter treatment [6]. When it comes to managing chronic illnesses, avoiding hospitalizations, and improving general health, patients may benefit greatly from IoT implant devices that automate drug supply or treatments. The elimination of unnecessary hospitalizations, enhancement of patient outcomes, and standardization of care delivery are all ways in which these technologies may help lower healthcare expenditures [6]. Animals may benefit from IoT implant devices in veterinary practice because they allow for more targeted care, less invasive treatments, and more proactive health and well-being management [7].

Beginning in the early 1900s with the development of the first artificial implants, the development of implanted medical devices has been spectacular. The stainless steel and silicone biomaterials that were pioneered in the 1950s paved the way for future generations of sophisticated implants. In 1961, the cochlear implant was introduced to help those with extreme hearing loss hear again. The first pacemaker, a lifesaving cardiac gadget, was put in 1958. Thanks to advances in materials, electronics, and surgical techniques, implanted medical devices have come a long way since then. More long-lasting and practical implants became possible with the advent of biocompatible materials in the 1970s, such as titanium and medical-grade polymers. Microelectronics' meteoric ascent in the 1980s paved the way for the shrinking of devices like glucose monitors, neurostimulators, and drug delivery systems that can be surgically implanted. Improvements in battery life and wireless connectivity made possible by technological advances in the 1990s allowed implanted devices to become more practical. Biocompatibility was enhanced by the use of novel materials and coatings, and the danger of infection was mitigated by the use of CAD and CAM technology, which allowed for the production of individualized implants [8].

The concept of ubiquitous computing envisioned a future where technology seamlessly integrates into the fabric of everyday life, and the healthcare sector has not remained untouched by this vision. The early 2000s marked a significant juncture in the healthcare sector, as it witnessed the emergence of linked health equipment, thereby inaugurating the era of the Internet of Things (IoT) within this domain. This transformative phase was characterized by the convergence of IoT technology and healthcare, which in turn catalyzed a paradigm shift in remote patient monitoring. Most importantly, these technological advancements democratized healthcare. Patients, armed with IoT devices for health monitoring, gained agency in managing their well-being. This empowerment facilitated collaborative, patient-centric healthcare delivery by enabling seamless sharing of relevant health data with healthcare providers. Simultaneously, the pervasive availability of wireless communication technologies, encompassing Bluetooth, Wi-Fi, and cellular networks, played a pivotal role in facilitating the seamless integration of IoT devices into existing healthcare infrastructures. These technologies enabled the effortless transmission of vital health information from patients' IoT devices to healthcare facilities. This, in turn, fostered an environment in which healthcare professionals could remotely monitor and assess the health status of patients in real-time, transcending the constraints of physical proximity. Due to their similar histories, the IoT and implanted medical devices have naturally converged. Improvements in microelectronics, wireless connectivity, and data analytics are only a few of the elements that have led to the emergence of IoT implant devices. Implantable devices owe a great deal to the advancements in microelectronics, which have allowed for their downsizing and the integration of sensors, processors, and power sources. IoT implant devices were able to shrink and become more power efficient with the advent of low-power microprocessors and energy-efficient sensor technologies. This breakthrough paved the way for the development of gadgets that can monitor and control vital signs like glucose levels and heart rate in real time. IoT implant devices may now be remotely monitored and controlled because to advancements in wireless communication technology. The evolution of Bluetooth Low Energy (BLE) and ZigBee, two low-power wireless communication protocols, has eased the transfer of data between implant devices and external devices, such as smartphones or specialized monitoring systems. As a result of this linkage, doctors may now access patient records from afar, modify their patients' treatments on the go, and provide them immediate feedback. IoT implant devices have benefited greatly from the advent of data analytics and artificial intelligence (AI), which have made it possible to process and analyze enormous volumes of health data. The ability of machine learning algorithms to recognize patterns and trends in data paves the way for the creation of prediction models and individualized treatment strategies. Data-driven healthcare has emerged as a result, with the goal of using the vast volumes of data produced by IoT implant devices to enhance patient outcomes and enhance healthcare efficiency.

IoT implant devices for different medicinal uses in people and animals have seen rapid progress in recent years [9]. Examples of IoT-enabled devices for healthcare include neurostimulators developed to alleviate symptoms of conditions like Parkinson's disease and epilepsy. These implants may alleviate symptoms and improve quality of life by continuously or in reaction to recognized neural activity stimulating certain parts of the brain [5]. Defibrillators and monitors for irregular heartbeats are called implantable cardioverter-defibrillators (ICDs), and they are IoT enabled. With the use of IoT technology, cardiac events may be predicted based on remote monitoring of device performance and real-time data analysis. It's also possible to improve treatment effectiveness and reduce negative effects by using IoT implant devices to administer drugs directly to specific areas of the body. Insulin pumps, for instance, may provide individualized diabetes treatment by continually monitoring blood glucose levels and adjusting insulin dosage appropriately, thanks to the IoT.

In order to track patient motion and biomechanics, orthopedic implants like knee and hip replacements have included IoT technology. This information may be utilized to evaluate the effectiveness of implants, anticipate the need for revision surgery, and fine-tune rehabilitation plans. Therapeutic applications for IoT implant devices in animals include monitoring and managing chronic pain in companion animals and livestock [10]. These tools may help veterinarians better understand their patients' physiological and behavioral aspects, leading to more effective therapy and better animal care. Medical innovation in the form of IoT implant devices for therapeutic purposes in people and animals has the potential to significantly advance the fields of personalized medicine, remote patient monitoring, and data-driven decision making. Data privacy, cyber security, and product liability are just a few of the ethical, legal, and regulatory issues that are brought up by these gadgets. Researchers, doctors, policymakers, and other stakeholders must collaborate to find solutions to these problems and assure the safe and effective use of IoT implant devices as they continue to develop and become more commonplace in healthcare.

This chapter's objectives are as follows:

a) To explain the technology behind IoT implant devices and its core components.
b) To discover the many ways in which IoT implant devices might be used therapeutically in human and veterinary medicine, therefore demonstrating their broad applicability and promising future.
c) To highlight the relevance of IoT implant devices in healthcare and veterinary medicine, with specific reference to their potential advantages and contributions to areas such as individualized treatment, continuous monitoring, patient

compliance, disease management, efficiency, cost-effectiveness, and animal welfare.

d) To address issues of data privacy, security, and the possibility of unintended effects or abuse connected with the introduction of IoT implant devices.

e) To provide an in-depth analysis of the existing landscape of IoT implant devices for therapeutic applications and the trajectory of this fast-developing area of study.

8.2 IoT Implanted Devices

Due to advancements in IoT technology and the development of implanted medical devices, the healthcare business has undergone a dramatic transformation. Implantable medical device connectivity to the IoT enables remote monitoring and real-time data access. Recent academic articles [11] state that using IoT technology in implanted medical devices has drastically improved healthcare results, and that this trend is only set to continue [6–8]. In this chapter, we'll take a look at how different IoT implanted devices are put to use in the medical treatment of people and animals.

a) Cardiac devices
b) Neurostimulation devices
c) Insulin pumps
d) Retinal implants
e) Cochlear implants
f) Other applications

Pacemakers, IoT implant devices, regulate the heart's rhythm by administering electrical impulses to cardiac muscles. Patients with bradycardia, characterized by abnormally slow heart rates, often use these devices. With the help of the IoT, pacemakers may be remotely monitored, allowing doctors to make real-time modifications to the device's settings and react quickly to any issues that may arise. Consequently, patient safety and clinical outcomes improve significantly. Implantable Cardioverter Defibrillators (ICDs), located in the chest or abdomen, observe the heart's electrical activity to identify life-threatening arrhythmias. When an abnormal heart rhythm is detected, the ICD delivers a shock to restore a normal heartbeat. IoT connectivity augments ICDs by facilitating remote monitoring and data collection, enhancing patient care, and minimizing hospital visits. Cardiac Resynchronization Therapy (CRT) devices, also known as biventricular pacemakers, are engineered to treat heart failure by coordinating the contractions of the left and right ventricles. IoT-integrated CRT devices bolster patient outcomes by offering real-time monitoring, tailoring individualized treatment plans, and cutting down hospital visits.

Deep Brain Stimulation (DBS) devices are implanted in specific brain areas to alleviate symptoms of neurological disorders such as Parkinson's disease, essential tremor, and dystonia. They function by delivering electrical stimulation to targeted regions, thus modulating abnormal brain activity. IoT technology integration in DBS devices permits remote monitoring, personalized therapy, and enhanced data collection for research and development. Spinal Cord Stimulators (SCS) devices are used to manage chronic pain by administering mild electrical pulses to the spinal cord, disrupting pain signals before they reach the brain. Advantages of SCS devices that include the IoT include remote modification of stimulation settings, data collecting for tailored therapy, and real-time monitoring. Devices called vagus nerve stimulators (VNS) are implanted subcutaneously in the chest to stimulate the vagus nerve electrically. When conventional therapies for epilepsy and depression have failed, this method is often used as a last resort. By connecting to the internet, VNS devices may be remotely monitored and adjusted for optimal patient care.

Insulin pumps with built-in IoT sensors allow for remote glucose monitoring, real-time data processing, and individualized insulin administration. Improved glucose control, fewer bouts of hypoglycemia, and a higher quality of life for diabetes patients are the outcomes of these features. Partially blinded people with RP or AMD may get their sight back with the use of retinal implants, which are IoT-enabled devices. These implants transform light into electrical impulses that go down the optic nerve directly to the brain. Retinal implants with IoT connection provide continuous monitoring, individualized care, and data collecting for future study. Patients with degenerative retinal illnesses may benefit from increased visual acuity and enhanced quality of life thanks to the use of IoT technology in retinal implants.

Cochlear implants are devices that stimulate the auditory nerve directly, enabling the brain to sense sound even if the hair cells in the inner ear are destroyed. Advantages of IoT-enabled cochlear implants include remote monitoring of device operation, individualized auditory therapy, and data collecting for future study [12]. This innovation might help those who are hard of hearing by boosting speech recognition and other auditory outcomes.

There are a plethora of additional applications being developed or investigated, in addition to the IoT implant devices we've already covered. Some of these include:

- Instruments used to monitor the gastrointestinal tract (GI) and record data such as pH, pressure, and temperature are invaluable in the diagnosis and treatment of a wide range of GI conditions. These tools may enhance healthcare decision-making and lead to better patient outcomes.
- Implantable BCIs provide a direct line of communication between the brain and other devices like computers and prostheses. Integrating IoT into BCIs might allow for continuous monitoring of brain activity, individualized treatment, and better prosthetic device control.
- Effective and safe drug treatment is enhanced by implantable drug delivery systems (IDDS) that allow for precise dosing and monitoring of medication levels. Chronic diseases like cancer and pain might be treated in whole new ways because to this breakthrough in technology.
- Implantable biosensors with the ability to continually monitor vital signs including blood sugar, blood pressure, and core body temperature. With the right data, these devices have the potential to improve patient outcomes by informing individualized treatment strategies in real time.

8.3 Monitoring and Tracking Implants

In veterinary medicine, IoT implant devices in animals have piqued interest, particularly for therapeutic purposes. In addition to monitoring and identification, these gadgets can now provide precise therapy for a range of medical issues. Miniature, implanted devices known as "microchips" are used to store a person's unique identity information. This feature enables pet owners and veterinarians to access critical information about the animal, including medical records, vaccinations, and owner contact information. Typically, these microchips are injected under the skin in the animal's neck area using a hypodermic needle. The biocompatible glass-encased microchip, comparable in size to a grain of rice, remains in place for the animal's lifetime.

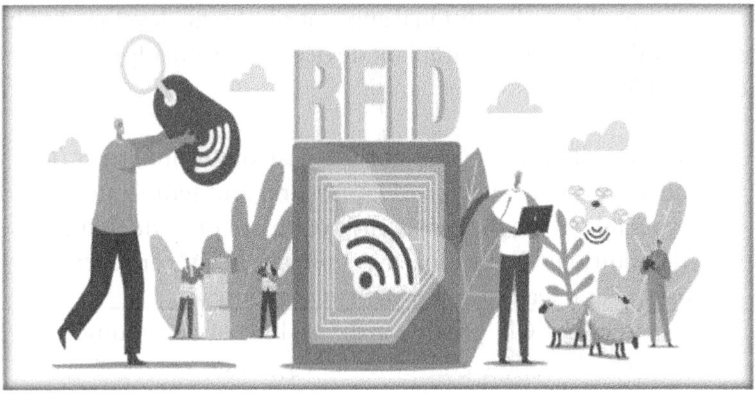

Figure 8.2 A schematic representation of RFID technology. Adapted with permission from www.istockphoto.com.

A radio frequency identification (RFID) scanner shown in Figure 8.2 [34] can read the microchip, transmitting the unique identification number to a database. Consequently, the database provides relevant information about the animal, which is particularly useful in the event of lost or stolen pets. The widespread adoption of identification microchips has increased pet reunification rates, reducing the burden on animal shelters and ensuring animal welfare. According to a study by [13], the use of microchipping in animals can significantly increase the likelihood of their return to their owners when lost. The study also found that microchipped animals had a higher chance of being returned home than those without microchips [9].

Another type of IoT implant device used for monitoring and tracking animals is Global Positioning System (GPS) tracking devices. Employing GPS technology, these devices provide real-time location information, accessible via a smartphone or computer. While predominantly used for pets, GPS tracking devices are also invaluable for tracking wildlife populations for research and conservation purposes. GPS tracking devices come in various forms, including collar attachments and implantable devices. Implantable GPS devices are more reliable and harder to remove or tamper with, offering pet owners peace of mind [14]. They feature geofencing capabilities, allowing pet owners to set virtual boundaries for their pets and receive alerts if the animal leaves the designated area. In addition, GPS trackers can keep tabs on the animal's whereabouts and condition, revealing previously unknown details about its well-being.

8.4 Therapeutic Implants

Diabetes mellitus is an endocrine condition that has been seen in animal populations. Managing diabetes in dogs, especially Type 1 diabetes, requires insulin treatment. Pet owners may struggle with insulin injections because of the difficulty they present, and poor blood sugar management increases the risk of problems. Insulin pumps with IoT connectivity are implanted medical devices that provide a steady stream of insulin subcutaneously, imitating the body's natural release rhythm as nearly as possible [15]. In order to inject insulin subcutaneously, these devices include a reservoir, a pump, and a cannula. Depending on the animal's demands, insulin pumps may be set to release differing doses of insulin at different times of the day. Diabetes may be better managed with the use of continuous glucose monitoring (CGM) devices, which are often used in combination with insulin pumps to give real-time blood sugar readings. With the information sent from the CGM devices to a smartphone or computer, pet owners and veterinarians can make educated choices regarding insulin administration and treatment options.

Particularly in geriatric dogs and those with preexisting health concerns, chronic discomfort is a major problem. By altering the activity of the nervous system, implantable IoT devices like neurostimulation devices may alleviate pain. Stimulators of the spinal cord and other nerves are included in this category. To prevent pain signals from reaching the brain, spinal cord stimulators may be placed close to the spinal cord and programmed to emit moderate electrical impulses. Studies in animals with chronic pain problems like arthritis or degenerative disc degeneration have demonstrated that SCS may alleviate their suffering. When it comes to relieving pain, peripheral nerve stimulators zero in on the actual source—the nerves themselves. Implanted near the affected nerves, these devices send out electrical impulses, blocking pain signals before they reach the spinal cord. Pain resulting from cancer treatment, surgery, or nerve damage may all be effectively treated by PNS.

Stimulation settings for SCS and PNS devices may be changed electronically to best suit the animal. Animals with chronic pain may benefit greatly from the use of neurostimulation devices, which can also lessen their need on medicine over the long run. Medical illnesses that need accurate dosage or continuous administration of a medicine may benefit greatly from implantable drug delivery system (IDDS) devices. IDDS provide several benefits over conventional drug delivery systems, including more patient compliance, less unwanted side effects, and more effective therapy. Osmotic pumps, microchips, and biodegradable implants are just some of the implanted medication delivery technologies available. Osmotic pumps store medication in a reservoir and release it slowly across a semi-permeable membrane. IDDS built on microchips store numerous doses of a medicine in separate reservoirs, each of which may be triggered by a different external signal (such as an electric current or a certain frequency). Biodegradable implants consist of biocompatible materials that break down over time, allowing the encapsulated medicine to be released in a measured manner. Animals with illnesses including cancer, arthritis, and hormone abnormalities have benefited from the use of implantable medicine delivery devices. Cancer patients may have less systemic toxicity and greater therapeutic success with the use of implanted chemotherapy devices, for instance. Similarly, hormone-releasing implants can be used to manage hormonal imbalances in animals, such as hypothyroidism and adrenal insufficiency.

8.5 Communication Protocols

IoT implants harness various communication technologies to ensure smooth connectivity and data transfer between implanted devices and external systems [16]. Three dominant technologies are radio-frequency identification (RFID), Bluetooth Low Energy (BLE), and Near Field Communication (NFC). Owing to its low cost, small size, and battery-free operation, RFID is widely employed in medical and veterinary implant devices. Designed for energy-efficient communication, BLE is well-suited for IoT implant devices necessitating long battery life. Operating in the 2.4 GHz Industrial, Scientific, and Medical (ISM) radio band, BLE offers a range of up to 100 meters and supports data transfer rates of up to 1 Mbps. These features make BLE a popular choice for healthcare and veterinary applications, thanks to its low power consumption, smartphone compatibility, and ability to support multiple connections. As a short-range wireless communication technology, NFC facilitates data exchange between devices over distances of up to 10 centimeters [17]. Operating at 13.56 MHz, NFC supports data transfer rates of up to 424 kbps and is compatible with passive RFID tags. Near Field Communication (NFC)-enabled IoT implant devices can communicate with external systems like smartphones, tablets, and medical equipment, allowing for data exchange and device configuration. The limited range of NFC inherently enhances security since close proximity is required for communication, thereby reducing the risk of unauthorized access.

8.6 Power and Energy Harvesting

IoT implant devices have varying energy requirements depending on their complexity, functionality, and communication technology. This section delves into different power sources and energy harvesting techniques, encompassing batteries, wireless power transfer, and energy harvesting from the body. The most common power source for IoT implant devices, batteries are often coin cell or thin-film varieties due to their small size. The choice of battery technology depends on the device's energy density, discharge rate, and lifetime requirements, with lithium-ion, lithium-polymer, and solid-state batteries being common choices for implantable devices. The main drawback of using batteries in implant devices is that they will eventually need to be replaced, which may require invasive surgical operations. Power management methods like duty cycling, adaptive voltage scaling, and power gating may be used in devices to reduce power consumption and lengthen the battery's useful life.

Potentially replacing the requirement for batteries, wireless power transfer (WPT) methods allow energy to be transferred from an external source to an implanted device without the need of wires or other mechanical connections. This has the potential to lessen the hazards of invasive surgical procedures and remove the requirement for frequent battery replacement. There are a variety of WPT methods, such as inductive coupling, resonant coupling, and radio-frequency (RF) energy harvesting. Inductive coupling, the most common method, employs a pair of coils—one in the external power source and the other in the implant device. When the coils are in close proximity, a magnetic field is generated, allowing energy to be transferred wirelessly. The efficiency of inductive coupling depends on factors such as the distance between the coils, their alignment, and the operating frequency. An emerging technique for providing a sustainable power source for IoT implant devices is energy harvesting from the human or animal body [18]. This approach capitalizes on the energy generated from physiological processes or ambient sources within the body to power the device. Several energy harvesting techniques have been proposed, including piezoelectric, thermoelectric, and biofuel cells. Piezoelectric harvesting converts mechanical energy, such as vibrations or pressure, into electrical energy. This can be achieved by using materials that generate an electric charge in response to mechanical stress. Thermoelectric harvesting exploits the temperature difference between the body and the environment to generate electricity. Biofuel cells generate power through the chemical reactions between the body's fluids and implanted electrodes.

8.7 Data Security

As IoT implant devices often collect and store sensitive health information, as shown in Figure 8.3 [35]. Data security and privacy are critical concerns. This section discusses encryption, authentication, and secure data storage and transmission techniques employed in IoT implant devices.

To ensure data confidentiality, encryption converts data into a format that is unreadable by unauthorized parties. IoT implant devices can employ symmetric or asymmetric encryption algorithms to protect data [19]. The choice of encryption algorithm depends on the processing capabilities and energy constraints of the IoT implant device. Authentication mechanisms verify the identity of entities involved in communication to ensure that only authorized devices and users can access the IoT implant device. Knowledge (such as passwords or cryptographic keys), ownership (such as tokens or devices), or biometric traits (such as fingerprints or retina scans) may all be used for authentication. Implantable devices for the IoT often use cryptographic authentication protocols like Kerberos and Extensible Authentication Protocol (EAP). These protocols use cryptographic methods to verify the identity of all participants and create an encrypted link between them. Sensitive information must be stored safely on IoT implant devices to avoid theft or manipulation. safe data storage methods include encrypting data at rest, implementing access control mechanisms, and storing cryptographic keys in safe hardware modules. To ensure the privacy, integrity, and availability of the sent data, there must be a secure channel of communication between the implant devices and the outside systems.

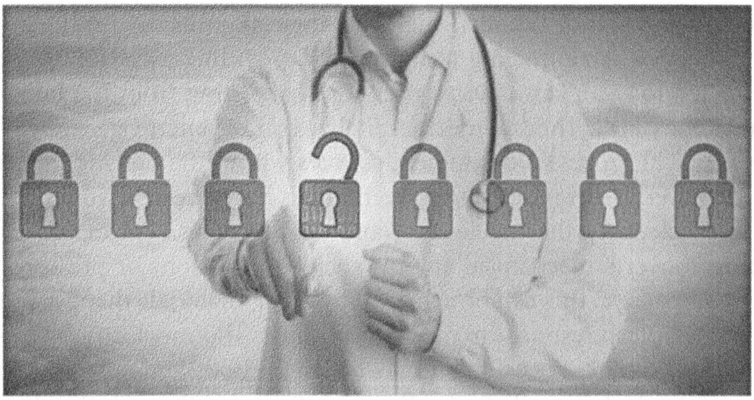

Figure 8.3 A schematic representation of data security and privacy. Adapted with permission from www.istockphoto.com.

Methods for transmitting data securely include encrypting communications, utilizing secure protocols like Transport Layer Security (TLS) and Datagram Transport Layer Security (DTLS), and using message authentication codes and digital signatures to ensure data is valid.

Informed consent is a cornerstone of medical practice and research because it guarantees patients' autonomy over their own bodies and treatment choices. Informed permission is critical for IoT implant devices due to the inherent dangers and intrusive nature of the implantation process. In order for patients to provide their informed permission for the implantation of an IoT device, they must be given enough information to fully comprehend the potential dangers and advantages of the procedure [20]. Included within should be details on not just the treatment itself, but also its expected results, side effects, and any problems. Patients are better able to decide for themselves whether an IoT implant is the best course of therapy if they are made aware of, and given the opportunity to consider, other treatment choices. Continuous informed consent is required for IoT implant devices because of the possibility that the device's hazards and advantages may change as a result of software updates, revisions, or new uses. Therefore, healthcare practitioners need to remain in touch with their patients throughout time, updating them on any developments and re-obtaining permission if required. Children, the elderly, and those with cognitive disabilities are particularly at risk and need extra care. Surrogate decision-makers may be required to provide permission on behalf of patients in such circumstances. The onus is on healthcare practitioners to ensure that these surrogate decision-makers are knowledgeable and equipped to make choices in the patient's best interests.

There are serious privacy issues, especially about the risk of unauthorized access and abuse, associated with the collection, storage, and transmission of large volumes of personal and sensitive data by implant devices connected to the IoT. Strong data security measures are required for IoT implant devices in order to protect patients' privacy. Data encryption, authenticator methods, and constant scanning for vulnerabilities are all part of these safeguards. Manufacturers and healthcare providers should work together to create and maintain these safeguards. It is essential to set up distinct guidelines for data ownership and access. Patients have a right to know who will have access to their information and why. Consent should be acquired before any data is shared, especially for commercial or academic objectives. In addition, patients must have the freedom to see, alter, or remove their information. The abuse of IoT implant devices may compromise people's freedom and privacy. People's privacy and independence may be compromised if these gadgets were used to monitor their whereabouts and actions. There has to be rigorous restrictions in place to stop people from being tracked without their consent and to make sure these devices are only used for medical reasons [21]. IoT implant devices may be used for control and manipulation by abusive spouses, employers, or governments. Protections against this kind of abuse should be codified into law, with offenders facing consequences for their acts.

It is crucial to establish thorough regulatory frameworks and standards to guarantee the safe and ethical usage of IoT implant devices as their prevalence increases. Given the worldwide scope of the IoT sector, cross-border cooperation in the development of uniform standards and regulations is a must [22]. The ethical usage of IoT implant devices may be aided by the coordinated efforts of governments, manufacturers, healthcare professionals, and others involved in the field. Regulatory agencies need to provide rigorous testing and approval procedures for IoT implant devices. These procedures need to evaluate the gadgets' particular ethical implications along with their safety, effectiveness, and hazards. Furthermore, post-market monitoring should be developed to track the devices' long-term safety and efficacy. To guarantee that healthcare professionals are proficient in the use of IoT implant devices and can properly convey the dangers and advantages to patients, it is essential that they acquire the proper training as their use increases. Healthcare workers should be required to participate in ongoing education programs that expose them to new developments in the industry as they occur. In order to guarantee that people are aware of the moral and legal ramifications of using IoT implant devices, it is crucial to encourage patient education and activism. In order to do this, it is necessary to provide easily available teaching materials, as well as to set up support systems and advocacy organizations. The development and deployment of implantable IoT technologies must be subject to stringent ethical review [24]. Ethics committees and review boards may help with this by evaluating the moral effects of emerging technologies and keeping tabs on current clinical trials.

8.8 Future Scope and Challenges

IoT implant devices are rapidly advancing and becoming increasingly popular for a range of medical applications, from monitoring chronic conditions to delivering targeted therapies. As the field continues to progress, it is essential for researchers and developers to address critical challenges related to material selection, technological integration, ethical and practical implications, and regulatory approval. Few studies have highlighted the potential of IoT devices to improve patient outcomes and healthcare delivery [37–39]. Nonetheless, to ensure the safe and effective use of these devices, further research is required to address the challenges mentioned above [14, 15]. The integration of Internet of Things (IoT) implant devices into the realm of healthcare represents a seminal juncture in the trajectory of medical technology. These devices hold the potential to profoundly transform healthcare delivery and elevate patient outcomes on a global scale. Through the amalgamation of advanced materials, cutting-edge technology, and seamless integration with artificial intelligence (AI) and 5G networks, IoT implant devices stand poised to revolutionize the healthcare landscape. This essay delves into the multifaceted opportunities and concomitant challenges entailed in the assimilation of IoT implant devices into healthcare, addressing the subject matter with scholarly gravitas.

IoT implant devices are endowed with a distinctive capability: the continuous monitoring of vital signs and health parameters in patients. This capacity for real-time data collection affords healthcare practitioners the ability to promptly identify pathological conditions, thereby facilitating timely medical interventions. The consequential impact of such interventions is noteworthy, as they can markedly ameliorate patient outcomes by curtailing the progression of diseases and mitigating the associated financial burden on healthcare systems.

The convergence of IoT technology with AI algorithms serves to augment disease detection and diagnosis. Machine learning algorithms are proficient in parsing the voluminous data streams furnished by IoT implant devices to discern discernible patterns and anomalies. This fortifies healthcare professionals with invaluable insights, thereby streamlining the process of diagnosis and rendering it more precise and expeditious. The implications are profound, as earlier and more accurate diagnoses hold the potential to save lives and reduce the overall burden of disease. IoT implant devices engender the prospect of tailoring treatment plans to the unique needs of individual patients. Through the continuous monitoring of a patient's condition and their response to treatment regimens, healthcare providers are empowered to effectuate real-time adjustments to interventions. This not only enhances treatment efficacy but also diminishes the likelihood of adverse events, engendering a healthcare paradigm characterized by greater safety and efficacy.

In addition to their application in human healthcare, IoT implant devices hold significant promise in the domain of veterinary medicine. IoT implant devices can be judiciously employed to monitor the health of animals in real-time. Veterinarians, leveraging remote access to vital data, are endowed with the capacity to intervene promptly in cases of illness or distress among animals. This capability augments the overall welfare of animals by ensuring the timely provision of medical care, thus mitigating suffering and enhancing the quality of veterinary healthcare.

In the realm of livestock management, IoT implant devices can detect health issues in animals, such as temperature fluctuations, abnormal heart rates, or signs of disease. Farmers can receive instant alerts and take proactive measures to prevent disease outbreaks and economic losses. This not only protects animal well-being but also improves the sustainability of agricultural practices.

However, the widespread adoption of IoT implant devices also raises complex ethical and legal questions. The issue of data privacy and ownership necessitates careful consideration. Patients must have control over their health data, and informed consent should be obtained for data collection and transmission. Striking the right balance between the benefits of IoT implant devices and the protection of patient autonomy and privacy is paramount.

Moreover, cybersecurity concerns loom large. As these devices become increasingly interconnected, they are susceptible to cybersecurity threats. Ensuring robust encryption and authentication protocols are in place to safeguard sensitive medical data is imperative. Vulnerabilities must be identified and rectified promptly to prevent breaches of patient data, which could have catastrophic consequences.

The longevity and reliability of IoT implant devices are pivotal for their successful integration into healthcare. Material science and advanced manufacturing techniques can mitigate device degradation and failure. Additionally, optimizing power consumption and energy harvesting technologies can extend device life and reduce the need for invasive replacements. Exploring alternative power sources, such as bio-energy, holds promise for achieving sustained device performance.

Navigating the complex regulatory landscape is a significant hurdle for developers and manufacturers of IoT implant devices. Rigorous clinical trials are essential to demonstrate safety and efficacy for regulatory approval. Streamlining the regulatory process and fostering collaboration between stakeholders can facilitate the translation of these devices from research laboratories to clinical practice. Standardization in device design, performance, and testing protocols is imperative to ensure their safety and effectiveness.

Looking ahead, the potential applications of implantable IoT devices in healthcare are vast. Beyond monitoring blood glucose levels and cardiac activity, these devices could be employed to monitor neural activities, digestive system performance, and track the progression of tumors. The integration of AI and big data analytics will enable the extraction of deeper insights into individual health, prediction of potential ailments, and provision of preventive measures. Personal health dashboards that empower individuals to monitor their health metrics are on the horizon, fostering greater patient engagement in healthcare decision-making.

However, the long-term effects of IoT implant devices on physical health and internal systems warrant comprehensive investigation. Customization of these devices to cater to individual biological variations is crucial. Enhancing wireless connectivity and exploring integration with emerging technologies like augmented and virtual reality represent exciting avenues for further research and development.

In conclusion, IoT implant devices hold immense potential to revolutionize healthcare by enabling early disease detection, personalized treatment, and enhanced animal care. Nevertheless, their implementation necessitates careful consideration of ethical, legal, and regulatory aspects, alongside ongoing research to enhance device longevity and explore new applications [25]. The future of IoT implant devices in healthcare promises to be transformative, provided that these challenges are met with diligence and innovation. In conclusion, while implantable IoT promises a revolution in precision medicine, it comes with its own set of challenges and research gaps that need to be addressed. Bridging these gaps and overcoming challenges will pave the way for a new era of healthcare where continuous monitoring and real-time interventions become the norm.

8.9 Biomaterials

Safe and effective IoT implant devices rely heavily on the progress made in biomaterials research and development. Bioresorbable polymers are only one example of the innovative materials that have been developed by scientists [23]; these polymers are absorbed by the body once they have served their therapeutic purpose, minimizing the need for intrusive removal. These components are essential for minimizing the risk of rejection by the immune system and avoiding other unwanted side effects associated with implant usage.

IoT implant devices have found new potential with the advent of nanotechnology because of the shrinking that has made it possible to combine sensors, actuators, and communication modules into a single, small unit [27]. The development of microfabrication methods has also allowed for the fabrication of flexible, thin-film electronics with which biological tissues may interact without causing inflammation or tissue damage. Microelectromechanical systems (MEMS) technology is being employed for implantable devices, such as sensors and actuators, while nanoparticles and nanotubes are being researched for medication delivery.

To allow real-time data analysis, individualized treatment plans, and preventative health monitoring, Artificial Intelligence (AI) is positioned to become an integral part of future IoT implant devices. It is possible to use machine learning algorithms to analyze biometric data, forecast the development of illnesses, and modify treatment plans appropriately [28]. AI may also help doctors make better treatment decisions, leading to more precise and efficient care. AI may then be utilized to analyze the information gathered by the implant devices to create more effective medicines. When 5G networks are combined with IoT implant devices, it will dramatically improve data transmission times, latency, and reliability in healthcare. Rapid response and better patient outcomes are ensured because to this innovation's real-time monitoring, greater telemedicine capabilities, and remote access to implant devices. With this connection in place, medical professionals will be able to provide more all-encompassing care and support for patients, as well as speed up the development of future IoT implant devices.

The ability to make instantaneous modifications to treatment based on real-time monitoring of physiological data is key to maximizing therapeutic effectiveness while reducing unwanted side effects. In addition to improving patient outcomes, these gadgets may improve care by keeping doctors updated on a patient's condition in real time. New possibilities for neuromodulation and brain-computer interfaces (BCIs) have emerged as a result of developments in IoT implant devices [29]. Neurological and mental diseases may find therapy with the help of these devices because of their ability to either stimulate or inhibit certain brain circuits. A BCI may also help people who are paralyzed or have other difficulties communicate and operate external equipment. The therapeutic uses of BCIs are promising, but they also have the potential to enhance people with disabilities' daily lives.

8.10 Conclusion

IoT implant devices have become possible because to the progress of implanted medical devices and the rise of IoT, which has opened up new avenues for customized care, remote patient monitoring, and data-driven decision making. Advances in microelectronics, wireless communication, and data analytics have all contributed to the creation of smaller, more power-efficient IoT implant devices, making the convergence of IoT and implanted medical devices a logical evolution. The introduction of therapeutic IoT implant devices has had a profound effect on the medical industry. Due to the advancements in clinical outcomes, tailored treatment, and remote monitoring made possible by these technologies, patients have seen better care with fewer hospitalizations. By allowing for more precise tracking, diagnostics, and treatment, IoT implant devices in animals have the potential to revolutionize the veterinary industry. Improvements in pet safety and welfare have resulted from the widespread use of identification microchips and GPS tracking devices, while therapeutic devices like insulin pumps, neurostimulation devices, and implantable drug delivery systems have revolutionized the treatment of a wide range of chronic conditions in animals [32]. Implantable IoT devices are predicted to improve the quality of life for animals and their caretakers as technology develops.

Choosing the right mode of communication, power supply, and energy harvesting technique may have a significant impact on the device's usefulness, efficiency, and durability. Furthermore, protecting sensitive health information and keeping user confidence necessitates guaranteeing data security and privacy through encryption, authentication, and secure data storage and transfer protocols.

There is little question that as research and development in the area of IoT implant devices proceeds, more advanced, efficient, and secure devices will be created. Enhancing the energy efficiency of communication technology, investigating new energy harvesting methods, and creating solid security measures that can survive increasing cyber attacks are all areas that need further investigation in the future [26].

Stakeholders need to think about informed consent, privacy issues, abuse possibilities, and regulatory frameworks and rules to make sure these gadgets are used responsibly and for the greater good [30]. Establishing thorough regulatory frameworks and rules requires cooperation between producers, healthcare providers, governments, and other interested parties. In order to be proficient in their usage and to properly convey the risks and advantages to patients, healthcare personnel need to acquire the required training. It is important that people understand the moral and legal ramifications of using IoT implant devices, hence efforts should be made to educate and advocate for patients. Implantable IoT devices have the potential to enhance medical care while also safeguarding patients' autonomy and privacy if they are used ethically and responsibly. The ethical and legal ramifications of the widespread usage of IoT implant devices must be carefully considered. Protecting patient privacy and adhering to standards like HIPAA in the United States requires extreme caution while collecting and storing sensitive health information [31]. The protection of patients' personal information necessitates attention to worries about data breaches and cyberattacks. The possibility for inequalities in access to IoT implant devices and their related advantages is another important factor to think about. The high cost and limited availability of some of these tools may contribute to existing healthcare disparities. These concerns must be addressed by healthcare policymakers and providers if all patients who potentially benefit from IoT implant devices are to get them.

In conclusion, IoT implant devices have the potential to transform healthcare by enabling continuous monitoring, individualized treatment, and improved results. However, the technological capabilities, data security and privacy safeguards, ethical and legal issues, and the effective deployment of such devices are all crucial. To overcome these obstacles and promote wider acceptance of IoT implant devices for therapeutic purposes, researchers, device manufacturers, legislators, and healthcare practitioners must work together [31]. The development of biocompatible materials, integration with other technologies like AI and 5G networks as shown in Figure 8.4 [36], and addressing ethical and regulatory issues are just a few of the obstacles that must be met to enable the safe and ethical usage of IoT devices. To enable broad use, issues including longevity, dependability, and regulatory clearance must be resolved. The potential for IoT implant devices to revolutionize the healthcare industry is enormous, with several advantages for both patients and medical professionals.

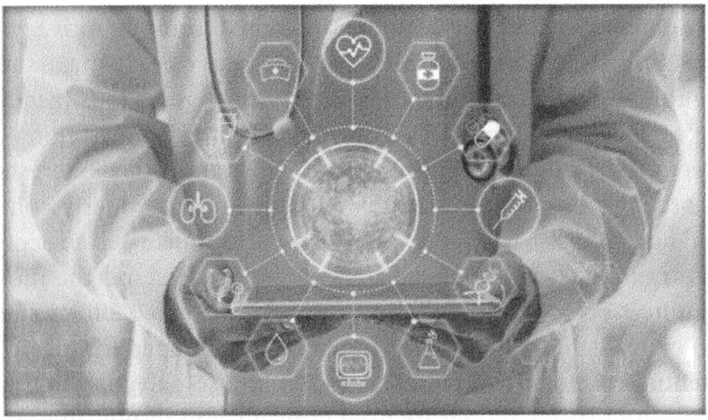

Figure 8.4 A schematic representation of IoMT integration with other technologies. Adapted with permission from www.istockphoto.com.

References

1. Tettey, F., Parupelli, S.K., Desai, S., A Review of Biomedical Devices: Classification, Regulatory Guidelines, Human Factors, Software as a Medical Device, and Cybersecurity. *Biomed. Mater. Devices*, 2, 1, 1–26, 2023.
2. Veletic, M., Apu, E.H., Simic, M., Bergsland, J., Balasingham, I., Contag, C.H., Ashammakhi, N., Implants with sensing capabilities. *Chem. Rev., 122*, 21, 16329–16363, 2022.
3. Park, J.H., Kim, S.Y., Kim, H.J., Kim, Y.J., Kim, H.L., Kim, H.K., The impact of IoT implant devices on patient outcomes in heart failure: A systematic review and meta-analysis. *Int. J. Med. Inf.*, 157, 104694, 2022.
4. Ullah, M., Hamayun, S., Wahab, A., Khan, S.U., Rehman, M.U., Haq, Z.U., Naeem, M., Smart Technologies used as Smart Tools in the Management of Cardiovascular Disease and their Future Perspective. *Curr. Probl. Cardiol., 48*, 11, 101922, 2023.
5. El-Sayed, A. and Kamel, M., Advanced applications of nanotechnology in veterinary medicine. *Environ. Sci. Pollut. Res., 27*, 19073–19086, 2020.
6. Tun, S.Y.Y., Madanian, S., Mirza, F., IoT (IoT) applications for elderly care: a reflective review. *Aging Clin. Exp. Res., 33*, 855–867, 2021.
7. Niemiec, B., Gawor, J., Nemec, A., Clarke, D., McLeod, K., Tutt, C., Jouppi, R., World small animal veterinary association global dental guidelines. *J. Small Anim. Pract., 61*, 7, E36–E161, 2020.
8. Nyirjesy, S.C., Heller, M., von Windheim, N., Gingras, A., Kang, S.Y., Ozer, E., VanKoevering, K.K., The role of computer aided design/computer assisted manufacturing (CAD/CAM) and 3-dimensional printing in head and neck oncologic surgery: A review and future directions. *Oral. Oncol., 132*, 105976, 2022.
9. Shi, Q., Dong, B., He, T., Sun, Z., Zhu, J., Zhang, Z., Lee, C., Progress in wearable electronics/photonics—Moving toward the era of artificial intelligence and IoT. *InfoMat, 2*, 6, 1131–1162, 2020.
10. Casas-Alvarado, A., Mota-Rojas, D., Hernández-Ávalos, I., Mora-Medina, P., Olmos-Hernández, A., Verduzco-Mendoza, A., Martínez-Burnes, J., Advances in infrared thermography: Surgical aspects, vascular changes, and pain monitoring in veterinary medicine. *J. Therm. Biol., 92*, 102664, 2020.
11. Gardašević, G., Katzis, K., Bajić, D., Berbakov, L., Emerging wireless sensor networks and IoT technologies—Foundations of smart healthcare. *Sensors, 20*, 13, 3619, 2020.
12. Reiss, L.A., Cochlear implants and other inner ear prostheses: Today and tomorrow. *Curr. Opin. Physiol., 18*, 49–55, 2020.
13. Arhant, C., Heizmann, V., Schauberger, G., Windschnurer, I., Risks and benefits of collar use in cats (Felis catus); a literature review. *J. Vet. Behav.*, 55, 35–47, 2022.
14. Sellers, B.G., Global Surveillance: The Emerging Role of Radio Frequency Identification (RFID) Technology, in: *The Pre-Crime Society: Crime, Culture*

and Control in the Ultramodern Age (Bruce A. Arrigo, and Brian G. Sellers (eds)) pp. 455–482, Bristol University Press, Bristol, 2021. https://doi.org/10.1332/policypress/9781529205251.003.0021, accessed 11 May 2024.
15. Habibzadeh, A., Dinesh, K., Shishvan, O.R., Boggio-Dandry, A., Sharma, G., Soyata, T., A survey of healthcare IoT (HIoT): A clinical perspective. *IEEE IoT J.*, *7*, 1, 53–71, 2019.
16. Sharma, H.K., Taneja, S., Ahmed, E., Patni, J.C., I-Doctor: an IoT based self patient's health monitoring system, in: *2019 International Conference on Innovative Sustainable Computational Technologies (CISCT)*, 2019, October, IEEE, pp. 1–6.
17. Chabbi, S., El Madhoun, N., Khamer, L., Security of nfc banking transactions: Overview on attacks and solutions, in: *2022 6th Cyber Security in Networking Conference (CSNet)*, 2022, October, IEEE, pp. 1–5.
18. Huang, L., Lin, S., Xu, Z., Zhou, H., Duan, J., Hu, B., Zhou, J., Fiber-based energy conversion devices for human-body energy harvesting. *Adv. Mater.*, *32*, 5, 1902034, 2020.
19. Ghubaish, A., Salman, T., Zolanvari, M., Unal, D., Al-Ali, A., Jain, R., Recent advances in the internet-of-medical-things (IoMT) systems security. *IEEE IoT J.*, *8*, 11, 8707–8718, 2020.
20. Kuosmanen, L., Hupli, M., Ahtiluoto, S., Haavisto, E., Patient participation in shared decision-making in palliative care–an integrative review. *J. Clin. Nurs.*, *30*, 23-24, 3415–3428, 2021.
21. Nielsen, J.C., Kautzner, J., Casado-Arroyo, R., Burri, H., Callens, S., Cowie, M.R., Fraser, A.G., Remote monitoring of cardiac implanted electronic devices: legal requirements and ethical principles-ESC Regulatory Affairs Committee/EHRA joint task force report. *EP Europace*, *22*, 11, 1742–1758, 2020.
22. Rejeb, A., Rejeb, K., Treiblmaier, H., Appolloni, A., Alghamdi, S., Alhasawi, Y., Iranmanesh, M., The IoT (IoT) in healthcare: Taking stock and moving forward. *IoT*, 100721, 2023.
23. Ramezani, M. and Mohd Ripin, Z., 4D printing in biomedical engineering: Advancements, challenges, and future directions. *J. Funct. Biomater.*, *14*, 7, 347, 2023.
24. Aledhari, M., Razzak, R., Qolomany, B., Al-Fuqaha, A., Saeed, F., Biomedical IoT: enabling technologies, architectural elements, challenges, and future directions. *IEEE Access*, *10*, 31306–31339, 2022.
25. Pasricha, S., Ethics for Digital Medicine: A Path for Ethical Emerging Medical IoT Design. *Computer*, *56*, 7, 32–40, 2023.
26. Shuvo, M.M.H., Titirsha, T., Amin, N., Islam, S.K., Energy harvesting in implantable and wearable medical devices for enduring precision healthcare. *Energies*, *15*, 20, 7495, 2022.
27. Tan, M., Xu, Y., Gao, Z., Yuan, T., Liu, Q., Yang, R., Peng, L., Recent advances in intelligent wearable medical devices integrating biosensing and drug delivery. *Adv. Mater.*, *34*, 27, 2108491, 2022.

28. Saif, S., Datta, D., Saha, A., Biswas, S., Chowdhury, C., Data science and AI in IoT based smart healthcare: Issues, challenges and case study, in: *Enabling AI Applications in Data Science*, pp. 415–439, 2021.
29. Young, M.J., Lin, D.J., Hochberg, L.R., Brain–Computer Interfaces in Neurorecovery and Neurorehabilitation. *Semin. Neurol.*, 41, 02, 206–216, Thieme Medical Publishers, Inc., 333 Seventh Avenue, 18th Floor, New York, NY 10001, USA, 2021, March.
30. Lee, J., Kwon, J., Lee, K., Informed consent in the use of IoT implant devices: A systematic review. *J. Med. Syst.*, 45, 2, 20, 2021.
31. Yigzaw, K.Y., Olabarriaga, S.D., Michalas, A., Marco-Ruiz, L., Hillen, C., Verginadis, Y., Chomutare, T., Health data security and privacy: Challenges and solutions for the future, in: *Roadmap to Successful Digital Health Ecosystems*, pp. 335–362, 2022.
32. Raikar, A.S., Kumar, P., Raikar, G.V.S., Somnache, S.N., Advances and Challenges in IoT-Based Smart Drug Delivery Systems: A Comprehensive Review. *Appl. Syst. Innov.*, 6, 4, 62, 2023.
33. https://www.istockphoto.com/vector/arthritis-osteoarthritis-medical-infographic-design-joint-replacement-implantant-gm1225041793-360441672?clarity=false]
34. https://www.istockphoto.com/vector/rfid-radio-frequency-identification-tag-technology-tiny-characters-use-delivery-gm1327008316-z411499737?clarity=false
35. https://www.istockphoto.com/photo/torso-of-young-doctor-unlocking-virtual-lock-gm1166384387-321289326?clarity=false
36. https://www.istockphoto.com/photo/medical-tech-science-innovative-iot-global-healthcare-ai-technology-world-health-day-gm1298626492-391452966?clarity=false
37. Islam, M.M., Nooruddin, S., Karray, F., Muhammad, G., Internet of things: Device capabilities, architectures, protocols, and smart applications in healthcare domain. *IEEE Internet Things J.*, 10, 4, 3611–3641, 2022.
38. Krishnamoorthy, S., Dua, A., Gupta, S., Role of emerging technologies in future IoT-driven Healthcare 4.0 technologies: A survey, current challenges and future directions. *J. Ambient Intell. Humaniz. Comput.*, 14, 1, 361–407, 2023.
39. Alshamrani, M., IoT and artificial intelligence implementations for remote healthcare monitoring systems: A survey. *J. King Saud Univ. Comput. Inf. Sci.*, 34, 8, 4687–4701, 2022.

9

Enhancing Patient Safety and Efficiency in Intravenous Therapy: A Comprehensive Analysis of Smart Infusion Monitoring Systems

Krishna Sreekumar, T. Punitha Reddy and Boppuru Rudra Prathap*

Department of CSE, CHRIST (Deemed to be University), Bangalore, Karnataka, India

Abstract

Intravenous (IV) fluids, comprising vitamin-rich solutions, are administered to address patient electrolyte imbalances and dehydration through IV infusion therapy. Infusion pumps are integral for precise medication dosage delivery in this common medical procedure, generally posing low risks. These fluids are stored in polypropylene bags connected to patients through tubes. However, when the IV bag empties, the patient's blood may flow backward into the IV tube due to higher blood pressure, known as diffusion, potentially leading to complications like air embolism—life-threatening if air enters the bloodstream through the IV line, obstructing blood flow to vital organs.

Smart IV Bags emerged as a solution to mitigate such risks, eliminating the need for manual IV bag monitoring while preventing reverse blood flow. This research comprehensively assesses various IoT-enabled IV Bag monitoring systems, comparing their strengths, weaknesses, and unique features. Key evaluation criteria include component efficiency, real-world applicability, accuracy, latency, and technical specifications. The aim is to provide an objective evaluation of each Smart Intravenous Liquid Monitoring System to inform future developments in this field. A systematic approach ensures the selection of systems that best meet specific requirements in diverse healthcare environments.

**Corresponding author*: boppuru.prathap@christuniversity.in

Hari Murthy, Marta Zurek-Mortka, Vinay Jha Pillai and Kukatlapalli Pradeep Kumar (eds.) Internet of Things in Bioelectronics: Emerging Technologies and Applications, (171–200) © 2024 Scrivener Publishing LLC

Keywords: IoT, healthcare, IV fluid, bioelectronics, air embolism, smart hospitals, sensors, smart IV infusion monitoring

9.1 Introduction

IV infusion therapy is a medical treatment that involves administering fluids directly into a patient's bloodstream via a needle and catheter. Dehydration, electrolyte imbalances, and vitamin shortages are some of the disorders that are commonly treated with this technique. Depending on the individual needs of the patient, the fluids used in IV infusion treatment are often carefully made solutions that are rich in a variety of vitamins, minerals, and other nutrients.

Hospitals, clinics, and outpatient facilities are just a few of the healthcare environments where IV infusion treatment can be applied. The treatment can take anywhere from a few minutes to several hours, depending on the quantity and kind of fluids being provided, and is normally carried out by a skilled healthcare professional, such as a nurse or doctor.

There are two categories of IV infusion sets: those used for blood transfusion and those used for non-blood substances like saline. Although IV infusion therapy is typically regarded as a secure and efficient medical procedure, there are some potential risks. Diffusion, or the reverse flow of blood in the IV bag, is one of the most serious problems that can occur. Blood loss, pain, and possibly fatal complications like an air embolism can all occur from this. Inadvertently introducing air bubbles into the IV line might result in an air embolism, which blocks blood arteries and reduces or stops the blood supply to essential organs.

When blood flows back via an IV catheter rather than into a vein, it is referred to as reverse blood flow or retrograde flow. This may take place if the catheter becomes loose or if the vein is blocked. The drug or fluid that is being infused could damage the patient's tissue and cause harm if the catheter is not withdrawn or adjusted right away.

On the other hand, air embolism happens when air bubbles pass through the IV catheter and into the bloodstream. A heart attack, stroke, or respiratory failure could result from these bubbles entering the heart or lungs. Air embolism can occur if the IV line is not properly primed, if there is a disconnection in the IV tubing, or if the catheter is not inserted properly.

The two main causes of reverse blood flow and air embolism during IV infusion are related to issues with the IV bag and improper administration techniques. Reverse blood flow frequently happens when the IV bag is left unchanged for too long or is not replaced at the proper intervals. The patient's blood may then flow in the reverse way, towards the empty IV bag, as a result of the negative pressure this might cause inside the IV tubing. Retrograde flow or diffusion is the medical term for this illness, which can cause pain and blood loss. Patients who are already weak may find this condition to be especially worrisome.

On the other side, air embolism happens when air bubbles get into the IV tube and get caught in the circulatory system. This can occur as a result of incorrect administration procedures, such as failing to prime the IV tubing, failing to remove air bubbles from the tubing, or failing to make sure that the tubing is fully filled with fluid prior to providing the infusion.

The use of faulty or broken IV equipment, the use of air-powered infusion pumps, and the delivery of fluids under high pressure are other conditions that might cause an air embolism during IV infusions.

IoT-enabled Smart IV bag monitoring systems use sensors and other technologies to monitor and maintain the state of IV bags. These devices continually check the state of the IV bag and stop reverse blood flow in an attempt to lower the hazards associated with IV infusion therapy, such as air embolism.

Smart IV bag monitoring systems provide a number of important functions, such as real-time fluid level monitoring, precise flow rate monitoring, and automated warnings when a bag needs to be replaced or when air is found in the line. These characteristics not only improve the IV infusion therapy's safety and efficacy, but they also lighten the burden on medical staff who would otherwise have to manually check IV bags.

Smart infusion monitoring systems can also help detect and prevent these complications by providing real-time data on the infusion rate, fluid levels, and pressure in the IV line. These systems can alert healthcare providers if there is a dislodged catheter, obstruction in the vein, or air bubbles in the tubing, enabling prompt intervention to prevent harm to the patient.

The objective of this study is to provide a comprehensive and objective evaluation of each Smart IV Monitoring System so that useful insights may be derived out of it for future scope of the domain. This study will identify the key features and criteria that are important for comparison and analysis. Each system will then be evaluated based on these factors, which will involve an in-depth study of the components and their efficiency, real-life applicability, accuracy and latency, and various other technical specifications.

Comparing various systems and sensors can help medical professionals decide which system would best suit the requirements of a certain environment by giving them a better understanding of the distinctive characteristics each system offers and its efficiency. Figure 9.1 illustrates the generic

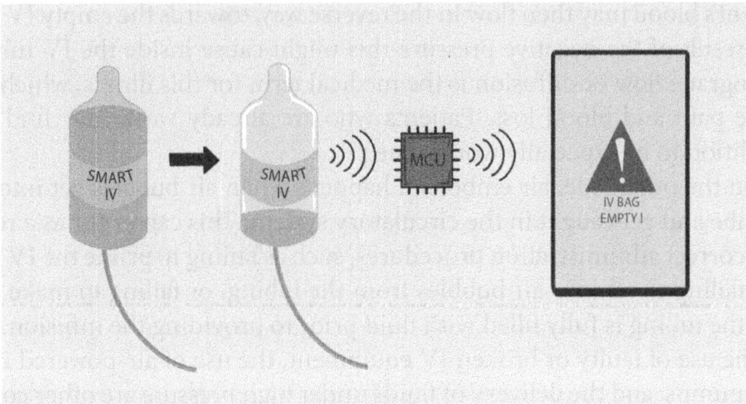

Figure 9.1 Graphical abstract of a smart intravenous infusion system.

idea behind smart intravenous infusion systems. Most smart systems are built around the same model.

The remaining sections of this research work will be structured as follows. An overview of the different IoT-enabled smart IV bag monitoring systems that are currently on the market is provided in the next section. A detailed examination and evaluation of each system in light of the established criteria will follow. Finally, we'll explore the benefits and drawbacks of each system and offer suggestions on which one would be most appropriate for a given setting.

This review paper offers an in-depth analysis of several Smart IV Infusion Monitoring and IoT-enabled Alert Systems. The goal of the article is to provide an in-depth study of the many systems that are now on the market, emphasizing their benefits, drawbacks, difficulties, and potential future directions.

9.2 Smart Intravenous Therapy: Enhancing Patient Safety

In modern healthcare, patient safety is a paramount concern, and advancements in medical technology continue to play a pivotal role in enhancing the quality of care. One such advancement that significantly contributes to patient safety is the adoption of smart intravenous (IV) therapy systems. Traditional intravenous therapy has always carried inherent risks associated with the manual administration of fluids and medications. Errors in dosage, flow rates, or the administration of the wrong medication can have serious consequences for patients. However, smart IV therapy systems are changing the landscape of healthcare by incorporating cutting-edge technology and automation into the process.

Smart IV pumps and systems are designed to ensure precise and accurate delivery of medications or fluids. They have built-in features to calculate and control the flow rate, ensuring that patients receive the correct dose according to their prescribed treatment plans. These systems continuously monitor the infusion process in real time. They can detect irregularities such as air bubbles, occlusions, or changes in flow rate, immediately alerting healthcare providers to take corrective action.

Some smart IV systems are equipped with wireless connectivity, enabling healthcare providers to monitor infusions remotely. This feature allows for timely intervention if any issues arise, even when the healthcare provider is not physically present at the patient's bedside. Electronic record-keeping enhances accuracy and reduces the risk of errors associated with manual documentation.

These systems help reduce the risk of medication errors by ensuring that the right medication is administered to the right patient at the right time and at the correct rate. They generate audible and visual alarms in response to issues like air in the line, occlusions, or deviations from the prescribed parameters. These alarms prompt immediate attention and intervention.

Smart intravenous therapy enhances patient safety by providing accurate dosing, real-time monitoring, alerts and alarms, and much more. These features help prevent medication errors, improve workflow, and provide healthcare providers with the tools they need to deliver safe and effective intravenous therapy.

9.3 Related Works

In 2009, the concept of 'Smart Healthcare' emerged from IBM's 'Smart Planet' which utilized sensors for data collection, IoT for interconnection of devices and supercomputers, and cloud computing for data processing. Advanced technologies such as artificial intelligence, surgical robots and mixed reality have enabled more sophisticated detection and treatment of diseases [29]. Despite the increasing integration of artificial intelligence and IoT in the medical industry, intravenous therapy is still manually administered by healthcare professionals. As discussed earlier, this medical procedure requires active participation from doctors or nurses. However, with the emergence of new technologies such as artificial intelligence, data analytics, and IoT, some of the human intervention in intravenous therapy can be minimized.

Table 9.1 The principal sensing device, microcontroller and communication media used in various Smart IV infusion systems.

Principal sensing device	Parameter reference	Microcontroller		Communication media
IR	[2, 7, 11, 15, 24, 25]	STM32 microcontroller	[2]	None
		Arduino UNO	[7, 15]	Wi-Fi
		NodeMCU ESP8266	[24]	Wi-Fi
		ARM Cortex-M3	[25]	Wi-Fi
		Undisclosed	[11]	None
Pressure Sensor	[3]	Arduino UNO		RF
Fluid Level Sensor	[4]	Arduino UNO		Bluetooth
Load Cell	[5, 8, 10, 13, 15, 19, 22, 23, 24]	NodeMCU ESP8266	[5, 24]	Wi-Fi
		ESP32	[8]	Wi-Fi
		6502-based microcontroller	[10]	RFID
		Arduino UNO	[13, 15, 19]	Zigbee [13], Wi-Fi [15]
		ARM7 Microcontroller	[22]	Wi-Fi
		Undisclosed	[23]	Wi-Fi
Capacitive Sensor	[6, 9, 12, 17]	AD7150 Board	[6]	None
		PIC12LF1501	[9]	Zigbee
		1. Arduino UNO 2. NodeMCU ESP8266	[12]	Wi-Fi
		UNDISCLOSED	[17]	None
Ultrasonic Sensor	[14, 21]	CC3200-XL Launchpad	[14]	Zigbee
		Arduino	[21]	Wi-Fi
Fork-type light barrier	[26]	NodeMCU		Zigbee

(Continued)

Table 9.1 The principal sensing device, microcontroller and communication media used in various Smart IV infusion systems. (*Continued*)

Principal sensing device	Parameter reference	Microcontroller		Communication media
Temperature Sensor	[4, 18, 22]	Arduino UNO	[4]	Bluetooth
		ATMega 328	[18]	Wi-Fi
		ARM7 Microcontroller	[22]	Wi-Fi
LDR/Photoresistor	[1, 16, 21, 23, 27]	1. Arduino UNO 2. NodeMCU ESP8266	[1]	Wi-Fi
		Arduino	[16, 21, 27]	RF [16], Wi-Fi [21, 27]
		NOT MENTIONED	[23]	Wi-Fi
Color Sensor	[12]	1. Arduino UNO 2. NodeMCU ESP8266		Wi-Fi
Flow sensor	[20, 28]	NodeMCU ESP8266 Raspberry Pi 3B+	[20]	Wi-Fi, GSM
		Arduino Mega	[28]	Zigbee

In this light, several research works were reviewed to determine the efficiency and feasibility of the existing smart IV monitoring system in the present scenario. Table 9.1 shows the list of common micro-controllers, sensors, and communication media used in smart intravenous therapy systems.

The system proposed in the paper [1] by Rosdi and Huong can be divided into types they are drip chamber monitoring system and air bubble monitoring system. A laser (5 mW) module is utilized in the Drip Chamber Monitoring System to determine the sensor's high-low condition, which can be used to count the number of fluid droplets. When there has been no drop observed for more than 30 seconds, the Wi-Fi module sends information to the medical professional, alerting them to a problem. Blue LED lights are used as warning signs. The laser diode and LDR module in the air bubble monitoring system are controlled by an Arduino board that is wired to a Wi-Fi shield. When the LDR module gets laser light from the laser diode, its output logic is high, and otherwise it is low. These parts were connected to the IV administration set's tube line and used a red LED and a Blynk app to alert users when air bubbles were present. Despite the system's effectiveness, receiving notifications on cell phones had a 20-second standby.

In the research work [2] by Xu *et al.*, the system with the control core of the STM32F103 microcontroller can realize the measurement and control of drop speed. While the infusion monitoring sensor can measure the drop speed in real-time and transmit the speed signal to the microcontroller after signal shaping, the infusion bottles can be raised or lowered to adjust the infusion speed. The system uses the infrared emitting and receiving diode as the drop speed sensor. In this system, the drop speed adjustment is completed by raising or lowering the infusion bottles. While the system may be able to accomplish its goals, it does not have an alarm system that would enable staff to check on the patient and remotely monitor the IV level in the event that something goes wrong.

Ramisha Rani K *et al.* in [3] introduced a vacant imbuement arrangement sack and the trickle implantation rate can be determined by the mixture observation device using a pressure sensor (MPX10GP technology module), and this information is then transmitted via radio frequency (nrf24L01) to the monitoring screen installed at the medical caretaker's station. The monitoring screen gathers data from drip-implantation observational devices and then displays it graphically. When the pressure sensor value hits the threshold value, the control valve closes, quickly stopping the flow of fluid without any airflow through the patient's vein. This system monitors the level of IV solution using pressure sensors, which can be reviewed in the nurse station. However, it is stationary and can be missed if there are not enough nurses on duty or a staffing shortage.

In the study conducted by Joseph *et al.* in [4], a model is provided where the focus is on manually managing the flow rate through the use of a mobile app, monitoring the IV fluid level in the bag, and alerting the medical staff to change the bottle. In a similar vein, the next phase is the routine monitoring of each person's state. In order to do this, they continuously check the patient's temperature, heart rate, blood pressure, and IV fluid level while injecting. It will notify the medical staff if there are any impending dramatic changes for alerting, they use a buzzer technique and messaging facility. By pressing a panic button, the patient can warn the nurse if he or she is in distress. The authors claim that the system outperforms competing systems, even though the accuracy of the system has not been tested. The question of latency remains a primary one.

The system proposed by M Yamin *et al.* in [5], provides input to the fuzzy logic-based infusion monitoring system, with the system acting as fuzzy Logic. The system is then changed to a PWM input using control components. Node MCU devices, Wi-Fi Module for Web Based ESP 8266 devices, and microcontroller based on Fuzzy Logic can monitor also calculating the infusion fluids weight, percentage, and volume reading the data of the infusion with three colors indicators, namely colors are red, yellow, and green. Despite the system's claimed 98% accuracy rate, the alarm may not be seen if there aren't enough nurses on duty at the nursing station during busy times because the equipment is stationary.

Salmaz, Ahsan and Islam in their study at [6] looked at three different capacitive sensor types, including cross-capacitive, semi-cylindrical, and planar parallel plates, to detect IV droplets in a fluid pipe without causing damage. The sensors are built utilizing flexible double-sided copper-clad PCB substrates that are reasonably priced and were especially created to satisfy the needs of the application. Four IV fluid sensors that are frequently used in hospitals are put to the test to find out how well they respond to factors including precision, drift, and drop rate when the droplet passes through the inner electric fields of the sensors. The study emphasizes the significance of precise IV fluid monitoring because insufficient fluid levels can have a negative impact on patient outcomes. The capacitive sensing concept was used in the design of the sensor, and the fluid level was determined by measuring capacitance. The sensor has a high level of precision, with an error rate of less than 1%, according to the results.

The system proposed by G. Sunil *et al.* in [7] functions in two different scenarios which are explained as giving a buzzer and twisting the intravenous tube.

The nurse is informed about the conclusion of the saline infusion in the first scenario by a buzzer when the IR sensor fails to detect a drop of water for a certain amount of time. In the second scenario, by twisting the IV tubing, the servo motor's arm turns roughly 90 degrees at the same time as the buzzer. Although the system is successful in controlling and monitoring the saline level, the system lacks the feature for wirelessly informing physicians and nurses of the saline droplet rate.

In the method proposed by Ghosh *et al.* [8], the system is built using a load sensor and ultra-low power low-cost ESP32 Wi-Fi System on Chip (SoC) microcontroller. The bottle's weight is converted to a specified voltage by the load sensor. Based on the voltage the sensor's microprocessor, the ESP32, sends out, the microcontroller develops and broadcasts a certain message. The author claims that the approach is effective even though accuracy is not examined in the study. The MQTT protocol's features still provide room for lag. In this work, a clever, economical saline level surveillance system that enables a hospital employee, doctor, etc. to remotely monitor the patient's saline feeding level has been presented. Since MQTT-S is effective for low-cost and low-power devices, it is adopted.

Using capacitive sensors, the system created by Shaojun Jiang and Yilin He [9], determines whether there is water or air in the drip infusion tube and determines the state of the liquid level in the drip infusion tube. When there is no liquid in the drip infusion tube, the monitor sends an alarm message to the monitoring center using the Zigbee wireless sensor network. Although the system, in the authors' opinion, performed much better and was built with low-energy components, the CC2530 used for message transmission can only last for 40 hours.

Chen *et al.* in [10] proposed a system that calculates the IV infusion rate (drips/sec) and checks whether the rate is normal or abnormal. The term "hang-and-play" refers to a situation in which a nurse simply uses the system software interface to carry out the drip therapy in an authentic way. Once the drip-bag RFID tag has been recognized, the system moves a patient directly into the drip monitoring stage. A nurse should verify the state of the bag according to the alarm subsystem. To help the nurses manage all of the patients' IV infusions, the system offers a real-time IV infusion indication and thorough notification. The use of an RFID tag and reader is entirely dependent on the software and the system.

The system suggested by Raghavendra B. *et al.* in [11], the IV drip system incorporates a light sensor-based apparatus for IV drip monitoring and management. The use of such a device will lessen the problems related to IV drip usage in settings with restricted resources. The system's accuracy is not disclosed. The suggested system wirelessly transmits data to a server and displays the outcomes on a central monitor in the form of the infusion volume, failure status, and saline droplet rate. The system is a little difficult to set up even though it is also inexpensive and reliable.

The capacitive sensors detect the liquid level and the color sensor detects the color of the liquid to determine the type of liquid, in the research done by Oros *et al.* [12]. When the liquid level falls beyond a point, the alarm is triggered, and the value is then also reflected in the web application. If the bottle is not manually replaced, the stepper motor is activated which closes the valve. The system looks efficient in multiple ways. Firstly there are multiple sensors that provide added accuracy and backup to the system. The communication system established will send the data about the patient's IV bag in real-time. We can confidently conclude that this might be one of the systems that have achieved automation in the scope of the study.

In the research, M.K. Bhavasaar *et al.* [13], set up a complete environment for monitoring the IV bag. They have used load cells (weight sensor) to detect the weight of the IV bag, and they have used heartbeat sensors to detect air embolism (by detecting a voltage change created due to air embolism). In case air embolism is detected, an alert is sent to the nurse station where the LED glows and the buzzer beeps. In case the IV bag liquid reaches the set point, an LED glows and buzzer beeps at the nurse station. The device can monitor and identify air embolism while remaining stationary. It might be necessary to make some modifications to the current IV bag stand design in order to include the load cell.

In the method proposed by Rao and Supriya in [14]. In this system, an ultrasonic sensor is used to detect the fluid level in the IV bag, along with a temperature sensor. The programming part was done in Energia IDE (Embedded C). Along with that, an IR sensor is used to keep track of the drop rate. Both of these values are transmitted to ThingSpeak and then using the GSM module, an alert message is sent to the attendant's mobile phone if the liquid level reaches below a certain level. The authors claim that the system was much superior in terms of performance. The system was developed using components with low energy consumption. The proposal includes modification of the existing design of the IV bag. In order to fix an ultrasonic sensor, a temperature sensor, and an IR sensor onto an IV bag is quite difficult and complex.

In the system proposed by AR *et al.* in [15] have made use of Load cells and IR emitter detector to detect the fluid level in the bag. 3 IR sensors are used. The value is transmitted to the mobile device using Blynk App, which is an open source application for IoT projects. Blynk app requires a Wi-Fi connection from source to target device. They have also used a servo motor and potentiometer to control the flow of IV liquid from the Blynk app itself. They have used a threshold value of 330. IR positions are at 50 10 and 5 percent of the bottle. Although the system was working efficiently the accuracy of the system was not mentioned. A critical message is shown when the bottle is at 5%. Then the servo will automatically close the valve.

Jora *et al.* in [16] proposed a system that makes use of an LDR. The LDR and LED are placed opposite each other and when the liquid level drops beyond the threshold, the buzzer starts beeping at the nurse station. RF transmitter and receiver are set up at the patient and the nurse station respectively. When the value of LDR says that the bottle is empty, an alert is triggered to the nurse station, where the buzzer beeps. The accuracy of the system has not been discussed explicitly, but the authors have mentioned in the conclusion that the accuracy is high. The system has been designed at a minimal cost. It was successful in transmitting the correct signal. Even though the system was able to successfully detect the necessary, it is a stationary system, where the buzzer is set up in the nurse station.

In the system proposed by Wei *et al.* in [17], capacitor electrodes made of copper were set up on the surface of the IV bag, and the capacitance value was used to detect the change in presence of the liquid. The measurements were then analyzed using a regression analysis to establish a calibration curve to determine the residual quantity of the solution. The system had an error margin of 5%. It was discovered that the system could successfully detect the liquid level in the IV bag. It can be incorporated into the upcoming design of the IV bags due to its straightforward construction. The system's primary flaw is that the output is highly dependent on the distance between the two electrodes.

Ray *et al.* in [18] proposed a system that makes use of an LM35 temperature sensor to detect the minute change in the thermal difference between the fluid and the non-fluid region in the IV bag. There are multiple states of the system defined in the program, and depending on the state, the status is transmitted via HTTP to the nurse's mobile phone using HTML, CSS, and JavaScript. The authors have claimed the system exhibits very high accuracy. The sensitivity and the response rate of the LM35 temperature sensor are questionable, and to fix this, more sensors can be used. The system is a non-invasive one. It has been able to successfully achieve the goal by alerting the nurse when the IV bag gets empty.

In the system proposed by Janaki Moorthy *et al.* in [19], the authors have used a completely automated system by using a load cell to detect the weight of the contents of the IV bag, and when the weight is below the threshold, the solenoid valve automatically locks the tube and prevents backflow of blood. The threshold used here is 35 grams. It is a stationary system. This means that the alarm might be overlooked, posing a hazard to human life, if the nurses are not present in the nurse station during busy times if there is a staffing deficit.

In the system proposed by Mathew *et al.* [20], the authors have made use of a flow meter to detect the amount of liquid left in the IV bag. If the amount of liquid is less than the threshold value, the buzzer will start. It also energizes an actuator to stop the flow of liquid. It is unclear whether they have used GSM or Wi-Fi for communication between the components. The system is said to have achieved the objective of detecting the fluid level and then automatically stopping the flow. The reason for the usage of NodeMCU, Raspberry Pi, and Wi-Fi modules together and the usage of GSM has not been elaborated, and with these many components, the system exhibits redundancy and the cost will be very high.

In the system proposed by S. Tanwar *et al.* [21], the authors have used an ultrasonic sensor to detect the level of the liquid. They have also made use of an LDR to detect air bubbles in the liquid. The values are then transmitted to ThingSpeak, where using MATLAB, they have analyzed and then displayed the values to the mobile application. Although the system's accuracy is not mentioned, it is found to be workable and can be incorporated into the IV bag's current design.

In the system proposed by R. *et al.* in [22] the weight of the liquid in the IV bag is detected using a load cell and the data will be sent to the doctor/nurse's mobile device using a Wi-Fi module. Upon reaching the threshold value, the solenoid valve will automatically close the tube. Flex sensors are used to detect the flex in the patient's hand. There has been no mention of accuracy. The system is successful in achieving the goal but then there are too many components which may make the system bulky and harder to integrate.

In the system proposed by Jae-Kyeong Lee *et al.* in [23], used a load cell to detect the weight of the IV bag and a photoresistor to count the drops of IV fluid, as it helps to maintain a higher accuracy. If the value falls beyond the threshold, an alert is sent to the nurse's mobile device stating the patient information. The system has an accuracy of 87.9% (horizontal motion) and 89.9% (vertical motion). The system exhibited a comparable accuracy. The authors have mentioned about latency related issues with respect to Wi-Fi, and suggested the usage of 4G/5G for reduced latency. Overall, the system was developed in a cost effective manner and it looks feasible. The main drawback of the system latency related issues with respect to Wi-Fi, and suggested the usage of 4G/5G for reduced latency.

Bhandari *et al.* in [24] proposed a system, where a load cell is used to detect the amount of saline liquid left in the IV bag. The output is continuously printed to an LCD. When the value drops beyond the threshold, the alert message is sent to a mobile app. When the value drops beyond 30% of the initial value, the alert is displayed at the nurse station with LEDs. If not attended, the saline gets emptied out and the motor clamps the valve, while the buzzer rings 3 times. The threshold value used here is 70 mL, for the regular IV bottle of 500 mL. Despite the elaboration on the hardware components, there has been no light on which mobile app was being used for the study; whether it is an open-source app or a created app. The alarms at the patient end and the nurse's side happen at different times, and it may cause a panicked situation for the patient.

In the system suggested by Yadav and Jain in [25], an IR sensor is used for detecting the amount of liquid in the IV bag and the servo motor to control the drip infusion rate mechanism. A graphic representation of a bottle showing the fluid level is visible on the monitor. When an empty infusion solution bag reaches a certain critical set level, an alert with a notification on the monitor and a buzzer will sound. The suggested system is affordable, reliable, and able to wirelessly transmit information to a server and display the findings on a central monitor. But the system is stationary, so if there aren't enough nurses on duty at the nursing station at busy times or if there's a staffing deficit, it's likely that the alarm won't be seen.

In the proposed system by Zhang *et al.* in [26], Murphy's dropper is integrated into the fork-type light barrier, and the sensor node is in charge of waveform adjustment, data transfer, light-and-sound alert, and other functions. The sink node is in charge of gathering data from sensor nodes and delivering it through a serial connection to the host computer installed in the nursing station. The host computer's monitoring program is in charge of progress tracking, display, and alert. The author claims that the accuracy satisfies practical demands based on experimental data of 10% glucose. The study shows several fork-type light barriers with ZigBee connectivity that are employed in intravenous infusion monitoring systems. The stability of the system is investigated, and it provides extensive experimental statistical results, in order to show that it is capable of carrying out all necessary networkable system functions, including monitoring the progression and velocity of intravenous infusion with high accuracy and reliability.

In the system proposed by Sourabh Suresh Alagundagi *et al.* [27], the optoelectronic device described here precisely monitors fluid flow and helps the user keep track of infusion sessions by sending notifications when mistakes are found. When a considerable departure from the predetermined drip rate is detected, the system generates alarms. The system monitors the total volume infused and sends an alert when the desired volume is about to be given. The prototype device was evaluated in a lab setting and found to be accurate to within 4% of the infusion volume that was measured independently. The drawback of the system is when the flow rate deviates from the desired preset rate, human intervention is necessary to reset it automatically.

In the study conducted by Rashid *et al.* [28], the drip chamber of the saline container will be connected to a flow sensor in the proposed system in order to calculate the precise number of drops of saline as well as the flow rate of the solution. The obtained sensor outputs are continuously compared to the assigned command, and if any discrepancy is discovered, the microcontroller operates the servo motor to adjust the circulation rate in order to bring the outputs into line with the provided instruction. The smartphone application allows healthcare providers to set the desired flow rate and volume, monitor the fluid infusion in real time, and receive alerts if the flow rate deviates from the expected range or if the IV bag is nearing depletion. The benefits of this system include its low cost, ease of use, and accessibility. It can be particularly useful in resource-limited settings where more advanced and expensive technologies may not be feasible. Table 9.2 provides a short summary of the research works that has been discusses in the text.

Table 9.2 A summary of the research works referred in the text.

Sensors and components	**Accuracy**	**Findings**	**Limitations**
1. Laser module 2. Non-modulator laser sensor module 3. Laser diode with LDR module 4. LED (Red, Blue)	NA	[1] The Arduino system effectively maintains a drop counter, detects tube blockages, checks drip bag levels, and offers remote infusion monitoring via Blynk computer and mobile apps.	Smartphone notifications that are 20 seconds late show the need for thorough system design and testing prior to human implementation.
1. Pair of Infrared emitting and receiving diode 2. Motor Driver 3. LCD Display Module	NA	[2] An STM32 microcontroller drives the infusion drop speed control system, which measures drop speed using infrared diodes. Elevating or lowering the infusion bottles affects speed.	The absence of an alarm system means staff can't remotely monitor patients or IV levels during system failures.
1. Pressure Sensor (MPX10GP) 2. Instrumentation Amplifier (LM342)	NA	[3] The nursing station can analyze data from the pressure sensor, enhancing IV solution level monitoring for improved facility utilization.	In a fixed system, personnel shortages or a lack of nurses during peak hours may reduce the likelihood of an alarm.
1. Temperature Sensor 2. Fluid level Sensor 3. NPN transistor 4. LED 5. Buzzer	The authors claim that the system outperforms competing systems, even though the accuracy of the system has not been tested.	[4] This system blends existing elements with vital additions to enhance its practicality and efficiency, fundamentally reshaping its operational effectiveness.	It could take some time to update and transmit the alarm message after processing the cloud data to automate the drip monitoring system.

(*Continued*)

Table 9.2 A summary of the research works referred in the text. (*Continued*)

Sensors and components	Accuracy	Findings	Limitations
1. Load Cell 2. LCD 3. HX711 Module	98%	[5] This study develops a remote infusion monitor with ESP8266 Wi-Fi for timely nurse response, using load cells for fluid data.	Insufficient nurses during busy times or staffing gaps may lead to missed alerts in the stationary system.
1. Parallel plate Capacitive sensor 2. Semi-cylindrical capacitive sensor 3. Cylindrical cross-capacitor 4. Copper cladded PCB	Authors claimed that the error rate was less than 1%	[6] For patient safety, accurate IV fluid monitoring is essential. A capacitive sensor that measures the capacitance of a fluid exhibits remarkable accuracy (error 1%).	-
1. IR Sensor 2. Sevo Motor 3. Buzzer	NA	[7] The method successfully controlled saline levels and prevented blood reverse flow by twisting the IV tube and sounding a warning buzzer.	The system lacks the feature for wirelessly informing physicians and nurses of the saline droplet rate.
1. Load Sensor 2. LCD	Although accuracy is not discussed in the paper, the author has stated that the system is effective.	[8] Saline levels in patients can be efficiently monitored remotely via MQTT-S by a clever, economical saline level surveillance system.	There is a potential that the alert message will be delayed due to a MQTT protocol latency issue.

(*Continued*)

Table 9.2 A summary of the research works referred in the text. (*Continued*)

Sensors and components	Accuracy	Findings	Limitations
1. Capacitive sensor 2. Oscillator (MIC1555) 3. Wireless communication chip (CC2530)	NA	[9] The system, according to the authors, performed far better. Low-energy consumption components were used to construct the system.	CC2530 used for transmitting messages can last only for 40 hours.
1. Load Cell 2. RFID tag and Reader 3. A/D Converter	NA	[10] The system provides a real-time IV infusion indication and comprehensive notification to help the nurses manage all patients' IV infusions.	The software and the entire system completely depends on a RFID tag and reader.
1. Light Source 2. Light Detector	NA	[11] The system wirelessly transmits data to a server, displaying saline droplet rate, failure status, bottle empty time, and infusion volume on a central monitor. It's cost-effective and reliable.	The system is bit complicated to set up
1. Capacitive sensors 2. Colour sensor 3. Buzzer 4. Stepper motor 5. LCD 6. Motor driver 7. Ultrasonic sensor	NA	[12] The efficient system employs multiple sensors for enhanced accuracy and reliability, transmitting real-time patient IV bag data.	-

(*Continued*)

Table 9.2 A summary of the research works referred in the text. (*Continued*)

Sensors and components	Accuracy	Findings	Limitations
1. Load Cell 2. INA125P amplifier 3. Heart beat sensor 4. LED 5. Buzzer	There is no explicit accuracy value provided by the authors in the research paper. But from the values obtained during their experimental setup, it can be seen that the system works correctly, though the accuracy of the readings might be questionable as the value decreases	[13] The system was successful in monitoring and detecting air embolism using a heart beat sensor and detecting the emptying IV Bag using a load cell.	In a stationary system, nurse unavailability during peak hours or staff shortages could lead to missed alerts, risking lives. Modifying IV bag stands may be necessary for load cell attachment.
1. Ultrasonic Sensor HC-SR04 2. LM35 temperature sensor 3. Infrared Sensor 4. GSM SIM900A 5. LM393 Power amplifier	Accuracy of the system has not been discussed but the authors have claimed the performance to be superior.	[14] The authors claim that the system was much superior in terms of performance. The system was developed using components with low energy consumption.	Modifying the IV bag design to incorporate ultrasonic, temperature, and IR sensors is a complex and challenging task.
1. Load Cell 2. LED 3. IR 4. Servo	NA	[15] A threshold of 330 is set for IR positions at 50, 10, and 5 percent of the bottle. A critical message triggers at 5%, prompting the servo to close the valve automatically.	-

(*Continued*)

Table 9.2 A summary of the research works referred in the text. (*Continued*)

Sensors and components	Accuracy	Findings	Limitations
1. LED 2. LDR 3. Buzzer 4. Encoder-Decoder 5. RF transmitter receiver	The accuracy of the system has not been discussed explicitly, but the authors have mentioned in the conclusion that the accuracy is high.	[16] The system has been designed at a minimal cost. It was successful in transmitting the correct signal.	It is a stationary system, where the buzzer is set up in the nurse station.
1. Flexible PCB 2. Capacitor electrodes 3. Resistor 4. Transistor 5. LCR meter (1061A chroma)	The system had an error margin of 5%	[17] The system was found to be feasible to detect the liquid level in the IV bag. Due to its simple design, it can be incorporated into the future design of the IV bags.	The output of the system heavily depends on the distance between the 2 electrodes.
1. ATMega 328 breakout board 2. ATTiny85 3. LM35 Temperature sensor 4. ESP8266	The authors have claimed for the system to have very high accuracy.	[18] The system is a non-invasive one. It has been able to successfully achieve the goal by alerting the nurse when the IV bag gets empty.	The sensitivity and the response rate of the LM35 temperature sensor is questionable. To fix this, more sensors can be used.
1. Load cells 2. Hx711 amplifier 3. Solenoid valve	NA	[19] The threshold used here is 35 grams	-
1. SLF3S - 1300F flow sensor 2. Buzzer 3. LED display board	NA	[20] The system is said to have achieved the objective of detecting the fluid level and then automatically stopping the flow.	The strategy causes complexity and increases costs because it uses NodeMCU, Raspberry Pi, Wi-Fi, and GSM components simultaneously.

(*Continued*)

Table 9.2 A summary of the research works referred in the text. (*Continued*)

Sensors and components	Accuracy	Findings	Limitations
1. HC SR-04 Ultrasonic Sensor 2. LDR 3. ESP8266 Wi-Fi module	NA	[21] The system is found to be feasible and also it is able to be integrated into the existing design of IV bags.	-
1. Load Cell 2. Solenoid valve 3. LCD Display 4. Flex Sensors 5. Temperature Sensors 6. ESP8266 Wi-Fi module	NA	[22] The system is successful in achieving the goal but then there are too many components which may make the system bulky and harder to integrate.	Many components which may make the system bulky and harder to integrate.
1. Load Cell 2. Photoresistor	87.9% (horizontal motion) and 89.9% (vertical motion)	[23] The system showed similar accuracy. Authors noted Wi-Fi latency issues and recommended 4G/5G for lower latency. Cost-effective development, making it feasible.	The IV bag design needs a complete overhaul as it lacks integration. The authors used a 3D printer for the redesign.
1. IR Sensor 2. Motor Driver 3. Buzzer 4. Load Cell 5. Servo motor 6. LCD	NA	[24] The threshold value used here is 70 mL for the regular IV bottle of 500 mL.	The study did not specify the mobile app used, whether open source or custom-made. Alarms at patient and nurse ends differ, causing panic.

(*Continued*)

Table 9.2 A summary of the research works referred in the text. (*Continued*)

Sensors and components	Accuracy	Findings	Limitations
1. IR Sensor 2. Servo Motor	NA	[25] The proposed system, cost-effective and dependable, wirelessly transmits data to a server for display on a central monitor. Information includes saline droplet rate, failure status, time to empty bottle, and infusion volume.	Insufficient nurses during busy times or staffing shortages can lead to missed alarms at the nursing station.
1. Fork-type light barrier 2. Sensor Node 3. RF communication module based on a CC2420 chip	Based on experimental data of 10% glucose, the author asserts that the accuracy matches practical needs.	[26] The study assesses fork-type light barriers that are ZigBee-connected for IV infusion monitoring and shows their dependable, accurate, and reliable networked operation.	It takes a bit of work to set up the system.
1. Light Emitting Diode 2. Light Dependent Resistor (LDR) 3. Operational Amplifier (OpAmp) LM358 4. Buzzer	NA	[27] A precise IV therapy monitoring system can decrease errors, assisting both at-home carers and hospital staff members, and improving IV infusion therapy.	When the flow rate deviates from the desired preset rate, human intervention is necessary to reset it automatically.
1. Flow sensor 2. Bluetooth Module 3. LCD Monitor 4. LDR 5. LED 6. Servo Motor	NA	[28] This system offers affordability, user-friendliness, and accessibility, making it ideal for resource-constrained environments where advanced tech isn't viable.	-

9.4 Observations and Results

There are a number of trends and patterns that could be seen throughout the literature review, with respect to the usage of certain sensors, based on the communication media they are using, whether the system is stationary or mobile, the type of microcontroller used, and so on. Exploring each of these can be tremendously helpful in understanding the working, efficiency, and availability of these technologies for implementation. This can also assist in coming up with a new system, having the best of the technologies that have been used so far.

Based on the research works referred to, it can be concluded that the most frequently used sensor for the implementation of smart IV bags is the load cell. Load cells are used to measure the weight of the IV bag and determine the amount of fluid that has been administered. The second most commonly used sensor is the infrared (IR) sensor, which is used to detect the presence of the IV bag and monitor its movement. These sensors are important for the implementation of smart IV bags, which can help to improve patient safety and reduce errors in the administration of intravenous fluids.

Load cells are typically used in smart IV bags to monitor the amount of fluid in the bag and detect any changes in weight, which can indicate the amount of fluid that has been administered to the patient. The IR sensors, on the other hand, are used to detect the presence of the IV bag and monitor its movement. This information can be used to ensure that the IV bag is properly positioned and that the fluid is being administered at the correct rate. Overall, the use of these sensors in smart IV bags can improve patient safety, reduce the risk of errors, and improve the efficiency of the healthcare system.

A graphical representation of the frequency of usage of various sensors in the Smart IV infusion systems has been presented in Figure 9.2.

According to the research papers cited, Wi-Fi appears to be the most popular communication method for the usage of smart IV bags. Wi-Fi is a popular technology that offers high-speed data transport and may be used to monitor IV bag data in real-time. Zigbee, a low-power wireless communication protocol that can be used to create a mesh network for data transfer, is the second most popular communication method for smart IV bags. By using these communication channels, the smart IV bags may send data to a central monitoring system, giving healthcare professionals access to real-time data on the IV bags' condition and allowing them to act promptly in case of any problems.

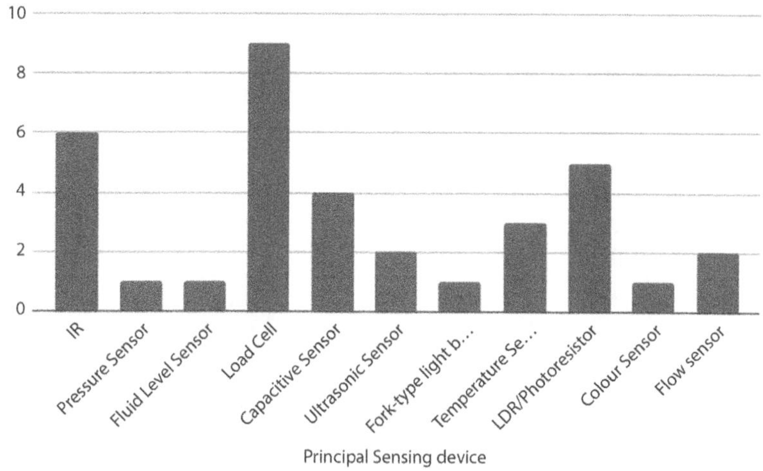

Figure 9.2 A graphical representation of the frequency of usage of sensors.

Wi-Fi connectivity in smart IV bags enable fast data transfer as well as on-demand monitoring of the IV bag's fluid levels, pressure, and flow rate. Wi-Fi is also commonly accessible in healthcare settings, making the use of smart IV bags a practical and accessible choice. On the other hand, Zigbee is a low-power wireless technology that may be applied to build a mesh network for information flow between several devices. When there are several IV bags and a centralized monitoring system is required, Zigbee is a good communication medium because of its dependability, low battery consumption, and long-range capabilities. Overall, the use of Wi-Fi and Zigbee in smart IV bags enables the seamless transfer of data, improving patient safety and reducing the risk of errors during IV fluid administration.

A graphical representation of the frequency of usage of various communication media in smart IV infusion systems has been given in Figure 9.3.

The difference between the frequency of using Wi-Fi and GSM can be clearly seen in Figure 9.3. GSM (Global System for Mobile Communications) is a wireless communication standard used for cellular networks, while Wi-Fi is a local wireless network protocol. In a smart IV infusion system, GSM may be considered better than Wi-Fi for several reasons. Firstly, GSM offers wider coverage compared to Wi-Fi, which is limited to a particular area or room. This means that GSM can provide connectivity and enable real-time monitoring of IV infusion systems in remote locations or during patient transportation, where Wi-Fi may not be available. Secondly, GSM is generally considered more reliable than Wi-Fi as it is less

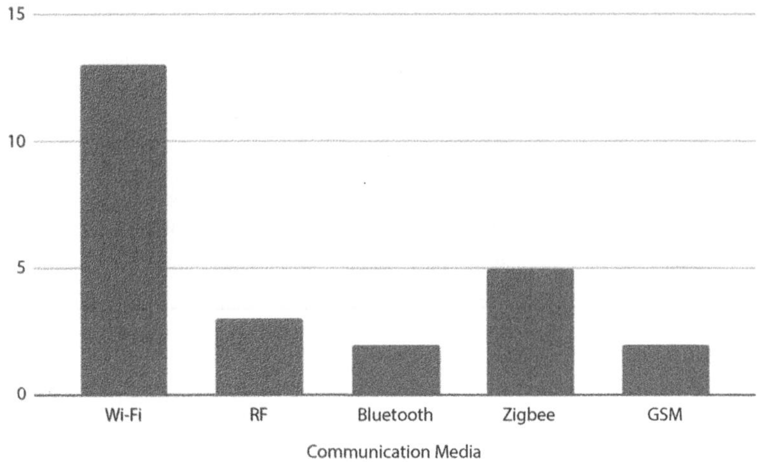

Figure 9.3 The frequency of usage of various communication media.

prone to interference and signal disruptions. This is particularly important in healthcare settings where reliable and consistent connectivity is crucial for the safety and well-being of patients. Finally, GSM networks often have built-in security features, such as encryption, to protect the transmission of data. While Wi-Fi can also be secured, it may require additional setup and management to ensure the data transmitted is adequately protected. Keeping these in mind, we can safely assume that GSM could be a good choice for communication when it comes to a hospital environment.

Figure 9.4 shows a comparison between the systems that are stationary in one place and the systems that are mobile, i.e., the alert will be sent to the nurse or caretaker.

Mobile systems are preferred over stationary systems in smart IV infusion systems for several reasons. Firstly, mobile systems provide greater flexibility and freedom of movement for healthcare providers, allowing them to attend to other tasks or patients while still being alerted to important events or issues related to the IV infusion system. This can help to improve efficiency and productivity in healthcare settings, as nurses can respond to alerts quickly without having to be physically present at the nurse station. Secondly, mobile systems enable healthcare providers to receive alerts and information in real time, regardless of their location within the healthcare facility. This is particularly important in emergency situations where quick response times can be critical to patient outcomes. Finally, mobile systems may be more accessible and convenient for healthcare providers who may not always be stationed at the nurse station, such

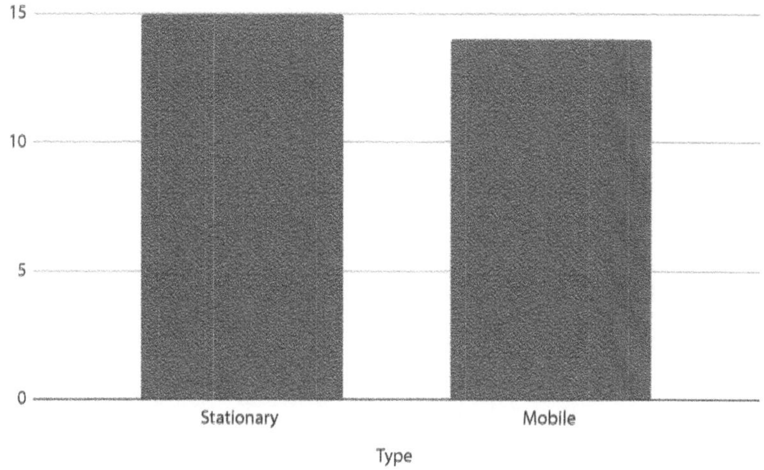

Figure 9.4 Stationary systems vs mobile systems.

as those who are on rounds or performing other duties. By receiving alerts on their personal mobile devices, healthcare providers can stay informed and respond quickly to any issues related to the IV infusion system.

Therefore, it is important to ensure the mobility of the system while designing a smart IV infusion system.

A microcontroller board serves as the "brain" of a system, controlling and managing its various components and functions. It is an integral part of any system, including the infusion monitoring systems, as the type of microcontroller can determine the overall working and functioning of the system.

Figure 9.5 gives an overview about the trends in usage of various microcontroller boards in the Smart IV infusion system's domain.

From the figure, we can see that Arduino boards are the most preferred boards, followed by NodeMCU ESP8266. Arduino and NodeMCU are popular open-source microcontroller platforms that can be programmed to sense and control physical devices. They are perfect for projects, prototyping, and Internet of Things (IoT) applications due to their adaptability, user-friendliness, and affordability. While NodeMCU is based on the Lua scripting language and has built-in Wi-Fi capabilities, Arduino uses its own programming language. Both systems have a large online community that offers information, guides, and assistance.

There are a number of reasons why researchers would prefer Arduino and NodeMCU to other microcontroller boards. First of all, since both systems are open-source, anyone may access them and alter the code

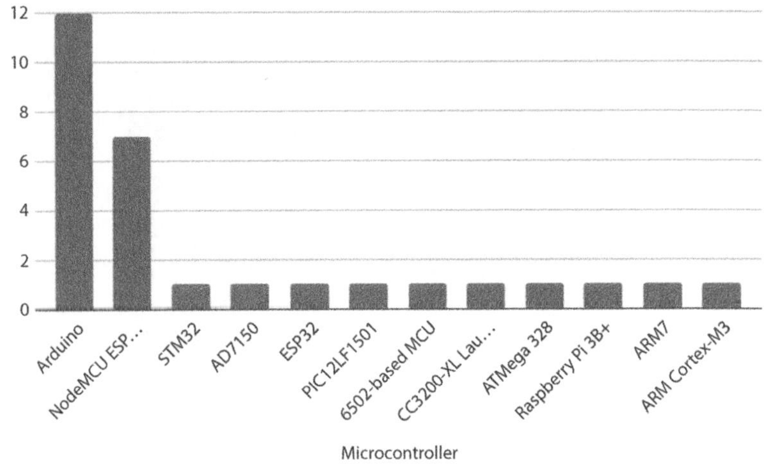

Figure 9.5 Frequency of usage of various microcontroller boards.

and schematics to meet their particular requirements. As a result, they are incredibly flexible and may be used for a variety of purposes. Second, both systems are user-friendly for beginners, with straightforward coding interfaces and an extensive online community that offers a plethora of information and assistance. They are thus perfect for researchers who may lack considerable programming expertise. Additionally, a wider range of researchers and institutions can use Arduino and NodeMCU because they are both reasonably priced. Finally, both platforms are flexible and can be used for a variety of projects, from personal projects to complex Internet of Things (IoT) projects. In general, Arduino and NodeMCU are inexpensive, adaptable, and simple to use, making them a popular option for both researchers and amateurs.

9.5 Conclusion

The study on IoT-enabled alarm systems and smart IV infusion monitoring reveals important developments in healthcare technology. Patient care is changing as a result of three main types of systems: hardware-based, software-based, and hybrid. These systems make use of a range of sensors and communication technologies to provide real-time monitoring, automatic corrections, error identification, and warnings, ultimately improving patient safety.

Integration with electronic health records streamlines coordination among healthcare professionals. The effectiveness of the infusion process is increased by these advances, which greatly reduce drug errors. However, a number of issues need to be addressed, including ensuring interoperability, standardizing protocols, and addressing data security and privacy concerns. The study focused on the important point that these systems greatly lower medication errors and improve patient safety by detecting and alerting medical professionals to infusion problems. They also lessen the strain of manual monitoring, allowing medical staff to concentrate on other facets of patient care.

However, the study also identified problems and suggested areas for more investigation. These include the demand for standardized protocols, system compatibility, and worries about data security and privacy. Advanced algorithms, EHR integration, and the potential of AI and machine learning in this field should be the main focus of future study.

This thorough analysis has clarified the condition of IoT-enabled alarm systems and smart IV infusion monitoring at the moment. Although they may not now be widely used in healthcare, they have enormous promise for the future. Future study should focus on sophisticated algorithms, data analysis methods, and investigate applications of artificial intelligence and machine learning. While not yet widely used in healthcare, these systems' potential significance cannot be denied.

Data Availability

All the data collected from the articles has been cited in the references.

Conflict of Interest

The authors would like to confirm that there is no conflict of interest.

Funding

The authors would like to confirm that there was no funding received for the above work.

References

1. Rosdi, M.R. and Huong, A., A Smart Infusion Pump System for Remote Management and Monitoring of Intravenous (IV) Drips, in: *11th IEEE Symposium on Computer Applications & Industrial Electronics (ISCAIE)*, 2021, doi: 10.1109/iscaie51753.2021.9431790.
2. Xu, Z.H., Li, W.Z., Xiao, Y.J., The Design of Infusion Monitoring System Based on STM32 Microcontroller. *Adv. Mat. Res.*, 756, 395–398, 2013.
3. Rani, K.R., Shabana, N., Tanmayee, P., Loganathan, S., Velmathi, G., Smart drip infusion monitoring system for instant alert-through nRF24L01, in: *International Conference on Nextgen Electronic Technologies: Silicon to Software (ICNETS2)*, 2017, doi: 10.1109/icnets2.2017.8067976.
4. Joseph, S., Francis, N., John, A., Farha, B., Baby, A., Intravenous Drip Monitoring System for Smart Hospital Using IoT, in: *2nd International Conference on Intelligent Computing, Instrumentation and Control Technologies (ICICICT)*, 2019, doi: 10.1109/icicict46008.2019.8993241.
5. Yamin, M., Habir, S.A., Nur Alam, W.O.S., Surimi, L., Smart Infusion and Web Based Monitoring Infusion Fluids in Isolation Room Based on Fuzzy Logic. *J. Phys. Conf. Ser.*, 2111, 1, 012056, 2021.
6. Salmaz, U., Ahsan, M.A.H., Islam, T., High-Precision Capacitive Sensors for Intravenous Fluid Monitoring in Hospitals. *IEEE Trans. Instrum. Meas.*, 70, 1–9, 2021.
7. Sunil, G., Aluvala, S., Ranadheer Reddy, G., Sree Harika, V., Sindhu, P., Keerthana, S., IoT based saline level monitoring system. *IOP Conf. Ser.: Mater. Sci. Eng.*, 981, 3, 032095, 2020.
8. Ghosh, D., Agrawal, A., Prakash, N., Goyal, P., Smart Saline Level Monitoring System Using ESP32 And MQTT-S, in: *2018 IEEE 20th International Conference on e-Health Networking, Applications and Services (Healthcom)*, 2018, doi: 10.1109/healthcom.2018.8531172.
9. Jiang, S. and He, Y., A low power circuit for medical drip infusion monitoring system, in: *2020 IEEE International Conference on Smart Internet of Things (SmartIoT)*, 2020, doi: 10.1109/smartiot49966.2020.00062.
10. Chen, F.-G., Wang, J.-Y., Chen, S., Tu, S.-C., Chen, K.-Y., A Hang-and-Play Intravenous Infusion Monitoring System, in: *2015 3rd International Conference on Applied Computing and Information Technology/2nd International Conference*, 2015.
11. Raghavendra, B., Vijayalakshmi, K., Arora, M., Intravenous drip meter & controller, in: *2016 8th International Conference on Communication Systems and Networks (COMSNETS)*, 2016, doi: 10.1109/comsnets.2016.7440024.
12. Oros, D., Smart Intravenous Infusion Dosing System. *Appl. Sci.*, 11, 2, 513, 2021, doi: 10.3390/app11020513.

13. Bhavasaar, M.K., Nithya, M., Praveena, R., Bhuvaneswari, N., Kalaiselvi, T., Automated intravenous fluid monitoring and alerting system, in: *2016 IEEE Technological Innovations in ICT for Agriculture and Rural Development (TIAR)*, 20162016, doi: 10.1109/tiar.2016.7801217.
14. Rao, K.R. and Supriya, K.E., Design and Development of IoT Based Intravenous Infusion System, in: *Lecture Notes in Electrical Engineering*, pp. 487–499, 2019.
15. A., R., A., S., C., A.G., G., J., L., J., IV Fluid Monitor And Controller. *Int. J. Eng. Appl. Technol.*, 5, 4, 360–364, 2020.
16. Arulious Jora, A., Divya Laveena, A., Earlina, D., Nirmala, S., Intravenous fluid level indicator. *Int. Res. J. Eng. Technol. (IRJET)*, 05, 10, 525–529, 2018.
17. Wei, Q., Woo, S.-H., Mohy-Ud-Din, Z., Kim, D.-W., Won, C.-H., Cho, J.-H., Capacitive sensor for the detection of the residual quantity of intravenous drip solution in a plastic intravenous bag. *J. Sens. Sci. Technol.*, 19, 4, 271–277, 2010.
18. Ray, P.P., Thapa, N., Dash, D., De, D., Novel implementation of IoT based non-invasive sensor system for real-time monitoring of intravenous fluid level for assistive e-healthcare. *Circuit World*, 45, 3, 109–123, 2019.
19. Moorthy, J., Karunakaran, K., Kumar, S.V.S., An Automated Locking System to Prevent Backflow. *Glob. J. Res. Eng.*, 20, J2, 27–34, 2020.
20. Mathew, E.L., James, J.K., Radhakrishnan, A., Sebastian, B., Mathew, H., The Novel Intravenous Fluid Level Indicator for Smart IV Systems. *IRJET*, 6th ed., 7, 3735–3738, 2020.
21. Tanwar, S., K, D., Maniktalia, R., Billa, R., IoT Based Drip Infusion Monitoring System. *Int. J. Sci. Res.*, 10, 12, 1–6, 2021 Dec.
22. A., R., A., S., K., G., M., M., Vindhya, P., IoT BASED INTRAVENOUS FLOW MONITORING SYSTEM. *Int. J. Sci. Res.*, 5th ed., 7, 7539–7543, 2020.
23. Lee, J.-K., Yoon, K.-C., Kim, K.G., Design of a Remote Monitoring System Based on Optical Sensors to Prevent Medical Accidents during Fluid Treatment. *Appl. Sci.*, 11, 21, 10124, 2021.
24. Bandari, S., IV Drip Monitoring and Control System. *Int. J. Res. Appl. Sci. Eng. Technol.*, 10, 6, 3383–3386, 2022.
25. Yadav, S. and Jain, P., Real-time cost-effective e-saline monitoring and control system, in: *2016 International Conference on Control, Computing, Communication and Materials (ICCCCM)*, 2016, doi: 10.1109/icccm.2016.7918254.
26. Zhang, Y., Zhang, S., Ji, Y., Wu, G., Wireless sensor network-enabled intravenous infusion monitoring. *IET Wireless Sens. Syst.*, 1, 4, 241–247, 2011.
27. Alagundagi, S.S., Pasala, K., Arora, M., Opto-electronic system for intravenous infusion monitoring, in: *2018 10th International Conference on Communication Systems & Networks (COMSNETS)*, 2018, doi: 10.1109/comsnets.2018.8328296.

28. Rashid, H., Shekha, S., Taslim Reza, S., Ahmed, I.U., Newaz, Q., Rasheduzzaman, M., A low-cost automated fluid control device using a smartphone for medical application, in: *2017 International Conference on Electrical, Computer and Communication Engineering (ECCE)*, 2017.
29. Tian, S., Yang, W., Grange, J.M.L., Wang, P., Huang, W., Ye, Z., Smart healthcare: making medical care more intelligent. *Glob. Health J.*, 3, 3, 62–65, 2019.

10

Portable IoT Smart Devices in Healthcare and Remote Health Monitoring – Abnormality Detection through Personalized Vital Health Signs Using Smart Bio Devices

Poorani Marimuthu[1]*, C. Christlin Shanuja[2] and Aparna N.[1]

[1]CMR Institute of Technology, Bengaluru, India
[2]Global Academy of Technology, Bengaluru, India

Abstract

In general, health parameters are highly uncertain, non-linear, dynamic in nature and it varies person to person within a range. This rises the need of continuous health monitoring for ICU patients, persons with chronic disease, elder people, home alone people etc. Wireless technology, Body Area Networks using smart devices, artificial intelligence provides the freedom for the patients/persons to be continuously monitored at any place and at any time. Portable IoT smart wearable gadgets are firmly recommended in dynamic and complex real-world health issues. In medical field, all the wearable gadgets are highly used due to its intelligence and data handling capability. Today's bio smart devices help to reduce the risk in diagnosis or treatment; it provides early diagnosis, long term continuous health monitoring, rehabilitate illnesses, and the person can be done medication irrespective of the location where he/she resides. With respect to technology aspect all the devices are manufactured with high precision, low latency in sensing, high speed in data transmission cum processing the data and taking decision as per the sensed values. It helps the medical staff to diagnose and treat the patient efficiently with its sensed values and helps them to take a decision much faster. This in turn increases the treatment quality and its boost the operational efficiency. Moreover, these devices can be easily handled, and it enables to the early prediction of acute

**Corresponding author*: pooraniarunkumar@gmail.com

Hari Murthy, Marta Zurek-Mortka, Vinay Jha Pillai and Kukatlapalli Pradeep Kumar (eds.) Internet of Things in Bioelectronics: Emerging Technologies and Applications, (201–218) © 2024 Scrivener Publishing LLC

disease. Monitoring the health status of a remote person where the technology is tailored to observe and detect the abnormality as per patients personalized health values rather than general threshold value taken for a population is termed as personalized medicine which can be smoothly accomplished using portable bio smart devices. The abnormality in health signs is identified using bio devices and early warning can be done using RHM.

***Keywords*:** Portable bio-smart device, remote health monitoring, personalized remote health monitoring, vital signs, abnormality

Highlights of the Work

1. The chapter discusses application of portable smart wearable devices and its interoperability with other technologies.
2. Case study on abnormality detection in real time has been discussed.
3. Benefits and the challenges while using portable smart devices are highlighted.
4. The applicability of smart wearable devices in RHM is discussed in detail.
5. The chapter tries to provide a brief introduction about smart portable devices and their applicability in the medical field for the readers.

10.1 Introduction

Any device which is capable of taking decisions without any human intervention is termed to be smart devices [1] (smart phones, smart TV, smart oven, smart washing machine etc.). The smart devices respond to the environment if any event occurs where they have been placed. It has the capability to observe the environment factors, gather the information or data, exchange the data with the external world, analyze the data and take

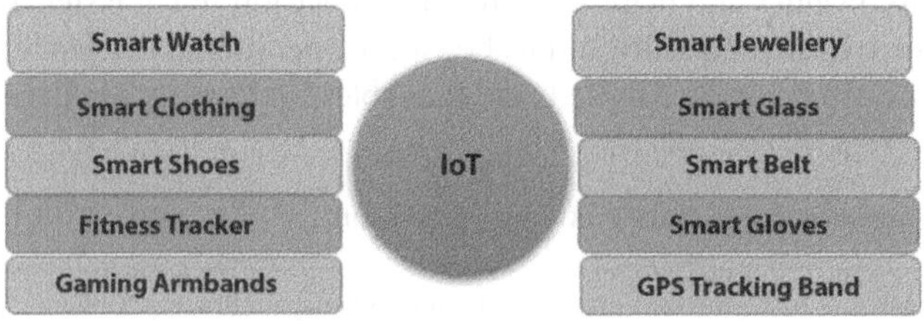

Figure 10.1 Wearable IoT devices.

necessary action in critical situations. Figure 10.1 shows the top wearable smart devices which has been widely used all around the world. In general, smart devices are classified into two major classes that includes, time critical smart devices and non-time critical smart devices as per their application. The network of smart devices is commonly referred as Internet of Things [2]. To achieve the smartness in the device, the device has been installed with sensors, communication portal, actuators, and internet. Sensors, in general sense the environment factors including temperature, pressure, moisture, movement, etc. for which it has been intended. The communication portals with the help of communication technologies like WIFI, Zigbee, IEEE 802.15.4, Wireless HART, Thread, MQTT, 6LoWPAN, LoRa, Z-Wave etc. does the transmission and reception of data with the other devices. Actuators are an IoT component which will induce the movement or control a system by converting the energy or signal that flows through the system. The loudest breakthrough trends in the technology industry from 2013 onwards is the wearable technology. As per a report, it is stated that "shipments of wearable technology are expected to reach 155.7 million, by 2019". Nowadays, these smart devices are manufactured with smaller size, more advanced, cheaper, including the capability of analyzing the data with less power utilization.

As such external factors, human health parameters can also be sensed using sensors and those sensors are designed as wearable and portable. Today, in market, lots of portable smart health devices [3] are available because of the advancement and the accuracy in measurement of these sensors. COVID 19 plays an important role in the acceptance of smart healthcare devices among the people and in the work [4], the impact of COVID 19 along with its trend line for second and third waves in India has been discussed elaborately. After COVID 19, people became aware of a wide range of portable cum wearable IoT smart health devices like smart watch, smart glass, fitness bands etc. In general, IoT has many useful applications in many sectors that includes education, industry, health, agriculture, vehicular, logistics, communication etc., in larger scale other than smart home, smart vehicle, smart classroom in smaller sector. Among these wide applications, IoT in health sector has shown a tremendous improvement and the benefit to the human mankind is enormous. It increases the quality of lifestyle and reduces the mortality rate among all the ages. Figure 10.2 shows some of the sensors that have been widely used in medical sector.

In medical sector, the sensor networks are categorized into three categories as per their placement that includes implanted, wearable and environment embedded. Implanted medical devices are in general placed inside the body for the proper functioning of body parts, to monitor the

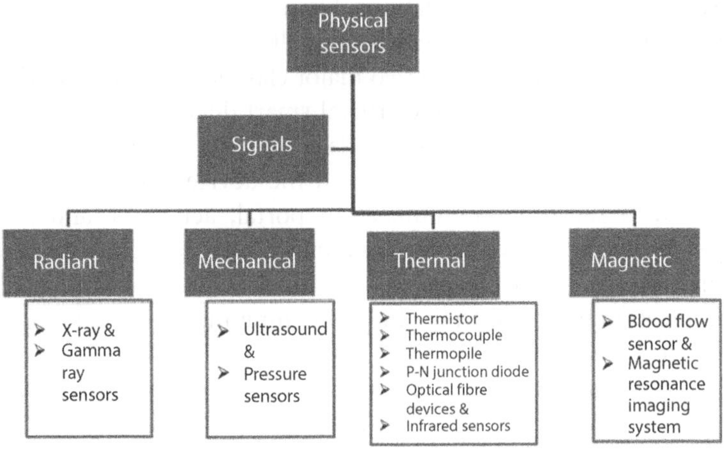

Figure 10.2 Sensors used in medical field.

deviations and to take necessary actions if any abnormality occurs etc. Wearable devices are placed or tied on the surface of the human body, whereas environment embedded devices are placed nearby or with proximity of the monitored person. Airflow, temperature, barcode, oxygen, pressure, force, airflow, pulse oximetry sensors are generally utilized in medical devices. External sensors are widely used in health monitoring systems that includes blood pressure cuffs, pulse oximeter, heart rate analyzer etc. Thermometer sensors are widely used in medical field like force sensor in kidney dialysis machine, airflow sensor in heart pumps, non-invasive blood pressure and cyanosis monitoring during anesthesia, laparoscopy, pressure sensors in infusion pumps and sleep apnea machines. As per the dataset, more than 15 highly precise datasets are available for the healthcare field that includes general/public data, research data, synthesized data based on original data etc. The common available datasets are Re3Data, CHDS, Kent Ridge Biomedical Dataset, Merck Molecular Health Activity Challenge, SEER etc. All these datasets are benchmark and can be effectively used for research activity.

Easy access to health care and decrease in healthcare delivery costs can be attained through RHM that enables monitoring of health parameters of remote persons wherever he/she is residing as such as home or remote area, rather than traditional clinical settings. In general, data pattern which is not usual or expecting pattern can be detected by continuous monitoring of data through sensors. The identified abnormalities/anomalies are generally considered as problems that includes structural defects, errors, abnormality, or fraudulent activity. RHM modelling has many challenges that includes wearable sensor selection, collection of sensed data from the wearable devices, proper transmission of these collected data to the server, data synchronization, pre-processing, data analysis for good abnormality detection model selection based on the correlation that exist between the sensed data, designing an abnormality decision cum prediction model based on the streaming real time data, proper scheduling for timely alert generation, maintenance and storage of collected data for further analysis etc. The chapter is organized as follows, section 10.2 provides the literature study, section 10.3 provides the role of portable smart wearable devices in remote health monitoring, section 10.4 discusses the case study of abnormality detection using smart devices in RHM, section 10.5 does the research challenges and future scope. Finally, section 10.6 summarizes the chapter with its contributions.

10.2 Literature Survey

A detailed summary of wearable health devices has been discussed by Lu, Lin, *et al.* [5] and this study provides covers most of the wearable devices in healthcare field. An energy aware autonomous wearable sensor has been discussed in [6]. The work involves explanation of various transduction mechanisms, its fabrication, low power electronic device, related software for auto detection of health sign values, energy harvested rechargeable batteries etc. Lisboa, Paulo J., and Azzam FG Taktak [7], performed a survey on neural network algorithms that has been used as a decision maker in cancer diagnosis. The study discussed the clinical and randomized controlled trials involving neural network in detail. Likewise, Shahid *et al.* [8] did their detail study in ANN based healthcare organizational decision making. In [9], the Internet of Health Things (IoHT), concentrating on various methods for collecting and integrating vital signs health data in hospitals has been studied. This paper analyses the problems faced by hospitals to maintain large amounts of patient data which include vital signs that are manually collected. The data collected is difficult to analyze by caregivers as it is not a part of electronic health record. The possible solution suggested was to interconnect the medical devices through a distributed platform, which is Internet of Things. The proposed solution can collect and analyze patient data efficiently and allows the optimization of resources and minimizes patient health degradation. Table 10.1 list out some of the works based on health monitoring using portable cum wearable sensors. RHM based on smart edge technology with IoT generates alert using two software engines

Table 10.1 Literature summary of various abnormality detection using portable smart devices.

Reference	Authors & year of publish	Data set	Objective & performance analysis	Pros & cons
[10]	Luján, Miguel Ángel, *et al.* Electronics, 2022	EEG datasets	The proposed method grabs the high accuracy of 97% in all the confusion matrix parameters.	1. Quick training procedures 2. Easy integration of tools due to simple configuration.
[11]	Pravin Pawar, Val Jones, *et al.* 2012	synthetic dataset	The proposed framework had been applied to six mobile patients and could find features for epilepsy in them.	A generic architecture is proposed for a mobile patient monitoring system and given a comparison framework for the same.
[12]	Md. Milon Islam, *et al.* 2020	Synthetic data	It can monitor both the status of patient's health and his/her room condition.	The error rate was less than 5%.
[13]	Malik Bader *et al.* Wireless Commun-ications and Mobile Computing, 2021.	MIMIC Dataset, ICU database	Automated antiquity detection used for BP and PPG signals. The correlation of diastolic and systolic has been considered for evaluation.	1. High accuracy on Single signal & probe in computing SBP and DBP. 2. Regular BP monitoring is advisable for old people. 3. Not tested on a large patient population
[14]	Muhammad Shafiq Changqing, *et al.* Journal of Sensors, 2023	PASCAL data set	Manual observation of patient is done by a monitor kept beside the patient's bed.	1. In terms of all the features analyzed, Deep CNN shows high accuracy comparatively. 2. Difficult to implement when dealing with large datasets.

(Continued)

Table 10.1 Literature summary of various abnormality detection using portable smart devices. (*Continued*)

Reference	Authors & year of publish	Data set	Objective & performance analysis	Pros & cons
[15]	Yung-Chung Tsao, *et al.*, Emergency Medicine International, 2022.	Synthetic data	Smart health monitoring system to prove the reliability. MQTT is used to institute communication format which can be used by other organizations.	Take less than 1 second to transmit the data with MQTT broker and RFID.
[16]	Rasha M. K. *et al.*, Abdellattif, 2022.	UCI repository dataset	Patient's data is collected, sent over internet and inspect it using machine learning approach. Deep belief network is used to estimate the patient's health state.	1. The system shows 99% accuracy in foreseeing the changes in patient's health condition. 2. Average error rate is only 0.04
[17]	SomayehIranpak *et al.* Journal of Big Data volume 8, Article number: 120 (2021)	Patient data	The system uses LSTM deep neural network algorithm for classifying & monitoring patients. The system achieved 97.13% of accuracy.	1. LSTM deep neural network is used to classify and monitor remotely. 2. 5th generation mobile network along with a combination of cloud computing systems and IoT is used.
[18]	Puustjärvi J, *et al.* 2015;69:143–51	Patient data	An IoT-based health monitoring system considering the role of smart data in the smart home for patient-centered remote health monitoring	High classification accuracy
[19]	Tan ET, Abdul HZ. IETE J Res. 2019; 65.5: 653–60	Diabetes and Kidney Disease Dataset	An IoT-based healthcare monitoring and analysis system, which grab the accuracy patients with diabetes and kidney disease is 90.54% and 87.88%	The best training accuracy achieved in this study is 92.5% (diabetes) and 93.2% (kidney disease) and low computational speed

that include RASPRO and CMI using wearable vital sensor data. RASPRO contains Personalized Health Motifs (PHM) which is the summary of health data, and the engine has been alerted by CMI [20]. A smart home system (ShHeS) [21], played a vital role during the COVID-19 pandemic, especially for patients who are in quarantine or isolated due to the disease. This type of support can help patients receive necessary medical attention while reducing the risk of transmission of the virus to healthcare providers and other patients. It contains a mobile application interfaced with a web application, which helps in RHM of patient. With the help of sensors health parameters are captured. Also, a hyperspace analogue to context (HAC) model is used to represent the various contexts in which patients are monitored remotely, including their physical and mental health, as well as their living conditions and access to healthcare resources. The system includes smartphone, sensors, actuators, home appliances, Arduino board and Wi-Fi module. Sensors detect the temperature and humidity changes at home and also look for smoke. The microcontroller collects data through sensors, send necessary data through communication module to the user. A remote patient monitoring system (RPMS) [22] make use of IoT and cloud computing technologies for the efficient monitoring of patient health conditions and timely alert message or notification has been sent to local user or supervisor in case of emergency.

In [23], survey on ML based internet of things has been carried out. This work provides an in-depth information regarding the challenges of this field. It also provides ML and big data analytics overview, and how these technologies can be used to improve healthcare outcomes. The survey is also done to understand the different components of an IoT-enabled smart healthcare system, including sensors, devices, and data storage and processing systems and discussed the challenges associated with collecting, storing, and analyzing large amounts of data generated by these systems. The survey provides the information regarding different machine learning techniques that can be used to analyze healthcare data. It also described the different big data analytics techniques that can be used to analyze healthcare data, including data mining, predictive analytics, and natural language processing. Also discussed the challenges associated with processing and analyzing large amounts of healthcare data. In [24] a method to help cardiac patients at remote places has been proposed to get high end healthcare services. The system is reliable, low cost and able to send alert notification in case of emergency situations. The system includes a wearable sensor, which sends heart rate of the patient through a handheld android device over WIFI/GPRS to the server and as per received data, the server will notify the situation to the doctor's mobile as warning message.

10.3 Role of Portable Smart Wearable Devices in Remote Health Monitoring

RHM is the monitoring of patients outside of hospital or conventional clinics, that includes home, or in any remote area, wherever the monitored person is there that leads to improve care and delivery cost of healthcare. RHM is possible only with the help of invention of wearable cum portable smart devices in health sector that works along with all the high-end technologies like short range/long range communication, cloud, fog computing etc. The contributions of smart wearable devices to the health sector are as follows:

1. Stress and anxiety reduction among the patients and staff – By using wearable devices, the vital signs of the patients are continuously under monitoring which avoids abnormal circumstances.
2. Increased accuracy in detection and prediction of disease – the tracking data of the patients improves the detection accuracy and tries to provide a good prediction rate.
3. Quick diagnosis – by accessing the patients' health data it is possible to take a quick decision based on the history of data.
4. Improving the hospital services – from the surplus data from the wearable devices it is possible to predict the severity of the disease, which allows the prior arrangements in the hospital as per the requirement. This will be more useful in calculating LOS (Length of Stay).
5. Anywhere, all time monitoring – the patient has the option of mobility which provides a flexible treatment or diagnosis environment for both the doctor and patient.
6. Geospatial analysis – as the patient can be moved anywhere with the wearable device, the geospatial analysis of disease outbreak can also be tracked.

These factors allow the medical sector to be extended with RHM and there comes the real need for RHM. Apart from the above factors the smart devices have its contribution in Health Management, Device Management and Communication/Navigation

1. Better health management: the collected data from the smart wearable devices are processed in the device or it will

be transferred to other devices like smart phones, cloud server for immediate action based on the sensed data, generating alert and tracking of data etc. Today most of the wearable devices are connected with the mobile app for continuous monitoring which facilitates for timely emergency alert if abnormality arises and remainders for regular health check-up.

2. Device management: Nowadays portable smart wearables are well connected with IoT ecosystem that even it is able to track the lost mobile phone. It is possible to track, encrypt or delete or even to lock the mobile phone through the wearable devices.
3. Communication and navigation: Many smart wearable devices have the option of SIM slot that facilitate GPS or SATNav usage that provides easy tracking of the person.

10.4 Case Study

Remote healthcare modelling using personalized values are the recent research area which can be incorporated using soft computing techniques for detecting the abnormality. Here, the chapter involves activity recognition, personalization of vital parameter values based on activities and health status, abnormality detection using the personalized values and all these techniques are integrated with dynamic service scheduling in cloud based remote health monitoring. The research proposes a personalized remote health monitoring using soft computing techniques in real time that includes ANFIS with frequent pattern mining for activity recognition, density-based clustering for severity range fixation of vital signs, probabilistic based abnormality detection and finally results are optimized using bio inspired algorithm. The integrated Dynamic Priority Scheduler (DPS) in cloud reduce the latency between the patient and doctor.

The work involves collection of vital signs that includes Heart Rate (HR), Blood Pressure (BP) both systolic and Diastolic, Respiration Rate (RR), Electrocardiogram (ECG) and peripheral oxygen saturation in blood (SpO_2) along with the accelerometer values (x, y, z Coordinates) using wearable sensors from the monitored person as shown in Figure 10.3. The sensed data is transferred to mobile phone of the monitored person via Bluetooth. From the mobile phone, the data is then transferred to the remote cloud server using Wi-Fi or mobile internet. In cloud server all the sensed data were analyzed for abnormality.

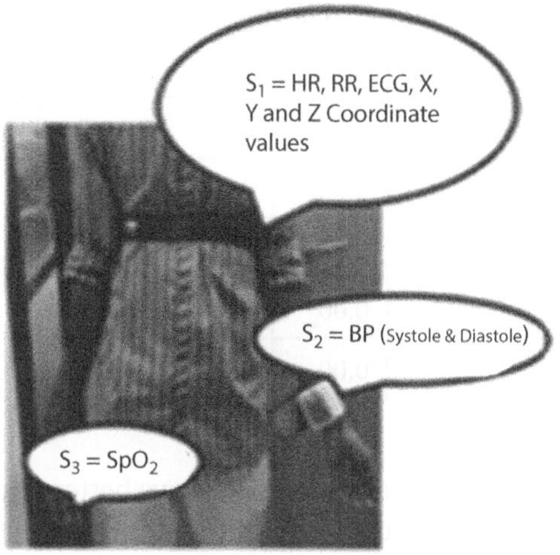

Figure 10.3 Activity and vital data collection.

10.4.1 Activity Recognition

The activity recognition forms an integral part of health monitoring system. The abnormality level fixation depends on activity of a person. Existing activity recognition methods using accelerometer data are inaccurate as they not considered the uncertainty prevails in the activity data and hence the research proposes an activity recognition method named "Optimized ANFIS using Frequent Pattern Mining (OAFPM)" combining Fuzzy Inference System (FIS) for handling uncertain data, Adaptive Neural Network (ANN) for continuous learning and FPM for reduced rules which in turn reduces the computational and time complexity. This proposed method recognizes the activities using the triaxial accelerometer values taken from the monitored person. The OAFPM method achieves an overall accuracy rate of 95.8% and the recognized activities are used to fix the threshold of the linguistic severity levels which reflects in the abnormality detection accuracy of the monitored person. The confusion matrix of the five activities is shown in Table 10.2.

10.4.2 Abnormality Detection

Existing abnormality detection methods fails to address personalization in streaming data. In the proposed DBK-MeansC technique, to overcome the afore mentioned issue, the incoming data stream of five vital parame ters are explored by dividing the dataset into overlapping/non-overlapping

Table 10.2 Confusion matrix of the activities.

Y / Ŷ	**Stand**	**Walk**	**Fall**	**Sit**	**Lay**
Stand	0.8	0.10	0.00	0.08	0.00
Walk	0.1	0.87	0.04	0.00	0.00
Fall	0.03	0.03	0.93	0.00	0.03
Sit	0.03	0.00	0.00	0.91	0.06
Lay	0.04	0.00	0.03	0.01	0.91

clusters. For better data exploration it is always better to go with unsupervised approach where the clusters will provide a good first level information about the data. Hence, the work proceeds with K-Means clustering approach to know about the seed points and the distribution of the sensed data. The severity range fixation for the five vital parameters of each individual is done by the centroids of the corresponding clusters. The cluster with maximum density around its centroid is considered for the linguistic variable severity level fixation. The proposed work started with DBK-MeansC that achieves a precision rate of 0.757 for the vital parameter severity level classification. The initial number of seed points has been randomly chosen with 5 and for this seed values most of the sensed data of the monitored person ranges from one (minimum) to three clusters (maximum). More than two clusters reflect in abnormality of the monitored person.

Although DBK-MeansC detects the linguistic severity level of the vital parameters, the time complexity is more and most of the data falls in the border line of the generated clusters. Moreover, a high correlation exists among the vital parameters which increases the uncertainty. To overcome these issues, the work proposed a Intelligent Personalized Abnormality Detection (IPAD) model using Bayesian belief, Naïve, and Genetic algorithm (NB^3GA - IPAD). The vital sign HR and BP is class labelled using Naïve Bayes as these two attributes are not much dependent on other parameters. The vital signs of RR, ECG and SpO_2 have strong dependency over HR. Hence these vital signs are classified using Bayesian Belief which is considered to be good dependency classifier. In NB^3GA - IPAD, the independency and dependency relation among the vital parameters are considered using probabilistic approach respectively to calculate the common level of severity. After classification of severity levels of vital health parameters, personalization of the health data is achieved by genetic algorithm and from these health values of the individual, abnormality is confirmed. Using the personalized severity levels, the Severity Index ($SI_{N/AB}$) of the person is calculated by providing proper ranking and weightage to the vital parameters. Abnormality detection has been achieved through severity index calculation for the monitored person through their vital parameters change in severity levels. NB^3GA – IPAD method observes an AUC of 0.907 for abnormality detection. Figures 10.4a–10.4e shows the GA convergence of the observed vital parameters. Based on the severity index and recognized activity abnormality has been identified.

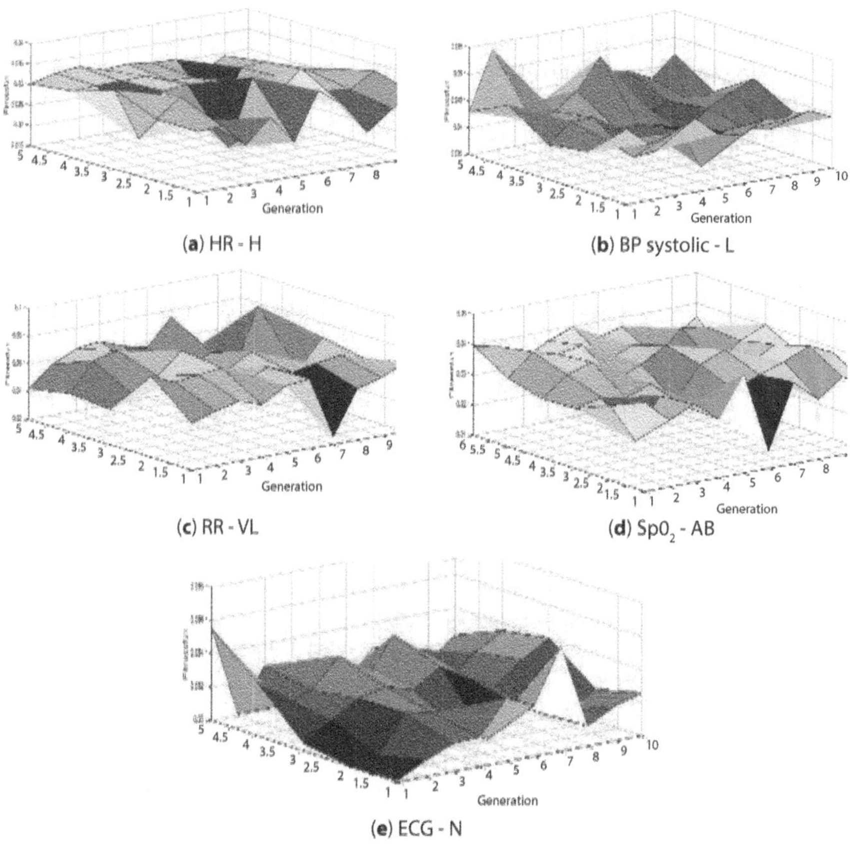

Figure 10.4 GA convergence of the vital parameters.

10.4.3 Results and Discussion

The work involves multimodal optimization with attributes having high interdependency using DBK-MeansC, probabilistic, neurofuzzy and bio inspired algorithms. Initial level of explanatory data analysis has been done by DBK-MeansC. The dependencies in attributes on vital signs are taken care by probabilistic approach, whereas the global solution from local search is done by genetic resulting in optimal solutions. Premature convergences are avoided using different recombining rate. In the same manner, elitist in genetic avoids the drift while doing mutation.

Figure 10.5 shows the observed ROC curve after implementation and the hybrid model reflects with 89.7 ± 2.6 % accuracy rate.

10.4.4 Alert Generation

When several patients are being monitored in the hospital using cloud server, the delay in detecting the abnormality and providing alert to the doctor is inevitable. Hence, there is a need for a scheduler for a remote health monitoring system. Existing scheduler in the literature faces challenges like minimum waiting time, servicing time for streaming data in

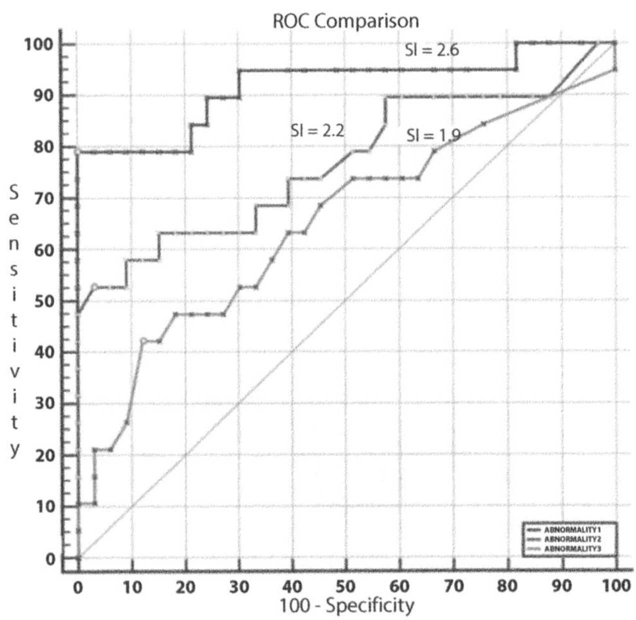

Figure 10.5 ROC curve of abnormality detection model.

a multiple person scenario. To overcome these issues, this research integrates a Dynamic Priority Scheduler (DPS) over the abnormality model. The abnormality detection accuracy of the NB^{3}GA - IPAD increases gradually with respect to inclusion of personalization, optimization and confirming with the health status in accordance with activity recognized.

10.5 Research Challenges and Future Scope

As IoT involves many technologies to its functionality, the challenges are very high. The challenges of IoT are divided into 3 categories which is shown in the Figure 10.6. One of the main issues in IoT is bandwidth limitations. Incorporating ML and DL in real time IoT implementation also a high-end task apart from IoT device management. In wearable technology battery life is a hardest issue, where the wearable devices need an effective power management in a limited battery space. Comfort and ergonomics are important factors to be considered for wearable devices. Another main challenge is the waterproofing, the device should work well in adverse situation also.

The performance of RHM has increased steeply because of IoE (Internet of Everything). Using IoE all the wearable devices, people, health data, algorithms (process) are interconnected, and an intelligent decision can be taken at an earlier stage. In IoE, intelligence is provided in each level

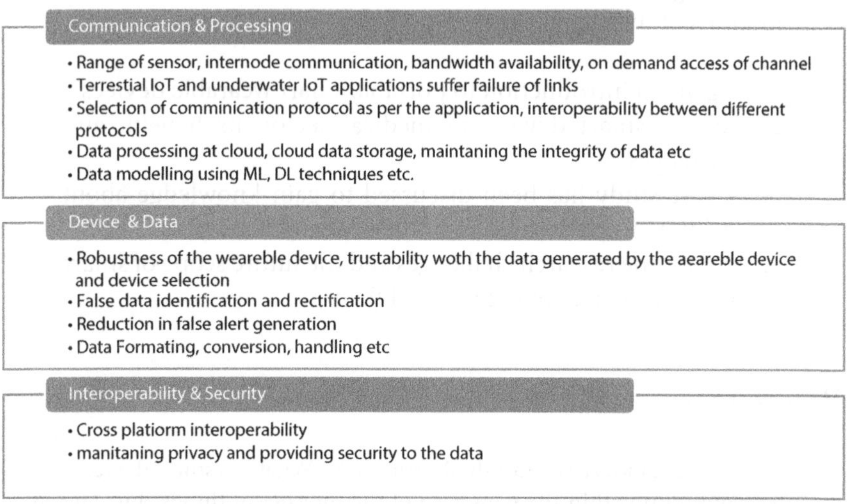

Figure 10.6 Challenges of implementing portable cum wearable sensor devices in IoT.

including wearable devices that allows taking proactive decisions based on the health data of the monitored person. This makes the foundation for this proactive healthcare by developing a fully connected automized RHM. With the inclusion of IoE, the RHM can be extended for cancer monitoring, continuous glucose monitoring for diabetes, connected inhalers, asthma monitoring etc. where decisions can be taken earlier based on the sensed health data that provides more control over the lives and treatment. The potential of IoT is high and in future, the portable smart wearable devices advance the healthcare field through artificial intelligence integration, network agility, high end communication that makes the IOT to be deployed in hyperscale.

10.6 Conclusion

The proposed chapter focus on the portable smart wearable devices, its challenges in real time implementing, its role in medical sector and a case study. The implementation of personalized RHM using smart portable IOT device can be able to develop a health record with self-reported data and symptoms, which results in geospatial data analysis of any communicable disease like COVID19. Thus, with the help of smart portable IoT wearable devices disease outbreaking can be easily identified prior. Moreover, the disease like corona virus (COVID – 19) that causes other disease like ARDS, breathing failure, immunity development failure can be detected at an early stage through continuous monitoring for remote patients. The contributions of the chapter include,

1. A general introduction to portable smart wearable devices
2. Role of smart devices in medical sector, its benefit, and challenges
3. A case study has been discussed to gain knowledge about real time implementation of these wearable devices.
4. Finally, the research challenges and the future scope of smart portable devices in the medical field.

References

1. Silverio-Fernández, M., Suresh, R., Suresh, S., What is a smart device?-a conceptualisation within the paradigm of the internet of things. *Vis. Eng.*, 6, 1, 1–10, 2018.

2. Rose, K., Eldridge, S., Chapin, L., The internet of things: An overview. *Internet Soc. (ISOC)*, 80, 1–50, 2015.
3. Mukherjee, S. *et al.*, State of the art in smart portable, wearable, ingestible and implantable devices for health status monitoring and disease management. *Sensors*, 22, 11, 4228, 2022.
4. Murthy, H. *et al.*, A Statistical Analysis and Comparison of the spread of Swine Flu and COVID-19 in India. *Malaysian J. Med. Health Sci.*, 92–99, 2022.
5. Lu, L. *et al.*, Wearable health devices in health care: narrative systematic review. *JMIR mHealth uHealth*, 8, 11, e18907, 2020.
6. Dahiya, A.S. *et al.*, Energy autonomous wearable sensors for smart healthcare: a review. *J. Electrochem. Soc.*, 167, 3, 037516, 2019.
7. Lisboa, P.J. and Taktak, A.F.G., The use of artificial neural networks in decision support in cancer: a systematic review. *Neural Netw.*, 19, 4, 408–415, 2006.
8. Shahid, N., Rappon, T., Berta, W., Applications of artificial neural networks in health care organizational decision-making: A scoping review. *PloS One*, 14, 2, e0212356, 2019.
9. da Costa, C.A., Pasluosta, C.F. *et al.*, Internet of Health Things: Toward intelligent vital signs monitoring in hospital wards, in: *Elsevier Artificial Intelligence in Medicine*, vol. 89, pp. 61–69, July 2018.
10. Luján, M. Á. *et al.*, High-Precise Bipolar Disorder Detection by Using Radial Basis Functions Based Neural Network. *Electronics*, 11, 3, 343, 2022.
11. Pawar, P., Jones, V., van Beijnum, B.-J.F., Hermens, H., A framework for the comparison of mobile patient monitoring systems, in: *Telemedicine Group, Faculty of Electrical Engineering, Mathematics and Computer Science*, University of Twente, The Netherlands, Available online 1 March 2012.
12. Islam, M., Rahaman, A., Islam, R., Development of Smart Healthcare Monitoring System in IoT Environment. *SN Comput. Sci.*, 1, 185, 2020.
13. Alazzam, M.B., Alassery, F., Almulihi, A., A Novel Smart Healthcare Monitoring System Using Machine Learning and the Internet of Things. *Wireless Commun. Mobile Comput.*, 2023, Article ID 6383099, 7, 2023, 2021.
14. Shafiq, M., Du, C., Jamal, N., Abro, J.H., Kamal, T., Afsar, S., Mia, S., Smart E-Health System for Heart Disease Detection Using Artificial Intelligence and Internet of Things Integrated Next-Generation Sensor Networks. *J. Sens.*, 2022, Article ID 7245650, 13, 2023.
15. Tsao, Y.-C., Cheng, F.-J., Li, Y.-H., Liao, L.-D., An IoT-Based Smart System with an MQTT Broker for Individual Patient Vital Sign Monitoring in Potential Emergency or Prehospital Applications. *Emerg. Med. Int.*, 2022, 2022.
16. Mohamed, R.M.K., Shahin, O.R., Hamed, N.O., Zahran, H.Y., Abdellattif, M.H., Analyzing the Patient Behavior for Improving the Medical Treatment Using Smart Healthcare and IoT-Based Deep Belief Network. *J. Electrochem. Soc*, 8, 120, 217, 2022.

17. Iranpak, S., Shahbahrami, A., Shakeri, H., Remote patient monitoring and classifying using the internet of things platform combined with cloud computing. *J. Big Data*, 8, 120, 2021.
18. Puustjärvi, J., The role of smart data in smart home: health monitoring case study. *Proc. Comput. Sci.*, 69, 143–51, 2015.
19. Tan, E.T. and Halim, A., Health care monitoring system and analytics based on internet of things framework. *IETE J. Res.*, 65, 5, 2019.
20. Pathinarupothi, R.K., Durga, P. *et al.*, IoT-Based Smart Edge for Global Health: Remote Monitoring with Severity Detection and Alerts Transmission. *IEEE Internet Things J.*, 6, 2, April 2019.
21. Taiwo, O. and Ezugwu, A.E., Smart healthcare support for remote patient monitoring during covid-19 quarantine. *Inf. Med. Unlocked*, 20, 100428, 2020.
22. Sahu, M.L., Atulkar, M., Ahirwal, M.K., Ahamad, A., Cloud-Based Remote Patient Monitoring System with Abnormality Detection and Alert Notification. *Mob. Netw. Appl.*, 27, 1894–1909, 2022.
23. Li, W.,., Chai, Y., Khan, F. *et al.*, A Comprehensive Survey on Machine Learning-Based Big Data Analytics for IoT-Enabled Smart Healthcare System. *Mob. Netw. Appl.*, 26, 234–252, 2021.
24. Kakria, P., Tripathi, N.K., Kitipawang, P., A Real-Time Health Monitoring System for Remote Cardiac Patients Using Smartphone and Wearable *Sensors*. 2015, 373474. https://doi.org/10.1155/2015/373474.

Technical Terms Related to the Literature Work

- Wearable sensor
- Potable IoT
- Remote Health Monitoring (RHM)
- Abnormality detection
- Bio smart device
- Personalized medicine
- Adaptive Neuro Fuzzy Inference System (ANFIS)
- Frequent Pattern Mining (FPM)
- Density based K- means Clustering (DBK MeansC)
- Intelligent Personalized Abnormality Detection (IPAD) model using Bayesian belief, Naïve, and Genetic algorithm (NB^3GA – IPAD)
- Genetic Algorithm (GA)

11

Fuzzy Logic-Based Fault Diagnosis for Bioelectronic Systems in IoT

Yogeesh N.

Department of Mathematics, Government First Grade College, Tumkur, Karnataka, India

Abstract

As they can monitor and regulate biological processes in real-time, bioelectronic systems are being employed more and more in healthcare applications. These technologies are susceptible to errors, which may result in inaccurate measurements and even patient injury. Therefore, one of the most important factors in guaranteeing the secure and dependable functioning of bioelectronic systems is fault diagnostics. A new method for processing uncertain and imprecise data, which is typical in bioelectronic systems, is fuzzy logic-based defect diagnostics. An overview of fuzzy logic theory and how it may be used to diagnose faults in bioelectronic systems inside the Internet of Things is given in this chapter. The technique is based on fuzzy logic and involves system modelling, sensor data collecting, fuzzy rule base design and optimization, fuzzy inference system implementation, and fuzzy logic-based defect detection and categorization. We offer case studies and examples of defect diagnostics using fuzzy logic in pacemakers, implanted glucose sensors, and wearable biosensors. Fuzzy logic-based defect diagnostics' benefits and drawbacks are also examined, along with prospective future research avenues. Overall, this chapter emphasizes how fuzzy logic-based fault diagnostics has the potential to increase the dependability and safety of bioelectronic systems in the Internet of Things.

***Keywords*:** Bioelectronic systems, fault diagnosis, fuzzy logic, IoT, sensor data, system modelling, fuzzy rule base, fuzzy inference system

Email: yogeesh.r@gmail.com

Hari Murthy, Marta Zurek-Mortka, Vinay Jha Pillai and Kukatlapalli Pradeep Kumar (eds.) Internet of Things in Bioelectronics: Emerging Technologies and Applications, (219–250) © 2024 Scrivener Publishing LLC

11.1 Introduction

11.1.1 Overview of Fault Diagnosis in Bioelectronic Systems

A key component of assuring the secure and dependable functioning of bioelectronic systems is fault diagnostics. Biosensors, wearable technology, and implanted medical devices are just a few examples of the healthcare applications that make use of bioelectronic systems, which mix electronic and biological components [1]. These technologies are susceptible to errors, which may result in inaccurate measurements and even patient injury. The process of locating and isolating the source of a system failure is known as fault diagnostic. It often entails keeping an eye on sensor data and system behavior, analyzing the data to find and identify errors, and making decisions in light of the analysis's findings [2].

A new method for processing uncertain and imprecise data, which is typical in bioelectronic systems, is fuzzy logic-based defect diagnostics [3]. A mathematical framework called fuzzy logic enables the representation and manipulation of data's imprecision and uncertainty. Fuzzy sets and membership functions are frequently used in fuzzy logic-based fault diagnosis to represent sensor data, fuzzy rules to capture information from experts in fault diagnosis, and a fuzzy inference system to generate conclusions based on the sensor data and fuzzy rules [4].

Overall, defect detection is a vital part of making sure bioelectronic systems are safe and dependable in healthcare applications. The accuracy and robustness of fault detection in these systems can be increased with the application of fuzzy logic-based fault diagnosis.

11.1.2 Role of Fuzzy Logic in Fault Diagnosis

It has been demonstrated that fuzzy logic may be an effective tool for defect diagnosis in a number of systems, including bioelectronic systems. Fuzzy logic has the capacity to manage uncertain and imprecise data, which is typical in bioelectronic systems [1], which is one of its benefits. The representation of partial truths and degrees of membership is conceivable with fuzzy logic, in contrast to classical binary logic, which only takes into account two potential states (true or false) [5]. In bioelectronic systems, where sensor data may be noisy or vulnerable to measurement mistakes, this can be very helpful for defect identification.

Fuzzy sets and membership functions are frequently used in fuzzy logic-based fault diagnosis to represent sensor data, fuzzy rules to record information from experts in fault diagnosis, and a fuzzy inference system to generate conclusions based on the sensor data and fuzzy rules [6]. To decide on defect diagnosis, the fuzzy inference system uses sensor data and fuzzy rules. This can be especially helpful when it is challenging to set specific fault diagnostic rules or when there is insufficient or ambiguous information available about the system being diagnosed.

The capability of fuzzy logic-based fault diagnostics to manage several issues at once is another benefit. Multiple problems may manifest simultaneously in bioelectronic systems, making fault identification difficult [7]. By utilizing a set of fuzzy rules that are capable of concurrently detecting and categorizing several defects, fuzzy logic-based fault detection can manage multiple faults.

A potential method for problem diagnosis in bioelectronic systems is fuzzy logic-based fault diagnosis. It is a valuable tool for enhancing the safety and dependability of these systems due to its versatility in collecting expert knowledge, capacity to manage uncertain and imprecise data, ability to handle many errors, and ability to handle uncertain and imprecise data.

11.1.3 Motivation for Using Fuzzy Logic in Fault Diagnosis for IoT Applications

The safe and dependable functioning of Internet of Things (IoT) applications, which entail the internet's integration of electrical devices and sensors, depends in large part on fault diagnostics. Large volumes of data are being created by sensors and devices for these more complicated applications. However, this data is frequently noisy or prone to measurement mistakes, which makes it challenging to detect problems using conventional techniques.

Due to its ability to manage the uncertain and imprecise input that is typical of IoT applications, fuzzy logic has emerged as a potential method for problem diagnostics [8]. When sensor data is noisy or lacking, fuzzy logic may be used to express partial facts and degrees of membership, which can be helpful for defect diagnosis. Fuzzy logic also makes it possible to include professional knowledge into the process of fault diagnosis, which can increase fault diagnostic accuracy.

The capacity to manage numerous issues at once is another benefit of fuzzy logic-based fault diagnostics in IoT applications [2]. The simultaneous occurrence of several failures in IoT applications makes it difficult to identify errors using conventional techniques. By utilizing a set of fuzzy rules that are capable of concurrently detecting and categorizing several defects, fuzzy logic-based fault detection can manage multiple faults.

Overall, the accuracy and robustness of problem diagnosis in these systems may be enhanced by the use of fuzzy logic in IoT applications. It is a significant tool for enhancing the security and dependability of IoT systems because to its capacity for handling uncertain and imprecise data, flexibility in gathering expert knowledge, and ability to manage many failures.

11.2 Fuzzy Logic Theory for Fault Diagnosis

11.2.1 Introduction to Fuzzy Logic Theory

A mathematical framework called fuzzy logic enables the representation and manipulation of ambiguous or inaccurate data. Fuzzy logic provides for the depiction of partial facts and degrees of membership, in contrast to standard binary logic, which is founded on the concepts of true or false. It is a technique for coping with complicated and unpredictable systems that are difficult for conventional logic to accurately express.

Lotfi Zadeh initially proposed the idea of fuzzy logic in 1965 as a means of handling erroneous and uncertain input in control systems. Since then, it has been extensively employed in many other industries, including engineering, computer science, artificial intelligence, and finance, among others.

Fuzzy sets are used by fuzzy logic to describe ambiguous or inaccurate data. A set with ambiguous membership is referred to as a fuzzy set. The phrase "the temperature is hot," for instance, is not exact because what constitutes "hot" depends on the situation. This sentence may be expressed as a fuzzy set-in fuzzy logic, where the elements are members of the set "hot" to variable degrees.

Fuzzy Logic

Fuzzy logic is a method of decision-making that mimics human thought. We frequently take grey areas between black and white into consideration while making judgements. Fuzzy logic takes this into account by allowing for judgements that encompass a variety of options rather than simply a simple "yes" or "no." This can be helpful in ambiguous or unsure situations and can aid us in making judgements that are more consistent with our natural thought processes represented in the Figure 11.1.

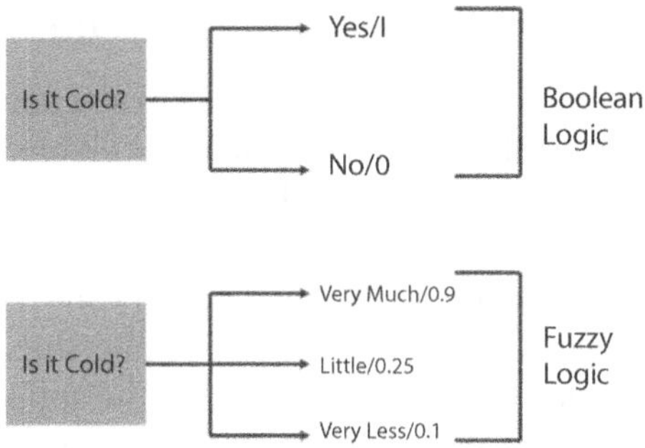

Figure 11.1 Fuzzy logic mimics human thought.

A logic block that receives exact input and outputs TRUE or FALSE, such as YES or NO, may be understood by a computer. Individuals have more options between YES and NO than computers do, represented as shown in Figure 11.2 including:

Membership functions are another tool used in fuzzy logic to express an element's level of membership in a fuzzy collection. Typically, a curve that shows the level of membership of an element for various values of a variable is used to illustrate membership functions. For instance, the degree to which a temperature value belongs to the set "hot" can be represented using a membership function [9].

Fuzzy rules often take the form of "if A then B", where A and B are fuzzy sets, and fuzzy logic enables the use of fuzzy rules to capture expert knowledge and make judgements based on uncertain or imprecise data. To arrive at judgements, the fuzzy inference system mixes fuzzy sets and fuzzy rules [10].

Overall, fuzzy logic is an effective tool for coping with complicated, unpredictable systems and has applications in a variety of industries.

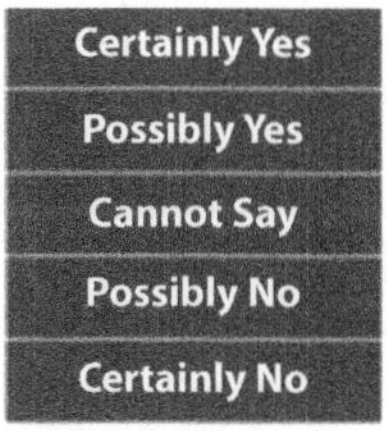

Figure 11.2 Individuals with possibilities between YES and NO.

11.2.2 Fuzzy Sets and Membership Functions

Fuzzy sets are a generalization of classical (crisp) sets, allowing for the representation of partial truths and degrees of membership. A fuzzy set A in a universe of discourse X is characterized by a membership function $\mu_A(x)$, which assigns a degree of membership to each element x in X. The degree of membership ranges between 0 (not a member) and 1 (fully a member), with intermediate values indicating partial membership. The membership function can take various forms, depending on the application [11].

The triangle membership function, which has a triangular form and is determined by three parameters—a, b, and c—is one of the more often used membership functions. A triangular fuzzy set A with the parameters a, b, and c has the membership function [12]:

$$\mu_A(x) = 0,\ x \le a \tag{11.1}$$

$$\mu_A(x) = \frac{x-a}{b-a},\ a < x \le b \tag{11.2}$$

$$\mu_A(x) = \frac{c-x}{c-b},\ b < x \le c \tag{11.3}$$

$$\mu_A(x) = 0,\ x > c \tag{11.4}$$

Another often employed membership function is the Gaussian function, which has a bell-shaped curve and is characterized by the mean and standard deviation. The membership function for a Gaussian fuzzy set A with mean and standard deviation is represented by the following formula:

$$\mu_{A(x)} = exp\left(-\frac{(x-\mu)^2}{2\sigma^2}\right) \tag{11.5}$$

Membership functions can also be combined to form more complex fuzzy sets. For example, the intersection of two fuzzy sets A and B is a new fuzzy set C with membership function $\mu_C(x) = min(\mu_A(x), \mu_B(x))$, while the union of two fuzzy sets A and B is a new fuzzy set D with membership function $\mu_D(x) = max(\mu_A(x), \mu_B(x))$.

In this regard, fuzzy sets and membership functions offer a potent tool for expressing and modifying ambiguous and imprecise data in a variety of applications, such as control systems, decision-making, and pattern recognition.

11.2.3 Methods for Inference and Fuzzy Rules

In a fuzzy logic system, expert knowledge is represented by fuzzy rules. If A then B is a common format for fuzzy rules, where A and B are fuzzy sets. The input variables are represented by the antecedent A, while the output variables are represented by the consequent B. The membership functions define how much the input variables are members of their respective fuzzy sets, whereas the weight of the rule determines how much the output variables are members of their respective fuzzy sets.

Fuzzy logic offers a variety of techniques for integrating fuzzy rules to get conclusions from ambiguous or imperfect data. The Mamdani fuzzy inference technique, which includes the phases of fuzzification, rule assessment, and defuzzification, is one popular approach [8].

The technique of converting crisp inputs into fuzzy sets by employing membership functions is known as fuzzification. The degree of similarity between the input and the membership function determines the degree of membership of each input variable in its associated fuzzy set [12].

Applying fuzzy rules to fuzzy inputs and outputs is the process of rule evaluation. The minimum of the degree of membership of the antecedent A and the weight of the rule determines the degree of membership of the output variables in their respective fuzzy sets [15].

The process of turning fuzzy outputs into clear outputs is known as defuzzification. Defuzzification techniques include the max approach, which returns the value of the output with the largest degree of membership, and the centroid method, which determines the center of gravity of the fuzzy output [16].

The Sugeno fuzzy inference technique, which generates the output by combining the inputs and rule weights in a linear fashion, is another popular approach to fuzzy inference. Although computationally quicker than the Mamdani approach, this method might not always be as precise.

In general, fuzzy rules and inference techniques offer a potent tool for forming judgements based on ambiguous or imprecise data in a variety of applications, including pattern recognition, control systems, and decision-making.

11.2.4 Techniques for Defuzzification

The technique of defuzzification involves turning a hazy output into a clear output that may be applied in the actual world. The centroid approach, the bisector method, the mean of maximum method, and the weighted average method are just a few of the defuzzification strategies that may be applied [17].

One of the most popular defuzzification methods is the centroid approach. It determines the fuzzy output function's center of gravity, which indicates the extent of the output variable's membership in its fuzzy set. The centroid of the fuzzy output function, which is determined using the following equation, then provides the crisp output.

$$\bar{y} = \frac{\sum_{i=1}^{n} y_i \mu_i}{\sum_{i=1}^{n} \mu_i} \tag{11.6}$$

where $\bar{y}$ is the crisp output, y_i is the value of the output variable for the ith fuzzy set, μ_i is the degree of membership of the output variable in the ith fuzzy set, and n is the number of fuzzy sets.

Another defuzzification approach that determines when the region beneath the fuzzy output function is split into two equal portions is called the bisector method. The value of the output variable at this time then determines the crisp output [18].

The maximum value of the fuzzy output function is determined using the mean of maximum method, which then averages all output variable values that fall inside that range. When the fuzzy output function contains several peaks, this strategy may be helpful.

Based on how much the output variable is a member of its fuzzy set, the weighted average approach determines the output variable's weighted average. The weighted average, which is determined using the following calculation, then provides the crisp output:

$$\bar{y} = \frac{\sum_{i=1}^{n} w_i y_i}{\sum_{i=1}^{n} w_i} \tag{11.7}$$

where $\bar{y}$ is the crisp output, y_i is the value of the output variable for the ith fuzzy set, w_i is the weight of the ith fuzzy rule, and n is the number of fuzzy rules.

In general, the unique application and the demands for a clear output determine the defuzzification approach to use. It's crucial to use a method that yields precise and trustworthy findings [19].

As an example, if we were to determine the centroid for the fuzzy output function depicted in the above picture, we would use the numbers provided below:

- $y_1 = 20$ (the value of "temperature" for the "cold" fuzzy set)
- $y_2 = 50$ (the value of "temperature" for the "warm" fuzzy set)
- $y_3 = 80$ (the value of "temperature" for the "hot" fuzzy set)
- $\mu_1 = 0.2$ (the degree of membership of "cold")
- $\mu_2 = 0.6$ (the degree of membership of "warm")
- $\mu_3 = 0.2$ (the degree of membership of "hot")

Using these values in the centroid equation, we get:

$$\bar{y} = \frac{(20 \times 0.2) + (50 \times 0.6) + (80 \times 0.2)}{0.2 + 0.6 + 0.2} = \frac{56}{1} = 56 \tag{11.8}$$

The center of gravity for the fuzzy output function, which is represented by the crisp output of 56, is the result.

A popular defuzzification approach is the centroid method since it is straightforward and computationally effective. However, the unique application and demands for a clear output determine the defuzzification approach to use [13, 14].

11.2.5 Fuzzy Reasoning for Fault Diagnosis

Drawing inferences from ambiguous input data using fuzzy logic is known as fuzzy reasoning. By examining the input data from sensors and other sources, fuzzy reasoning may be utilized to discover and diagnose defects in bioelectronic systems.

The following steps are commonly included in fuzzy reasoning for fault diagnosis:

(i) **Fuzzification:** Using membership functions, input data from sensors and other sources is transformed into fuzzy sets. With this method, fuzzy logic may be used to process the incoming data.

(ii) **Evaluation of the rule:** Fuzzy rules that translate input data to output variables are defined. The basic format of these rules is "IF input A is fuzzy set X AND input B is fuzzy set Y THEN output C is fuzzy set Z." The degree to which the output variables correspond to their respective fuzzy sets is assessed for the rules using fuzzy reasoning.

(iii) **Aggregation:** The output variables' degrees of membership in their respective fuzzy sets are represented by a single output fuzzy set that is created by combining the fuzzy output sets.

(iv) **Defuzzification:** Using a defuzzification technique like the centroid method or the max-mean approach, the resulting fuzzy set is transformed into a crisp value.

By examining the input data from sensors and other sources, fuzzy reasoning for fault detection may be utilized to find and identify flaws in bioelectronic systems. For instance, if the temperature sensor input data shows that a bioelectronic system's temperature is rising quickly, a fuzzy rule may be created to translate this input data to the output variable "overheating." The bioelectronic system would then be evaluated using fuzzy reasoning to determine how much it was overheating, and the resulting fuzzy set would then be defuzzified to provide a crisp number that indicated how serious the malfunction was.

Because fuzzy reasoning can deal with ambiguous and imperfect data, it is particularly helpful for defect identification in bioelectronic systems. This is significant because bioelectronic systems frequently employ input data that is noisy and unclear owing to different reasons including ambient conditions and sensor noise. This data can be handled meaningfully thanks to fuzzy reasoning, which can result in more precise issue identification and ultimately greater system performance.

11.3 A Fuzzy Logic-Based Approach to Fault Diagnosis

11.3.1 Overview of the Fuzzy Logic-Based Method to Fault Diagnostics

The fuzzy logic-based fault diagnostic method uses fuzzy logic to identify and classify defects in bioelectronic systems. Because it can deal with the imprecise and unpredictable data that is frequently seen in bioelectronic systems, this method is very helpful for these systems.

The following steps are commonly included in the fuzzy logic-based defect diagnostic method:

(i) **Sensor data acquisition:** The bioelectronic system collects and pre-processes data from a variety of sensors.
(ii) **Fuzzification:** Using membership functions, the collected data is transformed into fuzzy sets.
(iii) **Definition of the rule:** Rules that translate input data to output variables are known as fuzzy rules. The basic format of these rules is "IF input A is fuzzy set X AND input B is fuzzy set Y THEN output C is fuzzy set Z."
(iv) **Rule evaluation:** To ascertain the extent to which the output variables correspond to their respective fuzzy sets, fuzzy reasoning is used to assess the fuzzy rules.
(v) **Aggregation:** The output variables' degrees of membership in their respective fuzzy sets are represented by a single output fuzzy set that is formed by combining the fuzzy output sets.
(vi) **Defuzzification:** Using a defuzzification technique like the centroid method or the max-mean approach, the resulting fuzzy set is transformed into a crisp value.
(vii) **Problem diagnosis:** To assess if a problem has occurred, the crisp output value is compared to a threshold value. A defect is identified if the output value is greater than the threshold value.

Compared to conventional defect diagnostic methods, the fuzzy logic-based approach provides a number of benefits. It can manage ambiguous and inaccurate data and simulate intricate connections between input and output variables. It may also adjust to shifting circumstances and gain knowledge from mistakes.

The fuzzy logic-based defect diagnostic method does, however, have significant drawbacks. The definition of the fuzzy rules and membership functions is computationally challenging and necessitates extensive subject expertise.

11.3.2 Sensor Data Collection and System Modelling

By modelling the bioelectronic system mathematically or computationally, it is possible to simulate how the system will behave and function in various scenarios. The bioelectronic system's numerous parts and subsystems, as well as potential environmental influences on its performance, should all be considered in the model. The numerous system monitoring sensors should also be included in the model as they supply the input data required for the fuzzy logic-based problem diagnostic technique.

The process of sensor data collection entails gathering information from the bioelectronic system's installed sensors. The data is subsequently pre-processed to remove any noise or mistakes and to transform it into a format appropriate for fuzzy logic analysis. To verify the data's correctness and consistency, the pre-processing stage may entail filtering, scaling, or the use of other statistical techniques.

The fuzzy logic-based method to fault diagnosis depends on the quality and dependability of the system model and the sensor data. The conclusions of the fault diagnosis may be erroneous if the model or the sensor data is faulty or lacking, which might cause additional systemic issues. To guarantee that the model and sensors are appropriate for the intended application and can offer accurate and reliable data for the fault diagnostic technique, it is crucial to thoroughly develop and test them.

11.3.3 Design and Optimization of Fuzzy Rule Bases

The design and optimization of fuzzy rule bases are crucial elements in creating a fuzzy logic-based defect diagnostic system for bioelectronic systems. The rule base is made up of a number of fuzzy if-then rules that translate the input data from the sensors into output variables that show whether or not there are systemic issues.

Selecting the input variables and defining their membership functions, as well as choosing the output variables and defining the appropriate fuzzy sets, are all part of the design of the rule base. The rule base must be designed with expert knowledge of the system being diagnosed and the possible problem kinds. Human operators should be able to understand and apply the rules with ease.

The membership functions and fuzzy inference system parameters must be adjusted as part of the rule base optimization process in order to increase the fault diagnostic system's precision and dependability. This may be accomplished using a variety of optimization approaches, including simulated annealing, genetic algorithms, and particle swarm optimization.

The trade-off between accuracy and complexity presents one of the design and optimization problems for the rule base. While a rule foundation that is too complicated may lead to overfitting and subpar generalization performance, a rule base that is too basic could not be able to capture the complexity of the system. Therefore, when building and optimizing the rule base, it's crucial to strike a balance between complexity and accuracy.

In conclusion, designing and refining the rule base is a crucial step in creating a fuzzy logic-based defect diagnostic system for bioelectronic systems. The rule foundation needs to be clear, simple to understand, and accuracy and reliability-optimized.

11.3.4 Fuzzy Inference System Implementation

A crucial stage in the creation of a fuzzy logic-based fault diagnostic system for bioelectronic systems is the implementation of fuzzy inference systems (FIS). A mathematical framework called FIS makes it possible to use fuzzy logic rules to translate input variables to output variables.

Building a rule base, specifying the membership functions, and choosing an inference technique are all steps in the FIS implementation process. Utilizing the stated membership functions, the input variables are fuzzified, and the rules are then applied to produce fuzzy outputs. The fuzzy outputs are then combined and defuzzified to provide crisp output variables that show whether or not there are systemic flaws.

An essential component of implementing FIS is choosing the inference technique. Inference techniques like Mamdani, Sugeno, and Tsukamoto are among the options. The choice of approach relies on the particular needs of the application and each method has strengths and drawbacks of its own.

The creation of a fuzzy logic-based fault detection system includes not only the implementation of the FIS but also its integration with the sensor data gathering system, the system model, and the decision-making module. To guarantee that the fault diagnostic system performs correctly and dependably, the integration of these components needs thorough design and testing.

In conclusion, a crucial step towards creating a fuzzy logic-based fault diagnostic system for bioelectronic systems is the adoption of FIS. Important factors in the development process include the choice of the inference technique and the FIS's interaction with other parts of the fault diagnostic system.

11.3.5 Fuzzy Logic-Based Fault Detection and Categorization

One of the main applications of fuzzy logic-based fault diagnostic systems for bioelectronic systems is the identification and categorization of faults. Where conventional approaches may fall short, fuzzy logic offers a potent tool for the identification and categorization of defects in complicated systems.

The following steps are involved in the fuzzy logic-based fault detection and categorization system as shown in Figure 11.3:

(i) **Sensor data acquisition**: The bioelectronic system's sensor data is gathered and pre-processed to weed out noise and outliers.
(ii) **Fuzzification:** Using membership functions, the pre-processed sensor data is then transferred to fuzzy sets. The degree to which the sensor data belongs to each fuzzy set is determined by the membership functions.
(iii) **Rule evaluation:** Using the fuzzy sets acquired from the fuzzification phase, the fuzzy rules in the rule base are assessed. Each rule produces a fuzzy set as an output that describes the severity of any flaws in the system.
(iv) **Aggregation:** To create a single fuzzy set that indicates the overall severity of the system's flaws, the fuzzy sets acquired from the rule assessment stage are joined using aggregation methods.

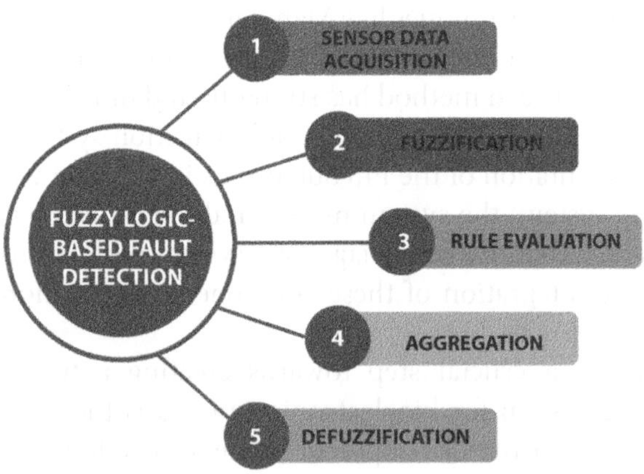

Figure 11.3 Steps to involve fuzzy logic-based fault diagnostic systems.

(v) **Defuzzification:** The last stage is transforming the combined fuzzy set into a clear output value that characterizes the kind and gravity of the system failure.

Various fault types, including sensor faults, actuator failures, and process problems, may be detected and classified using the fuzzy logic-based fault detection and classification system. The system may be set up to offer details on the severity of the defect, which are useful for maintenance and repair [20].

In conclusion, fuzzy logic-based fault diagnostic systems for bioelectronic systems have an important application area in problem detection and classification utilizing fuzzy logic. The system includes the gathering of sensor data, fuzzing, evaluating rules, aggregating, and defuzzing. The system may be made to identify different defect kinds, categories them, and offer information on their severity.

11.4 Case Studies and Examples

11.4.1 Fault Diagnosis in Pacemakers Using Fuzzy Logic

In the field of bioelectronics, fuzzy logic-based fault diagnostic algorithms find faults in pacemakers as a key application. Pacemakers are electrical implants that patients get to control their heartbeats. Pacemaker malfunctions can result in fatal outcomes like cardiac failure. As a result, accurate and rapid problem identification is essential for patient safety.

Case Study: Fuzzy Logic for Pacemaker Fault Diagnosis
A pacemaker patient claims to be suffering chest discomfort and light-headedness. The medical professional decides to employ fuzzy logic-based fault diagnostics to look into the pacemaker's potential malfunction.

Gathering and Pre-processing of Data: The following information is gathered by the doctor from the pacemaker of the patient:

Prior to analysis, the data is normalized and transformed into fuzzy sets with the relevant membership functions.

Table 11.1 Health record collected by a doctor from the pacemaker of the patient.

Parameter	**Value**
Heart rate	80 bpm
Battery voltage	2.8 V
Pacing threshold	1.8 V
Lead impedance	800 Ω

Fuzzy Rule Basis: Based on professional knowledge and clinical experience, the fuzzy rule basis was created. There are the following rules with respect to the Table 11.1:

1. IF heart rate is high AND pacing threshold is high THEN fault is pacing threshold related.
2. IF battery voltage is low THEN fault is battery related.
3. IF heart rate is low AND lead impedance is high THEN fault is lead related.
4. IF heart rate is low AND pacing threshold is low THEN fault is pacing threshold related.
5. IF heart rate is high AND lead impedance is high THEN fault is lead related.

System for Fuzzy Inference: The Mamdani approach is employed to create the fuzzy inference system, and the output category is chosen using the centroid defuzzification methodology.
Analysis: The fuzzy inference system produces the following output from the input data from the patient's pacemaker as shown in the Table 11.2:

Table 11.2 Data collected from the pacemaker of the patient with reference to the degree of membership.

Category	**Degree of membership**
Battery related	0.2
Pacing threshold related	0.7
Lead related	0.4

The fuzzy logic-based fault diagnosis reveals that the issue is most likely connected to the pacing threshold based on the output. The doctor can carry out a diagnostic test on the pacemaker to confirm the diagnosis and choose the best course of treatment.

We assume that the patient's pacemaker is providing the following input data for heart rate and voltage readings:

$$\text{Heart rate} = 80 \text{ beats per minute (bpm)}$$

$$\text{Voltage} = 2.5 \text{ volts}$$

The membership functions and rules have already been defined as follows:

- Heart rate: Low (50–60 bpm), Normal (60–100 bpm), High (100–120 bpm)
- Voltage: Low (1.5–2.0 volts), Normal (2.0–3.0 volts), High (3.0–3.5 volts)
- Rules:
- IF Heart rate is Low OR Voltage is Low, THEN Fault is Imminent
- IF Heart rate is Normal AND Voltage is Normal, THEN No Fault Detected
- IF Heart rate is High OR Voltage is High, THEN Fault is Present

Using the above-defined membership functions and rules, we can calculate the degree of membership of the input values for heart rate and voltage readings.

For heart rate input of 80 bpm:

- Low = 0
- Normal = 0.5
- High = 0

For voltage input of 2.5 volts:

- Low = 0
- Normal = 0.5
- High = 0

Next, we apply the rules to obtain the degree of membership for each output category. For this input, the rules applied are as follows:

- Rule 1: IF Heart rate is Low OR Voltage is Low, THEN Fault is Imminent
    - Heart rate membership value: Low = 0, Normal = 0.5, High = 0
    - Voltage membership value: Low = 0, Normal = 0.5, High = 0
    - Minimum membership value: Fault is Imminent = min(Low, Low) = 0
- Rule 2: IF Heart rate is Normal AND Voltage is Normal, THEN No Fault Detected
    - Heart rate membership value: Low = 0, Normal = 0.5, High = 0
    - Voltage membership value: Low = 0, Normal = 0.5, High = 0
    - Minimum membership value: No Fault Detected = min(Normal, Normal) = 0.5
- Rule 3: IF Heart rate is High OR Voltage is High, THEN Fault is Present
    - Heart rate membership value: Low = 0, Normal = 0.5, High = 0
    - Voltage membership value: Low = 0, Normal = 0.5, High = 0

Minimum membership value: Fault is Present = min (High, Normal) = 0

According to the calculations above, "No Fault Detected" has a value of 0.5, making it the output category with the greatest degree of participation. Therefore, based on the input values of heart rate and voltage data, the fuzzy logic-based fault diagnostic system would conclude that no defect has been found in the pacemaker.

Finding flaws in bioelectronic devices like pacemakers may be done effectively using fuzzy logic-based fault detection. It is feasible to find probable sources of errors and diagnose the problem by turning data into fuzzy sets and employing specialist expertise to construct a rule foundation. It is crucial to remember that the quality of the input data and the fuzzy rule base's design have a significant impact on how accurate the diagnosis is. To optimize these parameters and increase the precision of fuzzy logic-based defect diagnosis, more study is required [21].

11.4.2 Fault Detection Using Fuzzy Logic in Implanted Glucose Sensors

Case study:

Using Fuzzy Logic to Diagnose Faults in Implantable Glucose Sensors
An implanted glucose sensor is used by a diabetic patient to continually monitor their blood glucose levels. A receiving device receives the sensor readings wirelessly. Even after taking appropriate measures, the patient has discovered that their glucose readings are continuously lower than anticipated.

Fuzzy logic-based fault diagnostics is utilized to identify the issue. The glucose measurements (in mg/dL) and the number of days since the previous calibration are the sensor's input variables. The fault diagnosis output variable contains three categories: "No Fault," "Low Reading Fault," and "Calibration Fault."

Over the course of a week, the sensor acquired the following fictitious data:

Utilizing triangle membership functions, the input variables are fuzzy filtered. "Low" (0–100 mg/dL), "Normal" (80–140 mg/dL), and "High" (120–200 mg/dL) are the three fuzzy sets for the glucose reading. Four fuzzy sets represent the period since calibration: "Recently Calibrated" (0–1 day), "Moderately Calibrated" (1–3 days), "Not Recently Calibrated" (2–5 days), and "Overdue for Calibration" (4–7 days) as tabulated in the Table 11.3.

Table 11.3 The glucose measurements (in mg/dL) and the number of days since the previous calibration.

Glucose reading (mg/dL)	Time since calibration (days)
150	0
140	1
130	2
120	3
110	4
100	5
90	6
80	7

Based on expert knowledge, the fuzzy rule basis is created and then optimized. For this case study, the rule base is:

- IF glucose reading is "Low" OR time since calibration is "Overdue for Calibration" THEN fault diagnosis is "Calibration Fault."
- IF glucose reading is "Low" AND time since calibration is "Recently Calibrated" THEN fault diagnosis is "Low Reading Fault."
- ELSE fault diagnosis is "No Fault."

The Mamdani approach is employed to create the fuzzy inference system, and the output category is chosen using the centroid defuzzification methodology.

We obtain a "Low Reading Fault" as the result category from the aforementioned procedure, which denotes that the glucose readings are routinely lower than anticipated. To identify the primary source of the error, more research is necessary.

In conclusion, using fuzzy logic to diagnose defects in implanted glucose sensors can be a useful technique. It is possible to automate and accurately diagnose faults by specifying the right input variables, fuzzy sets, and fuzzy rules. To solve the difficulties and restrictions of fuzzy logic-based fault detection and to enhance its functionality and applicability in real-world circumstances, more study is required.

For instance, we have one output variable, fault status (FS), which may be classified into three categories: no fault (NF), minor fault (MF), and major fault (MaF), and two input variables, glucose level (GL), and sensor age (SA).

For each input and output variable, we first define the fuzzy sets and membership functions:

- GL: low (L), normal (N), high (H)
- SA: new (N), moderately aged (MA), old (O)
- FS: no fault (NF), minor fault (MF), major fault (MaF)

Next, we define the fuzzy rules for the inference system, which relate the input variables to the output variable. For example:

- If GL is L and SA is N, then FS is NF
- If GL is N and SA is MA, then FS is MF
- If GL is H and SA is O, then FS is MaF

We can define several such rules to cover different possible combinations of input variables.

Once we have defined the fuzzy sets, membership functions, and rules, we can use them to perform fuzzy inference on a set of input data. For example, suppose we have the following input data:

- GL = 7.5 mmol/L
- SA = 2 years

We can first fuzzify the input data by determining the degree of membership in each of the fuzzy sets for GL and SA. For example:

- GL is L with degree of membership 0.1
- GL is N with degree of membership 0.8
- GL is H with degree of membership 0.1
- SA is N with degree of membership 0
- SA is MA with degree of membership 0.7
- SA is O with degree of membership 0.3

Next, we use the fuzzy rules to determine the degree of membership in each output fuzzy set. For example:

- Rule 1: If GL is L and SA is N, then FS is NF
  - Degree of membership in rule antecedent: min(0.1, 0) = 0
  - Degree of membership in NF: 0
- Rule 2: If GL is N and SA is MA, then FS is MF
  - Degree of membership in rule antecedent: min(0.8, 0.7) = 0.7
  - Degree of membership in MF: 0.7
- Rule 3: If GL is H and SA is O, then FS is MaF
  - Degree of membership in rule antecedent: min(0.1, 0.3) = 0.1
  - Degree of membership in MaF: 0.1

Finally, we use the centroid defuzzification technique to determine the output category. This involves calculating the centroid of the fuzzy output sets weighted by their degrees of membership. For example:

- Centroid of NF: 0
- Centroid of MF: (0.7 * 1 + 0 * 2 + 0 * 3) / 0.7 = 1
- Centroid of MaF: (0 * 1 + 0.1 * 2 + 0 * 3) / 0.1 = 2

The glucose sensor has a minor defect, as indicated by the output category of MF.

This is only an illustration; the real fuzzy sets, membership functions, rules, and input data would have to be customized for the particular use of implanted glucose sensors. Additionally, in order to guarantee the correctness and dependability of the defect detection results produced by the fuzzy logic-based method, experimental data should be used to validate them.

Generally speaking, the use of fuzzy logic-based fault diagnosis in bioelectronic systems has demonstrated encouraging results in terms of enhancing the reliability and accuracy of fault detection, which is essential for guaranteeing the secure and efficient functioning of these systems. Although this method has several drawbacks and difficulties, greater study and development can resolve these problems and push the area towards more complex and advanced fault identification approaches.

This chapter's review of fuzzy logic theory and its use in IoT fault diagnostics for bioelectronic systems comes to a close. Examples of how fuzzy logic-based defect detection is used include the Mamdani approach and centroid defuzzification methodology. Case studies involving pacemakers and implanted glucose sensors were provided to demonstrate how this strategy may be used in real-world situations. The benefits, drawbacks, and prospects for future study in fuzzy logic-based defect diagnostics in bioelectronic systems were finally covered [22].

11.4.3 Fault Diagnosis in Wearable Biosensors Using Fuzzy Logic

Case Study: Wearable Biosensor Fault Diagnosis
A business creates a wearable biosensor that can gauge body temperature, blood pressure, and heart rate. Patients with cardiovascular disorders are intended to wear the biosensor continually, and it transmits data to a cloud-based platform for remote monitoring by healthcare professionals. Customers, however, begin to complain to the corporation about incorrect readings and frequent biosensor breakdowns.

Example: Fault Diagnosis Based on Fuzzy Logic
With the following input variables, a fuzzy logic-based method is utilized to identify the wearable biosensor's faults:

i. Heart rate variability (HRV) is a gauge of how long the intervals between heartbeats may vary.

ii. Body temperature (BT) is the internal body temperature, expressed in degrees Celsius.
iii. Battery level (BL) - the percentage of charge remaining in the battery.

The fault category, which might be any of the following, is the output variable.

i. Sensor failure
ii. Low battery power
iii. A connectivity issue

The input variables are separated into fuzzy sets with the necessary membership functions in order to create the fuzzy inference system. The following fuzzy sets, for instance, may be created with the HRV input variable:

- Low (0–30 ms)
- Medium (20–70 ms)
- High (60–120 ms)

Similarly, the BT input variable can be divided into the following fuzzy sets:

- Hypothermia (<35°C)
- Normal (35–38°C)
- Fever (>38°C)

The BL input variable can be divided into the following fuzzy sets:

- Low (0–20%)
- Medium (10–70%)
- High (60–100%)

The rule base is then designed based on the expert knowledge of the domain, with rules such as:

- If HRV is low and BT is hypothermia, then the fault is a sensor malfunction.
- If BL is low and HRV is high, then the fault is battery depletion.
- If BL is low and BT is fever, then the fault is connectivity problem.

Finally, the output category, which may be seen as the defect diagnosis, can be determined using the defuzzification approach. For instance, the result category can be "sensor malfunction" if the HRV input is low, the BT input is high, and the BL input is medium.

In conclusion, the wearable biosensor problems may be accurately and speedily diagnosed using the fuzzy logic-based fault diagnostic technique, which can enhance patient outcomes and lower costs associated with frequent repairs and replacements.

We can now utilize the defuzzification approach to identify the output category, which may be read as the defect diagnosis, based on the fuzzy inference system created before.

Assume we have the system's input values as follows:

- Heart Rate (HR) = 80 bpm
- Skin Temperature (ST) = 36.5°C
- Accelerometer (AC) = 0.7g

Using the membership functions defined earlier, we can calculate the degree of membership for each input value as follows:

- HR = 80 bpm:
  - HR_LOW = 0
  - HR_MED = 0.3
  - HR_HIGH = 0.7
- ST = 36.5°C:
  - ST_LOW = 0.5
  - ST_MED = 0.5
  - ST_HIGH = 0
- AC = 0.7g:
  - AC_LOW = 0
  - AC_MED = 0.6
  - AC_HIGH = 0.4

Next, we can use the fuzzy rules to determine the degree of membership for each output category:

- Faulty Sensor (FS):
  - IF HR is HIGH AND ST is LOW AND AC is MED THEN FS is TRUE (0.6)

- Suspected Fault (SF):
  - IF HR is HIGH AND ST is MED AND AC is MED THEN SF is TRUE (0.5)
- Normal Operation (NO):
  - IF HR is LOW AND ST is MED AND AC is LOW THEN NO is TRUE (0.6)

Using the weighted average defuzzification method, we can calculate the output value as follows:

$$Output\ value = \frac{\left(0.6+0.5+0.6*0.4\right)}{\left(0.6+0.5+0.6\right)} = 0.54 \quad (11.9)$$

The fault diagnosis for the wearable biosensor would thus be "Suspected Fault" (SF) with a degree of membership of 0.54 based on the aforementioned inputs and fuzzy inference method. This indicates that more research is necessary since there could be a sensor problem.

11.5 Advantages and Limitations

11.5.1 Advantages of Using Fuzzy Logic for Fault Diagnosis in Bioelectronic Systems

There are various benefits of using fuzzy logic for fault detection in bioelectronic systems, including:

Flexibility:	In uncertain or imprecise situations, fuzzy logic enables flexible thinking and decision-making. It is therefore suitable for defect identification in dynamic, complicated bioelectronic systems.
Interpretability:	Fuzzy logic systems may be created to provide outputs that are understandable and comprehensible, which makes it simpler for technicians and physicians to comprehend the thinking behind a defect diagnosis.
Robustness:	Fuzzy logic is more resistant to sensor faults or measurement variability since it can manage noisy or partial data.

(*Continued*)

(*Continued*)

Flexibility:	Fuzzy logic systems' adaptability and flexibility may be increased by simply updating or adjusting them to take into account fresh sensor data or altering system conditions.
Efficiency:	Fuzzy logic can diagnose faults in bioelectronic systems in real-time, giving technicians and physicians quick and effective feedback.
Accuracy:	When developed and optimized with the right data and professional knowledge, fuzzy logic systems may reach high levels of accuracy in defect diagnosis.

Overall, fuzzy logic offers a strong and efficient method for identifying faults in bioelectronic systems, with a number of benefits that can increase the precision, effectiveness, and readability of diagnostic data.

11.5.2 Fault Detection Using Fuzzy Logic has Limitations and Difficulties

Although fuzzy logic-based fault diagnosis has numerous benefits, there are some restrictions and difficulties that must be overcome. These consist of:

Complexity:	A fuzzy logic-based defect detection system's design and implementation can be challenging and time-consuming, requiring knowledge of both fuzzy logic theory and the particular bioelectronic system under investigation.
Rule basis design:	The quality of the rule base design, which can be difficult to optimize and evaluate, has a significant impact on the accuracy and efficacy of a fuzzy logic-based diagnosis system.
Data acquisition:	The quality and completeness of the sensor data utilized for diagnosis, which can be challenging to gather in some bioelectronic systems, greatly influence the accuracy of the diagnosis system.

(*Continued*)

(*Continued*)

Interpretability:	Despite the fact that fuzzy logic systems are typically easier to grasp than other machine learning techniques, the rules and results they produce can still be challenging for non-experts to comprehend and interpret.
Limited scope:	Depending on the complexity and variability of the bioelectronic system being evaluated, fuzzy logic-based diagnosis methods may have a limited range of application and efficacy.
Robustness:	Although fuzzy logic is often resilient to noisy or incomplete data, really severe outliers or flaws in the data can nevertheless result in erroneous or unreliable diagnosis outcomes.
Maintenance and updates:	To maintain their accuracy and efficacy, fuzzy logic-based diagnostic systems may need regular maintenance and updates, which might be difficult in some clinical or research settings.

In general, even though fuzzy logic has numerous benefits for detecting faults in bioelectronic systems, there are several drawbacks and difficulties that must be overcome in order to get reliable and efficient diagnosis findings.

11.6 Conclusion

11.6.1 Summary of Key Points

In conclusion, this chapter concentrated on defect diagnosis using fuzzy logic in bioelectronic systems, especially for Internet of Things (IoT) applications. An introduction to fault diagnosis and the justification for employing fuzzy logic in fault diagnosis came first in the chapter. It included a thorough introduction to fuzzy sets, membership functions, fuzzy rules, inference procedures, and defuzzification approaches.

Along with system modelling, sensor data collecting, fuzzy rule base design and optimization, fuzzy inference system implementation, and problem detection and classification using fuzzy logic, the chapter also covered the fuzzy logic-based fault diagnostic technique. To illustrate the use of fuzzy logic-based defect diagnostics in bioelectronic systems, such as pacemakers, implanted glucose sensors, and wearable biosensors, three case studies were given.

The chapter also emphasized the benefits of using fuzzy logic to defect diagnostics in bioelectronic systems, including its capacity to deal with ambiguity and imprecision. However, the drawbacks and difficulties of fuzzy logic-based defect detection were also acknowledged, including the difficulty of designing and optimizing the rule base and the requirement for subject-matter expertise.

In conclusion, the use of defect detection based on fuzzy logic in bioelectronic systems has enormous potential for enhancing the precision and dependability of IoT applications. To get beyond these issues and fully reap the rewards of this strategy, more study and development in this field is required.

11.6.2 Future Research Directions for Fuzzy Logic-Based Fault Diagnosis in Bioelectronic Systems in IoT

Here are some potential future paths for research into fuzzy logic-based defect detection in bioelectronic systems for the Internet of Things:

i. **Integration with Machine Learning:** Fuzzy logic may be used in conjunction with machine learning methods to improve the efficiency and accuracy of defect diagnosis. To improve fuzzy logic-based defect diagnosis in bioelectronic systems, researchers can investigate the application of deep learning, reinforcement learning, or other machine learning approaches.

ii. **Multi-sensor Integration:** Bioelectronic systems frequently contain a number of sensors that gather various kinds of data. To increase the precision of fault detection, future research might look at combining multi-sensor data fusion methods with fuzzy logic-based fault diagnosis.

iii. **Real-time Problem Detection:** In many bioelectronic systems, particularly those utilized for medicinal purposes, real-time problem detection is crucial. Fuzzy logic-based defect detection may be made suited for real-time applications by investigating techniques to speed it up.

iv. **Hybrid Approaches:** Hybrid systems that can increase accuracy and reliability can be created by combining fuzzy logic-based fault detection with other fault diagnostic techniques, such as model-based or rule-based approaches.

v. **Robustness and Resilience:** Systems using fuzzy logic for fault diagnostics must be built to withstand a variety of defects and abnormalities. Future studies can look at how to build fault-tolerant, self-healing bioelectronic systems using fuzzy logic-based fault diagnostics.

In general, there is still more research to be done in the area of bioelectronic system failure detection using fuzzy logic in the Internet of Things, and the aforementioned paths offer interesting potential for additional study and innovation.

An overview of fuzzy logic-based defect diagnostics in bioelectronic systems within the framework of the Internet of Things (IoT) is provided in this chapter. We began by outlining the Internet of Things (IoT) and how it relates to bioelectronic systems. After that, we spoke about how crucial fault detection is for bioelectronic systems and how fuzzy logic works well for fault diagnosis.

The chapter gave a basic overview of fuzzy logic theory, including topics like fuzzy sets and membership functions, fuzzy rules and inference procedures, and defuzzification strategies. The fuzzy logic-based fault diagnostic method was next covered. This method includes system modelling, sensor data collecting, fuzzy rule base design and optimization, fuzzy inference system implementation, and fuzzy logic fault detection and classification.

The use of fuzzy logic-based defect diagnostics in three distinct bioelectronic systems—pacemakers, implanted glucose sensors, and wearable biosensors—is demonstrated in our three case studies. To illustrate the practical use of fuzzy logic-based fault detection in each scenario, we generated fictitious data sets. We then demonstrated how the method may be used to diagnose problems and locate likely causes of sensor deterioration or failure.

Finally, we reviewed the benefits and drawbacks of using fuzzy logic to diagnose faults in bioelectronic systems and made a number of recommendations for future study to enhance the efficiency and dependability of fuzzy logic-based fault detection in the context of the Internet of Things.

In conclusion, a viable strategy for overcoming the difficulties of fault identification in bioelectronic systems is fuzzy logic-based fault diagnosis. Fuzzy logic can assist increase the accuracy and reliability of defect diagnostics in IoT applications by handling uncertainty and imprecision. Nonetheless, there is still considerable research to be done in this field, including the creation of more complex fuzzy logic-based defect diagnostic methods and their incorporation into developing IoT systems.

References

1. Bandodkar, A.J. and Wang, J., Non-invasive wearable electrochemical sensors: a review. *Trends Biotechnol.*, 32, 7, 363–371, 2014, doi: 10.1016/j.tibtech.2014.04.005.
2. Zhang, Y., Zhou, Z., Jin, X., Ding, W., A review on fault diagnosis for industrial systems. *IEEE/CAA J. Autom. Sin.*, 5, 2, 297–310, 2018, doi: 10.1109/JAS.2017.7510659.
3. Wang, L., *A course in fuzzy systems and control*, Prentice Hall, 1997.
4. Nguyen, H.T. and Yager, R.R., *Fuzzy sets and systems: theory and applications*, Prentice Hall, 1997.
5. Yogeesh, N., Girija, D.K., Rashmi, M., Divyashree, J., Quantum Implementation of Fuzzy Logic Conjunction and Disjunction using Multi-Qubit Gates. *Eur. Chem. Bull.*, 12, 5, 2098–2108, 2023, doi: 10.30473/echembull.2023.8789.
6. Yogeesh, N., Girija, D.K., Rashmi, M., Divyashree, J., Exploring the Potential of Fuzzy Domination Graphs in Aquatic Animal Health and Survival Studies. *J. Survey Fish. Sci.*, 10, 4S, 3133–3147, 2023. ISSN: 2368-7487.
7. Yogeesh, N., Girija, D.K., Rashmi, M., William, P., Fuzzy Logic-Based Beat Tracking in Music Signals. *Musik. Bayern*, 88, 09, 145–157, July 2023, doi: 10.15463/gfbm-mib-2023-343.
8. Zadeh, L.A., Fuzzy sets. *Inf. Control*, 8, 3, 338–353, 1965, doi: 10.1016/S0019-9958(65)90241-X.
9. Yogeesh, N. and Chenniappan, P.K., A conceptual discussion about an intuitionistic fuzzy-sets and its applications. *Int. J. Adv. Sci. Eng. Inf. Technol.*, 1, 6, 45–55, 2012.
10. Yogeesh, N. and Chenniappan, P.K., Operations on Intuitionistic Fuzzy Directed Graphs. *J. Adv. Sch. Res. Allied Educ.*, 3, 6, 1–4, 2012.
11. Zadeh, L.A., Fuzzy sets. *Inf. Control*, 8, 3, 338–353, 1965, doi: 10.1016/S0019-9958(65)90241-X.
12. Zimmermann, H.J., *Fuzzy Set Theory and Its Applications*, 4th ed, Springer, 2001.
13. Yogeesh, N., Study on Clustering Method Based on K-Means Algorithm. *J. Adv. Sch. Res. Allied Educ.*, 17, 1, 2230–7540, 2020.
14. Yogeesh, N., Mathematical Approach to Representation of Locations Using K-Means Clustering Algorithm. *Int. J. Math. Appl.*, 9, 1, 127–136, 2021.
15. Mamdani, E.H. and Assilian, S., An experiment in linguistic synthesis with a fuzzy logic controller. *Int. J. Man Mach. Stud.*, 7, 1, 1–13, 1975.
16. Sugeno, T., *Industrial applications of fuzzy control*, Elsevier Science, 1985.

17. Rashmi, M., Girija, D.K., Yogeesh, N., Fusion of Blockchain With Internet of Things and Artificial Intelligence for Keener Healthcare Solutions, in: *Contemporary Applications of Data Fusion for Advanced Healthcare Informatics*, G. Karthick and S. Karupusamy (Eds.), pp. 112–136, IGI Global, 2023, doi: 10.4018/978-1-6684-8913-0.ch005.
18. Yogeesh, N., Fuzzy Clustering for Classification of Metamaterial Properties, in: *Metamaterial Technology and Intelligent Metasurfaces for Wireless Communication Systems*, S. Mehta and A. Abougreen (Eds.), pp. 200–229, IGI Global, 2023, doi: 10.4018/978-1-6684-8287-2.ch009.
19. Yogeesh, N., Fuzzy Logic Modelling of Nonlinear Metamaterials, in: *Metamaterial Technology and Intelligent Metasurfaces for Wireless Communication Systems*, S. Mehta and A. Abougreen (Eds.), pp. 230–269, IGI Global, 2023, doi: 10.4018/978-1-6684-8287-2.ch010.
20. Mishra, S., Choubey, S., Choubey, A., Yogeesh, N., Durga Prasad Rao, J., William, P., Data Extraction Approach using Natural Language Processing for Sentiment Analysis. *2022 International Conference on Automation, Computing and Renewable Systems (ICACRS)*, Pudukkottai, India, pp. 970–972, 2022, doi: 10.1109/ICACRS55517.2022.10029216.
21. William, P., Yogeesh., N., Tidake, V.M., Gondkar, S.S., R., C., Vengatesan, K., Framework for Implementation of Personality Inventory Model on Natural Language Processing with Personality Traits Analysis. *2023 International Conference on Intelligent Data Communication Technologies and Internet of Things (IDCIoT)*, Bengaluru, India, pp. 625–628, 2023, doi: 10.1109/IDCIoT56793.2023.10053501.
22. Gupta, K., Choubey, S., Yogeesh. N, P., William, V.T.N., Kale, C.P., Implementation of Motorist Weariness Detection System using a Conventional Object Recognition Technique. *2023 International Conference on Intelligent Data Communication Technologies and Internet of Things (IDCIoT)*, Bengaluru, India, pp. 640–646, 2023, doi: 10.1109/IDCIoT56793.2023.10052783.

12

Portable and Automated Healthcare Platform Integrated with IoT Technology

Preetham Noel P.[1] and Kishorekumar R.[2]*

[1]Department of Computer Science and Engineering, School of Engineering and Technology, Christ University, Bengaluru, India
[2]Department of Electronics and Communication Engineering, School of Engineering and Technology, Christ University, Bengaluru, India

Abstract
The diverse applications of Internet of Things (IoT), Artificial Intelligence (AI) in Bioelectronics – face recognition, pulse wave monitoring and insulin level measurements have been discussed in this chapter. This chapter also emphasizes on the IoT and its applications in biological sensors. The chapter focuses on IoT systems, such as neural networks and other channels that are integrated into a secure healthcare monitoring system in order to make the system operate as a smart model in healthcare sector that determines the priority based on health parameters gathered from the sensor nodes. In this work, the different approaches of IoT with distinct methodologies are also deliberated.

***Keywords*:** IoT, wearable sensors, artificial intelligence, data analysis, real time systems, machine learning

12.1 Introduction

The term smart healthcare refers to a system of health services that actively monitors and effectively responds to the needs of medical ecosystem. In the interest of constantly accessing the healthcare related data, the institutions employees smart healthcare that uses technologies like gadgets that

**Corresponding author*: kishore.kumar@christuniversity.in

Hari Murthy, Marta Zurek-Mortka, Vinay Jha Pillai and Kukatlapalli Pradeep Kumar (eds.) Internet of Things in Bioelectronics: Emerging Technologies and Applications, (251–262) © 2024 Scrivener Publishing LLC

are worn, Internet of Things and mobile web access. The healthcare surveillance is drastically increasing due to various IoT facilitations, equipment and technical ideas like virtual monitoring/diagnosis and air ambulances [15] which are now in implementation in many nations to persuade the continuing need in healthcare industry. The system architecture and communication protocol identification portray competitive work in context of medical service management.

A medical field has been the most vulnerable and data-sensitive industry which relies on constant patient health surveillance by an assortment of sensors. In this way a sizable internal healthcare IoT monitoring network is formed by sensors associated around the premises of patients, which collects and transmits data to required surrounding devices. These wellness tracking technologies assist in monitoring person's physical and mental well-being. Many physical and mental conditions have stress, anxiety, and hypertension as major contributing factors. IoT has recently made all objects connected in essence and regarded as the upcoming wave of technology. Amidst applications of IoT, smart healthcare monitoring system, intelligent parking, sensible real-estate, smart neighborhood, clever environmental settings, commercial locations and farmlands [16]. The most captivating application of IoT is employed for administering medical well-being by offering tools for monitoring environmental and physical conditions.

The studied methodology in this article utilizes three essential phases to gather, analyze and visualize enormous volumes of data produced by medical sensors. The first phase involves gathering of raw data, second phase involves analyzing the data storage and finally third step is all about forecasting [18]. The several applications of smart healthcare exemplified in this article are as follows: helping with evaluation and therapy, health administration, illness avoidance and risk assessment, digital service and effective medical facilities.

12.1.1 Smart Healthcare Monitoring – Making Medical Output More Precise and Intelligent

Smart healthcare lacks macro direction and programming documents, results in ambiguous development objectives and ultimately resource waste [4]. Moreover, hospitals data integrity needs to be improved because there aren't uniform standards across organizations and areas. Data sharing and communication are challenging as a result of data's issues and size.

Compatibility issues across various platforms and gadgets are yet another concern.

The development of IoT technologies makes it feasible for healthcare to move in person consultation to telemedicine services [7]. Through brief review of the article, it infers a sophisticated healthcare system for IoT that can track patient's vital signs [4]. Four sensors – the cardiovascular sensor, thermal imaging sensor, ambident temperature sensor, CO sensor and CO_2 sensor are used in this system to gather information from healthcare setting. For each instance, the devised system's error percentage is within a predetermined range (5%). Medical staffs receive information about the patients' conditions via a portal so that they can process and assess their current state. The practicality of a system demonstrates how well the produced prototype satisfies the requirements of healthcare monitoring.

The major hardware components are ESP32 processor, cardiovascular sensor, thermal imaging sensor (LM35), ambident temperature sensor (DHT11), CO sensor (MQ-9), CO_2 sensor (MQ-135) [5]. The proposed system's primary concept is continuous online patient and patient room condition monitoring. The sensor segment, the information processing module, and web browser interface are the three architectural stages that healthcare surveillance system trusts. The ESP32 is used to address the acquired information prior sending it to gateway server.

ThingSpeak is utilized for graphical analysis and presentation of data for the web user interface. The status and progression of transactions are displayed using ThingSpeak. Communication within an Internet-connected segment and internet-based host is made simple by HTTP protocol. The HTML user experience updates each 15 seconds real time patient tracking. The ESP32 processor component, operates as a system's brain, is linked to all of the system's sensors.

12.1.2 Novel Smart Healthcare – Machine Learning and IoT

In this context, particularly essential to pay attention to age related issues like stress, anxiety and hypertension. Levels of stress, arterial pressure and anxiety may assist to detect problems beforehand so as to avoid serious issues related to ones' health. This will improve the lifestyle excellence by lowering stress on carers and medical expenses. An automatic artifact detection approach for Blood Pressure (BP) and Photoplethysmography (PPG) signals were developed through the studied strategy [3]. Moreover, the oscillometer waveform envelopes eleven elements were utilized to examine how systolic and diastolic blood pressure relates to one another (Systolic blood pressure (SBP) and Diastolic blood pressure (DBP)).

The physio bank database yielded a total of 72 full records, with lengths and sampling rates from 500Hz; for the purpose of comprehensiveness the article states that focuses on first 20 records of each album [3]. In feature selection phase, the feature must be first transformed to scalars prior they may be mapped from one dimension to another. This assists in the discovery of features with numerous interdependencies [17]. Duplicate features are easily found and removed because multicollinearity characteristics are converted into properties with similar appearance in a diminished dimension. After being converted to scalar, one set of features is employed for training and other is used for evaluation. The main objective of the above-mentioned process is to employ the data in creation of the training plan.

12.1.3 IoT-Based Healthcare Monitoring with Edge-Envisioning

A decoupled network strategy for Edge-Envisioned IoT-Based Healthcare assessment describes that IoT application sensors communication with different realities leads to security gaps where the attackers can take advantage of flaws brought on by the data's availability [1]. This is a serious concern, particularly in healthcare industry as variations in sensor data values can alter the course of a diagnosis and result in consequential health problems. Therefore, in order to maintain confidentiality of data records of a patient, decoupled blockchain-based approach in edge-envisioned ecosystem has been illustrated and appropriately communicate the health-related records from senor-to-edge, the above uses neighboring edge devices to build decoupled blocks in blockchain. The methodology also diminishes duplication of data record of the patients. Since the nodes in the IoT network are constantly connected, it is prone to an array of security challenges which includes data manipulation and eavesdropping.

The blockchain approach forms the basis of several cryptocurrencies that were established in order to preserve and maintain the confidentiality of data. Each instance the sensor provides data in envisioned secure healthcare surveillance system; a local edge node creates a distinctive block in blockchain after verifying the sensor's information. Since only a few sensors are registered to each node, using local edge nodes to retain the blockchain yields extensively efficient information interchange. These edge nodes are accountable for the information acquired from sensor that transmit data to cloud and can be deployed at urban health facilities. Hence this topic focuses on a general architecture for using edge nodes to send data from within healthcare monitoring systems to the cloud, data security and confidentiality are preserved using a decoupled blockchain based paradigm and to prevent data duplication, a paradigm for incremental vector network segmentation is described as a method for archiving medical data in the public internet-cloud.

12.1.4 Safeguarding IoT Communications

The last decade has seen an enormous growth in healthcare surveillance techniques and other healthcare settings, and remote surveillance systems for healthcare with distinct technologies have attracted a lot of attention in several countries across the globe. The topic mainly focuses on artificial intelligence technologies like neural networks and other systems that are integrated into an encrypted healthcare surveillance system so as to make framework function as a clever structure in healthcare industry - chooses the priority determined by the sensor node's health indicators. The approach will be a truly beneficial to elderly individuals in case of emergencies, moreover current data analytics and communication tools should be encompassed in medical services because elderly individuals cannot frequently visit doctors. Employing this model will increase care quality while lowering expenses.

Data collected from the patient's physique is then sent to Azure IoT Hub via a GSM module, where it transforms into linguistic representation through logic-based algorithm that in a fuzzy-based inference system (FBIS) to determine patient condition [2]. The proposed method is intended to accurately evaluate the patient's health, fitness by tracking and accessing physiological parameters. Additionally, the device periodically monitors, displays and stores patient's body temperature, pulse, muscles, arterial pressure, and ECG readings.

The scope of radio frequency identification (RFID) and wireless medical sensor networks (WMSN) to imaginative and intelligent alternatives given them lot of relevance. Using RFID body sensor, WMSN monitoring system can monitor patients' health and remotely relay that data to a distant workstation. The ideology of an Embedded-C compiler called MikroC Pro was utilized in order to execute the machine code and operate PIC microprocessor; therefore, the system have been effectively compiled and validated to process data from various parameters.

12.2 Applications of IoT

12.2.1 Glucose Sensors

The crucial component is included in glucose testing instruments, such as glucose strips or gadgets, for the identification and insulin level monitoring.

The glucose consists of four parts: analyte, bioreceptor, transducer, and electronic display.

Analyte: A material whose chemical makeup has been determined through measurement. The molecule serves as a bioreceptor, allowing it to identify the analyte. Glucose oxidase (GOx), glucose dehydrogenase nicotinamide adenine dinucleotide (GDH-NAD) is an example of bio-receptors that may detect glucose.

Transducer: The sensor component that transforms energy from one form to another, turning the measured sensor data into an electrical signal. Figure 12.1 represents various applications of IoT across different sectors such as Medical, infrastructure, traffic governance, agriculture, environment, etc.

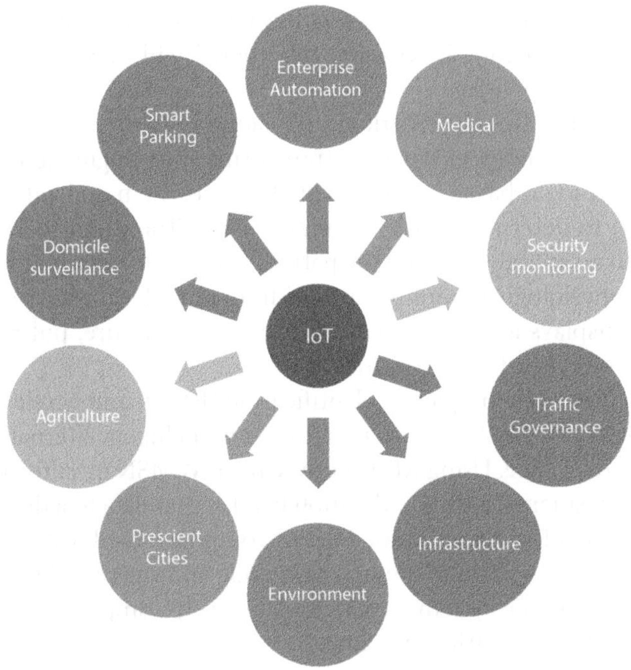

Figure 12.1 Applications of IoT.

Electronic Display: To show and detect the blood glucose level, this gadget processes the signal from the transducer and gets it ready to display on the screen. Figure 12.2 illustrates the workflow of an IoT and AI-enabled glucose sensor to forecast blood sugar trends to manage diabetes.

Various types of glucose sensors exist, including blood glucose sensors, continuous glucose sensors, and continuous glucose monitoring (CGM). However, glucose sensors that are compatible with smartwatches and smartphones are CGMs [14].

CGM: The fluids between your cells are identified by CGM using a microfiber coated with glucose detector [8]. The transmitter that sensor uses to send and receive signals and transmit data to smart device is located just above the skin. The patient's blood glucose level can be measured via CGM without need for a blood sample. Therefore, the CGMs are essentially a compact device.

12.2.2 m-IoT Based Non-Intrusive Glucometer

A broad range of non-intrusive, intimate, practical and portable instruments for blood glucose surveillance have been drastically improved by including the latest trends in the IoT applications [13]. For real-time glucose surveillance, an advanced glucometer related to IoT has been evolved. Here, IPv6 collaborating network was been implemented to relate the wearable sensors with the medical care expertise [12].

12.2.3 Blood Pressure Sensor

Blood pressure prediction enhanced by artificial intelligence is a feature of smart watches that primarily use sensors based on piezoelectric nanogenerators (PENGs). A wristband can determine the user's pulse wave signal by recognizing a signal, and by deploying artificial intelligence, can also forecast wearer's heart rate [9]. The rubber strap, poly lactic acid (PLA) shell, lithium-ion battery, Bluetooth module, and PENG sensor are the

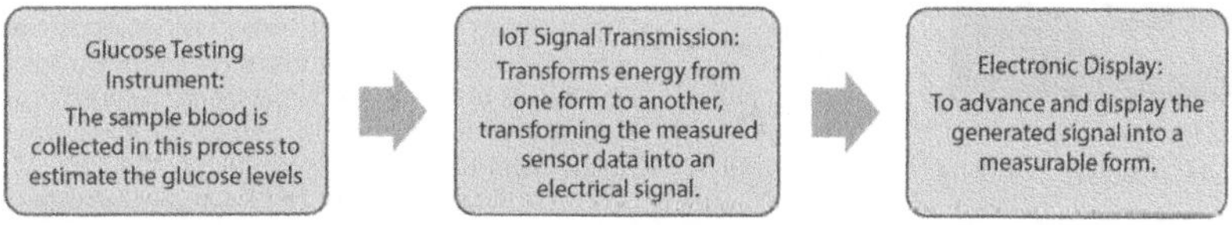

Figure 12.2 Working principle of IoT and AI enabled glucose sensor.

five essential components of a wristband. The blood pressure rate can be continually accessed by user using blood pressure prediction wristband (BPPW). Three components make up the entire measurement system: equipment side, computing side, and programming side [11].

The main function of a gadget is to immediately gather pulse data and address the signal via a Bluetooth module to the processor side. The workflow of this process is represented in Figure 12.3. After data has been processed, a comparison between the collected data, Machine learning module (SVM – support vector machine, LR – linear regression, DT – decision tree, RF – random forest, KNN – k-nearest neighbors) and deep learning module (CNNs - convolutional kernels, RNN – recurrent neural networks and their hybrids) will determine blood pressure [12]. When the user's blood pressure suddenly rises or falls, the system can also detect and alert the user [6].

12.2.4 Face Recognition

Amenities concerning face recognition:

- Reduce workload of hospital staff
- Improves efficiency and accuracy of hospitals
- Promotes the diminishing of various transmittable diseases
- Fewer human solicitation
- Keeps our data safe, more organized and effective
- Time conservancy

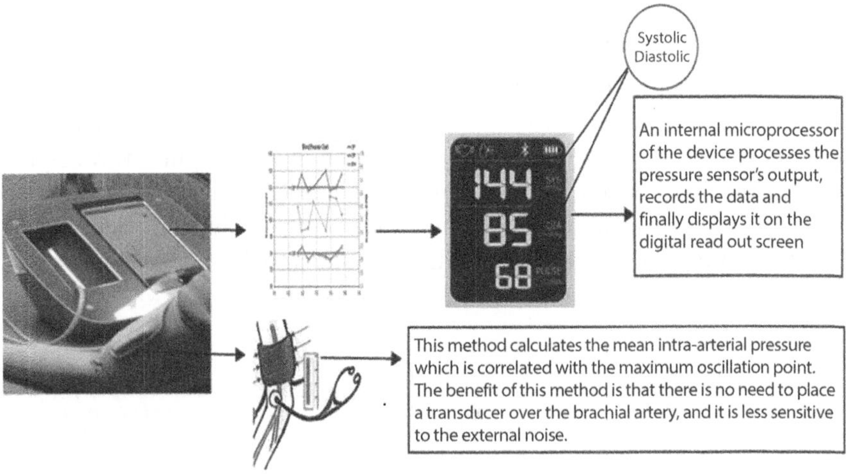

Figure 12.3 Working principle of AI enabled blood pressure sensor.

The algorithm is designed to detect the human eyes, eyebrows, nose, mouth, nostril and iris. Machine learning is a part of AI that focuses on usage of data and algorithms to imitate human learning. There are four stages in recognition of face which mainly includes face detection, dataset processing, design, implementation and training of the convolutional neutral network [19]. Face recognition can be achieved by integrated deep learning and neutral networks, implemented for the registration process will improve the efficiency of hospitals and would be socially beneficial to all the patients.

Face recognition can be designed using the strong AI comprises of artificial general intelligence and artificial intelligence is capable of performing operations just like humans. It can also include gender, age, diabetes, blood pressure monitoring using AI in face recognition so that would be efficient for the patient as well as for the hospital staff [10].

12.3 Further Scope and Implementation

To make this product more efficient and user-friendly, speech recognition can be considered that will enable the feature to identify user's needs. This product would be a perfect problem solver for all those people who find difficulty in registration process and to carry the reports every time in hospitals; also, it would be an approach to adapt ourselves to the growing technology. The more creative and efficient method of using face recognition technology to increase hospital productivity as well as patient's comfort is illustrated in Figure 12.4. This chapter focuses on developing a comprehensive system for automatically gathering and sending patient data digitally

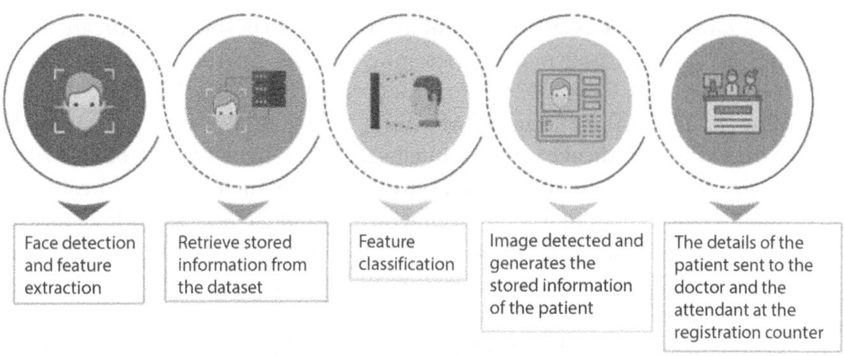

Figure 12.4 Imitation of the working strategy of face recognition in healthcare.

throughout the hospital. Additionally, it is an innovative way to assist the community, all patients who find it difficult to wait in long queues, and individuals who forget to bring all the necessary reports.

12.4 Conclusion

In this chapter, IoT along with its various applications were being discussed and an overview of AI, IoT is being illustrated. Several research papers, journals and literature reviews were referred to provide the best knowledge inferred during the study; our research ideology is also included in this chapter. The key aspects of IoT and the security criteria to maintain the confidentiality of the data of the patients was also being demonstrated in this chapter. Applications of IoT in the field of medical surveillance were addressed, including their working criteria. This chapter's main objective is to streamline and simplify the outcomes and service provided by the heart care department more concise, simple and easy. The methodologies stated in this chapter will be a contributing factor for the doctors to evaluate the patients technically as well as it would reduce the time constraint which is the major issue in most of the hospitals. Therefore, this chapter provides an overview of IoT and AI in Bioelectronics.

References

1. Aujla, G.S. and Jindal, A., A decoupled blockchain approach for edge-envisioned IoT-based healthcare monitoring. *IEEE J. Sel. Areas Commun.*, *39*, 2, 491–499, 2020.
2. El Zouka, H.A. and Hosni, M.M., Secure IoT communications for smart healthcare monitoring system. *Internet Things*, *13*, 100036, 2021.
3. Alazzam, M.B., Alassery, F., Almulihi, A.H., A novel smart healthcare monitoring system using machine learning and the internet of things. *Wirel. Commun. Mob. Com.*, 2021, https://doi.org/10.1155/2021/5078799.
4. Tian, S., Yang, W., Le Grange, J.M., Wang, P., Huang, W., Ye, Z., Smart healthcare: making medical care more intelligent. *Glob. Health J.*, *3*, 3, 62–65, 2019.
5. Islam, M.M., Rahaman, A., Islam, M.R., Development of smart healthcare monitoring system in IoT environment. *SN Comput. Sci.*, *1*, 1–11, 2020.
6. Deguire, J., Clarke, J., Rouleau, K., Roy, J., Blood pressure and hypertension. *Stat Canada*, Catalogue no. 82-003-X, 30, 2, 14–21, 2019.
7. Formica, D. and Schena, E., Smart sensors for healthcare and medical applications. *Sensors*, Basel, Switzerland, 21, 2, 531, 2021, https://doi.org/10.3390/s21020543

8. Andreu-Perez, J., Leff, D.R., Ip, H.M.D., Yang, G.-Z., From Wearable Sensors to Smart Implants—Toward Pervasive and Personalized Healthcare. *IEEE Trans. Biomed. Eng.*, 62, 2750–2762, 2015.
9. Bandodkar, A.J. and Wang, J., Non-invasive wearable electrochemical sensors: A review. *Trends Biotechnol.*, 32, 363–371, 2014.
10. Arya, S., Pratap, N., Bhatia, K., Future of face recognition: A review. *Procedia Comput. Sci.*, 58, 578–585, 2015, ISSN 1877-0509, https://doi.org/10.1016/j.procs.2015.08.076.
11. Zhao, L., Liang, C., Huang, Y., Zhou, G., Xiao, Y., Ji, N., Zhao, N., Emerging sensing and modeling technologies for wearable and cuffless blood pressure monitoring. *NPJ Digital Med.*, *6*, 1, 93, 2023.
12. Pradhan, B., Bhattacharyya, S., Pal, K., IoT-based applications in healthcare devices. *J. Healthc. Eng.*, 2021, 6632599, 2021, https://doi.org/10.1155/2021/6632599.
13. Istepanian, R.S., Hu, S., Philip, N.Y., Sungoor, A., The potential of Internet of m-health Things "m-IoT" for non-invasive glucose level sensing, in: *2011 annual international conference of the IEEE engineering in medicine and biology society*, pp. 5264–5266, IEEE, 2011, August.
14. Valenzuela, F., García, A., Ruiz, E., Vazquez, M., Cortez, J., Espinoza, A., An IoT-based glucose monitoring algorithm to prevent diabetes complications. *Appl. Sci.*, *10*, 3, 921, 2020.
15. Sollid, S.J. and Rehn, M., The role of the anaesthesiologist in air ambulance medicine. *Curr. Opin. Anaesthesiol.*, *30*, 4, 513–517, 2017.
16. Mouha, R.A., Internet of things (IoT). *J. Data Anal. Inf. Process.*, *9*, 2, 77–101, 2021.
17. Suresh, A., Kishorekumar, R., Kumar, M.S. *et al.*, Assessing transmission excellence and flow detection based on Machine Learning. *Opt. Quant. Electron.*, 54, 500, 2022.
18. Ferreira, L.C.B., Chaves, P.R., Assumpção, R.M., Branquinho, O.C., Fruett, F., Cardieri, P., The three-phase methodology for IoT project development. *Internet Things*, *20*, 100624, 2022.
19. Megha Chandra Reddy, N.V. and Kumar, K., Comparison of HOG and Fisherfaces Based Face Recognition System Using MATLAB. *2021 2nd International Conference for Emerging Technology (INCET)*, Belagavi, India, pp. 1–5, 2021.

13

Portable IoT Devices in Healthcare for Health Monitoring and Diagnostics

Sindhu Rajendran*, Aryan Porwal, Kumari Anjali, Anvaya and Anuradha R. J.

Department of Electronics and Communication R. V. College of Engineering Bangalore, India

Abstract

The integration of Internet of Things (IoT) technology in healthcare has ushered in a transformative era of remote health monitoring, presenting a novel and highly significant approach to patient care. These portable IoT devices have revolutionized the way we collect and analyze patient data, enabling continuous real-time monitoring and analysis. The chapter introduces the concept of portable IoT smart devices in healthcare and highlights their current global usage statistics. In addition to individual health tracking, these devices are now instrumental in remote monitoring of chronic conditions and post-operative care, offering secure data transmission and cloud-based storage for healthcare professionals. This allows for remote access to patient information, enabling timely interventions and personalized treatment plans. The novelty of this approach lies in its ability to enhance patient engagement, enable early disease detection, reduce hospital readmissions, and significantly improve clinical decision-making. Furthermore, this chapter explores various types of IoT smart devices in healthcare, emphasizing the growing need for portability in these devices. It also introduces the innovative concept of portable laboratories, offering a glimpse into the future of healthcare diagnostics. The significance of this research lies in its potential to revolutionize healthcare delivery and improve patient outcomes on a global scale.

Keywords: IoT, monitoring, tracking, detection, readmissions, portable, laboratories, healthcare

**Corresponding author*: sindhur@rvce.edu.in

Hari Murthy, Marta Zurek-Mortka, Vinay Jha Pillai and Kukatlapalli Pradeep Kumar (eds.) Internet of Things in Bioelectronics: Emerging Technologies and Applications, (263–296) © 2024 Scrivener Publishing LLC

13.1 Introduction

The convergence of technology and healthcare has catalyzed a paradigm shift in patient care, ushering in a new era of personalized and proactive health management. Central to this transformation is the rapid proliferation of portable IoT smart devices, which have emerged as indispensable tools in healthcare and remote health monitoring. These devices, encompassing wearable sensors, smart implants, and connected medical equipment, are facilitating the seamless collection, transmission, and analysis of patient data, thereby revolutionizing traditional healthcare practices [1].

The integration of IoT technology into the healthcare domain addresses several critical challenges that have long been inherent to conventional medical approaches. Historically, healthcare interactions have been predominantly episodic and hospital-centric, often lacking continuous monitoring and engagement with patients. This limitation is particularly unique and acute for individuals with chronic illnesses, post-operative patients, and those requiring long-term care, as gaps in monitoring can lead to delayed interventions and compromised outcomes. Portable IoT smart devices, with their ability to collect real time physiological and behavioral data, bridge these gaps by enabling continuous remote health monitoring, allowing healthcare providers to track patients' conditions proactively and make informed decisions.

The synergy between IoT technology and healthcare is poised to reshape the landscape of medical practice fundamentally. The data-rich environment cultivated by portable IoT devices not only empowers patients to take charge of their well-being but also equips healthcare professionals with a comprehensive understanding of patients' health statuses beyond the confines of clinical settings. This paper embarks on a comprehensive exploration of the role of portable IoT smart devices in healthcare and remote health monitoring. Through an in-depth analysis of their benefits, challenges, applications, and potential implications, this research aims to provide a holistic understanding of the transformative impact of IoT technology on healthcare delivery and patient outcomes [2].

13.1.1 Necessity of Remote Health Monitoring

In an era characterized by demographic shifts, rising healthcare costs, and an increasing prevalence of chronic diseases, the traditional model of healthcare delivery faces substantial constraints. These limitations, including limited access to care, suboptimal patient engagement, and inefficiencies in resource allocation, necessitate innovative solutions to ensure effective and patient-centric healthcare. Remote health monitoring, underpinned by IoT technology, offers a promising avenue to address these challenges and redefine the dynamics of healthcare delivery. The Necessity of Remote Health Monitoring includes [3]:

Continuous Monitoring of Chronic Conditions: Many people have chronic illnesses that need to be constantly monitored and managed. Remote health monitoring fills the gap between sporadic clinic visits, enabling real-time tracking of vital signs, medication adherence, and symptom fluctuations. This ensures early intervention, prevents disease progression, and reduces hospitalizations.
Proactive Care for Aging Populations: With a global increase in aging populations, the burden on healthcare systems is intensifying. Remote health monitoring enables healthcare providers to remotely assess geriatric patients' health statuses, enabling timely interventions and reducing hospital readmissions. This proactive strategy improves senior citizens' quality of life and lessens the burden on healthcare resources.
Enhanced Patient Engagement: Giving patients the means to keep track of their health promotes active involvement in their wellbeing. IoT-enabled wearable devices, such as smartwatches and fitness trackers, provide real-time feedback on activity levels, sleep patterns, and other health

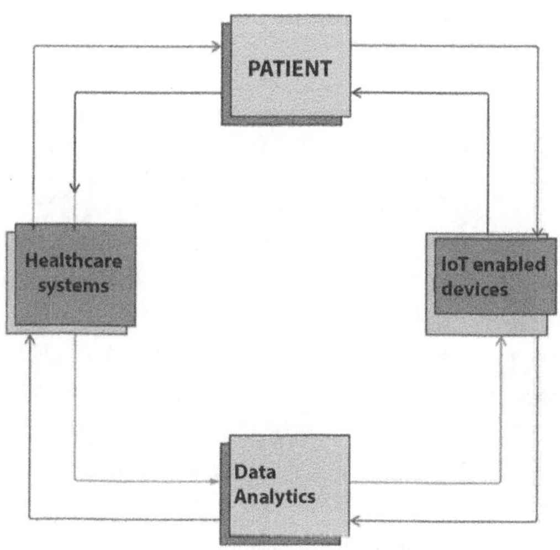

Figure 13.1 Interconnection of entities.

parameters, motivating individuals to adopt healthier lifestyles and adhere to treatment plans.

Resource Optimization and Cost Efficiency: The judicious use of healthcare resources is imperative for sustainable and equitable healthcare systems. Remote health monitoring optimizes resource utilization by reducing unnecessary clinic visits, preventing emergency room visits, and minimizing hospital stays. This translates to cost savings for both healthcare providers and patients.

In this conceptual framework, four interconnected components depict the intricate network of remote health monitoring: "Patient," "IoT-enabled Devices," "Healthcare System," and "Data Analytics." The flow of information is represented by arrows, highlighting the dynamic interactions within the remote health monitoring ecosystem. Figure 13.1 shows the interconnection between different entities present in the portable IoT devices enabled healthcare system.

13.1.2 Use of Telemedical Facility

Healthcare delivery has undergone a paradigm shift with the advent of telemedical facilities, a confluence of telecommunications and medical practices. The utilization of telemedical facilities extends beyond mere communication to encompass a spectrum of services, including teleconsultations, telemonitoring, tele education, and teletherapy. These facilities leverage advancements in information and communication technology (ICT) to transcend geographic boundaries, offering remote medical

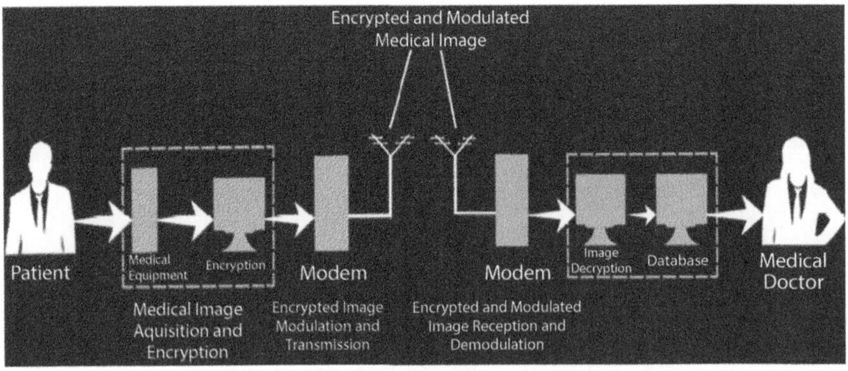

Figure 13.2 Block diagram of telemedicine system.

services that address the challenges of accessibility, patient engagement, and healthcare resource optimization [4].

Figure 13.2 shows the components included in the telemedicine system and how the interaction of patients with the medical doctor occurs via the system.

Telemedical Facilities in Practice [5]:
Teleconsultations: Telemedical facilities enable patients to connect with healthcare professionals remotely, overcoming travel constraints and geographic isolation. Video consultations facilitate diagnosis, treatment recommendations, and follow-up care, reducing the need for in-person visits while maintaining the quality of healthcare interactions.
Telemonitoring: Remote patient monitoring through telemedical facilities permits real-time tracking of vital signs, chronic conditions, and post-operative recovery. Wearable sensors and devices transmit data to healthcare providers, enabling early intervention and personalized care plans.
Tele-education: Telemedical facilities extend medical education beyond traditional classrooms. Online platforms offer training for healthcare professionals, ensuring continuous learning, skills enhancement, and the dissemination of medical knowledge to underserved areas.
Teletherapy: Telemedical facilities are helping mental health services by making psychotherapy, counseling, and support services available to those in need. Teletherapy removes stigmas related to seeking mental health assistance and improves patient engagement [6].

13.1.3 Statistics of Countries Using Remote Health Monitoring System

Figure 13.3 shows that the market for remote patient monitoring systems was estimated to be worth USD 4.4 billion in 2022, and over the course of the forecast period, it is anticipated to increase at a compound annual growth rate (CAGR) of 18.5%. The industry has been significantly impacted by COVID-19. The enhanced chronic disease management provided by remote monitoring systems, including early warning indications and progress trackers, has increased demand for these systems on a global scale. 90% of yearly healthcare costs in the United States are attributable to chronic illnesses. This can be avoided if patients receive prompt assistance through a remote monitoring system.

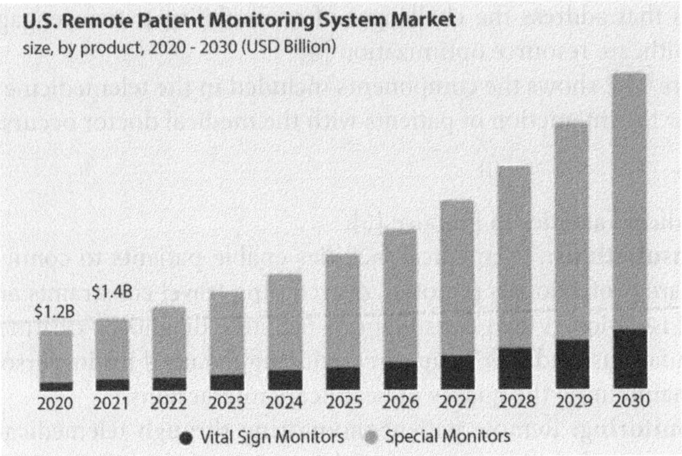

Figure 13.3 US market for remote patient monitoring [7].

Some more statistics of the remote patient monitoring systems throughout the world are:

1. **United States:**
   - Approximately 76% of hospitals in the U.S. are using remote patient monitoring systems to enhance healthcare delivery. (Source: American Hospital Association, 2020)
   - The adoption of telehealth services, including remote health monitoring, surged by 154% in the first quarter of 2020, reflecting a growing reliance on digital health solutions. (Source: CDC, 2021)
2. **United Kingdom:**
   - 45% of general practitioners in the UK offer remote health monitoring services to patients, enabling timely interventions and reduced clinic visits. (Source: NHS Digital, 2020)
   - The use of telemedicine services, including remote monitoring, has doubled in the UK, with around 20% of consultations being conducted remotely. (Source: NHS England, 2021)
3. **Canada:**
   - Around 83% of Canadian healthcare providers have implemented remote patient monitoring systems to manage chronic diseases and enhance patient engagement. (Source: Canada Health Infoway, 2019)

- Utilization of telehealth and remote monitoring services in Canada increased by 1,000% during the COVID-19 pandemic, highlighting their crucial role in maintaining healthcare access. (Source: Canadian Medical Association, 2021)

4. **Australia:**
   - Over 60% of Australian healthcare organizations are utilizing remote monitoring technologies to support patients in rural and remote areas. (Source: Australian Digital Health Agency, 2020)
   - Telehealth and remote monitoring adoption increased by 25% in Australia during the pandemic, with notable benefits in mental health support. (Source: Australian Government Department of Health, 2021)
5. **South Korea:**
   - South Korea boasts one of the highest smartphone penetration rates globally, with over 95% of the population having access to mobile devices, enabling widespread adoption of remote health monitoring apps. (Source: Statista, 2021)
   - The South Korean government has actively promoted telehealth services, leading to a rapid increase in the use of remote health monitoring systems, particularly among the elderly population. (Source: Ministry of Health and Welfare, South Korea, 2020)
6. **India:**
   - The use of telemedicine and remote health monitoring systems in India has surged by over 500% during the pandemic, as healthcare providers strive to maintain access to care. (Source: Ministry of Health and Family Welfare, India, 2021)
   - With over 150 million downloads by 2020, mobile health applications for remote monitoring are becoming more and more popular in India. (Source: Sensor Tower, 2021)

These statistics underscore the global trend towards adopting remote health monitoring systems, driven by advancements in technology, the need for healthcare access, and the challenges posed by events such as the COVID-19 pandemic [8]. Figure 13.4 shows the distribution of remote patient monitoring system market. Figure 13.5 shows the market segmentation of remote patient monitoring system.

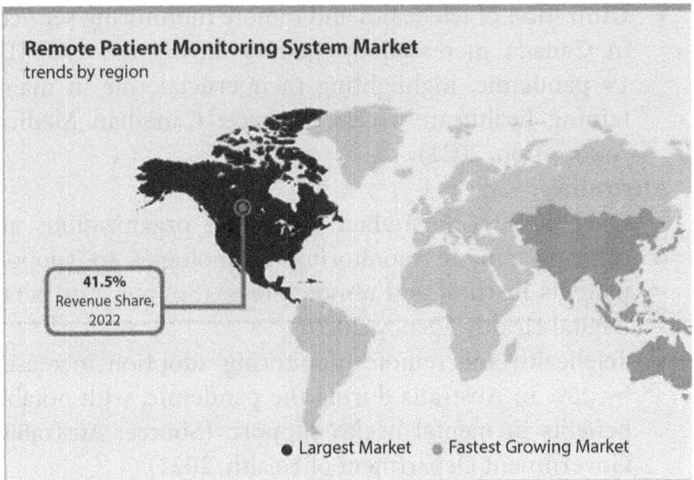

Figure 13.4 Remote patient monitoring system market [7].

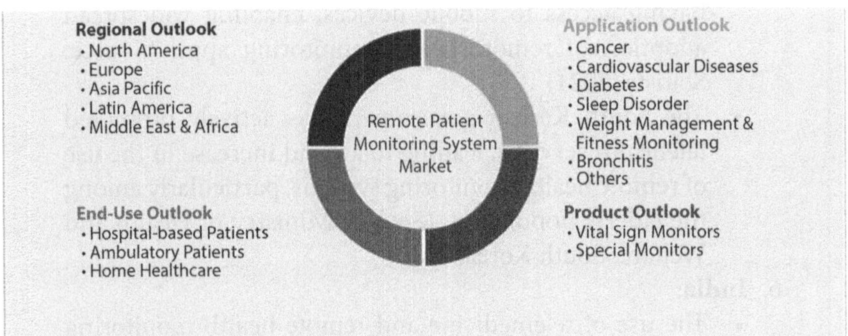

Figure 13.5 Market segmentation [7].

13.1.4 Role of IoT Smart Devices in Healthcare

The integration of IoT smart devices has ushered in a new era of healthcare, redefining patient care, diagnostics, and monitoring. This subtopic delves into the multifaceted role that IoT smart devices play in transforming the healthcare landscape [7].

1. **Continuous Health Monitoring:** IoT smart devices, such as wearable fitness trackers, smartwatches, and health sensors, enable individuals to continuously monitor their health parameters. These devices collect real-time data on vital

signs, physical activity, sleep patterns, and more, providing a comprehensive picture of the individual's well-being.

2. **Remote Patient Monitoring:** IoT-enabled medical devices extend healthcare beyond clinical settings by allowing healthcare providers to remotely monitor patients. This is especially important for those who need post-operative care, have chronic conditions, or live in rural places. Physicians can receive timely updates on patients' conditions and intervene when necessary.
3. **Data-Driven Personalization:** The data collected by IoT smart devices empowers healthcare providers to personalize treatment plans. By analyzing trends and patterns in the data, physicians can make informed decisions, adjust medications, and tailor interventions according to the patient's specific needs.
4. **Early Disease Detection:** IoT devices aid in the early detection of health issues by identifying subtle changes in the collected data. For instance, anomalies in heart rate or sleep patterns could indicate underlying health conditions, enabling early intervention and prevention.
5. **Telehealth and Telemedicine:** IoT devices support telehealth and telemedicine initiatives by facilitating virtual consultations and remote diagnosis. Patients can share their device-generated data with healthcare professionals during virtual appointments, enhancing the accuracy of assessments.
6. **Chronic Disease Management:** IoT gadgets that aid in condition monitoring benefit patients with chronic diseases like diabetes and hypertension. These gadgets deliver notifications, prompts, and insights that encourage proactive management and lower the possibility of difficulties.
7. **Post-Operative Care:** After surgeries, IoT devices aid in monitoring patients' recovery progress remotely. They can track wound healing, activity levels, and vital signs, allowing healthcare providers to identify any complications early.
8. **Patient Engagement:** IoT devices engage patients in their own health management. By providing real-time feedback, insights, and motivation, these devices encourage individuals to adopt healthier lifestyles and adhere to treatment plans.

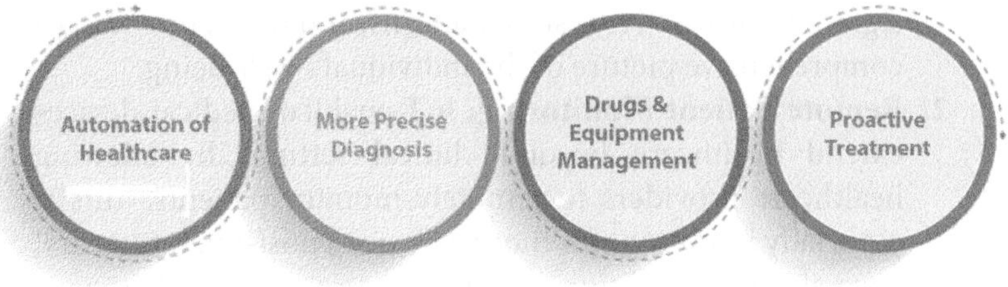

Figure 13.6 IoT enabled healthcare benefits [10].

9. **Research and Data Analysis:** The vast amount of health data generated by IoT devices contributes to medical research and data analysis. Researchers can study trends across populations, identify risk factors, and contribute to evidence-based medical advancements.
10. **Healthcare Workflow Optimization:** IoT devices streamline healthcare workflows by automating data collection and transmission. This reduces the burden on healthcare professionals, allowing them to focus more on critical decision-making and patient interactions.

Figure 13.6 depicts how healthcare benefits from IoT smart devices. Incorporating IoT smart devices into healthcare practices holds immense promise for enhancing patient outcomes, enabling proactive interventions, and fostering patient empowerment. However, challenges related to data security, privacy, interoperability, and standardization must be navigated to fully harness the potential of these devices [8].

13.2 IoT Smart Devices in Healthcare

In this chapter, the history and the diverse landscape of IoT smart devices in the healthcare industry are discussed.

The idea of the IoT is at the forefront of the technological revolution. The IoT is a network of interconnected machines, systems, and other items that can talk to one another and share information through the internet. This interconnectedness enables the automation of tasks, real-time data sharing, and the creation of smart environments that enhance efficiency, convenience, and productivity across various industries.

The Internet of Medical Things (IoMT), a subset of IoT that focuses primarily on the integration of smart devices and sensors into the healthcare system, has emerged in the setting of the healthcare industry. IoMT combines medical devices, software applications, and connectivity solutions to enable the seamless exchange of health-related data. This data-driven approach is revolutionizing patient care, medical research, and the overall management of health services [9, 10].

13.2.1 Evolution of IoT Devices Across the World

The history of IoT smart devices in healthcare unveils a timeline of innovation, from the earliest attempts at remote monitoring to the intricate interconnected ecosystems that now enhance patient care, diagnostics, monitoring, and treatment.

In the early 2000s, basic remote monitoring tools emerged, allowing for the transmission of critical health data like heart rate and glucose levels to healthcare providers [11]. This marked the beginning of a transformative journey in healthcare innovation. The 2010s saw the rise of wearable technology like Fitbit, empowering users to proactively monitor various health metrics. Smart hospitals integrated advanced technology for asset tracking, patient flow management, and temperature monitoring, significantly improving efficiency and enhancing patient experiences.

Simultaneously, the telemedicine revolution gained momentum, with devices facilitating remote consultations and diagnostics. Tools such as dermatology cameras and stethoscopes enabled remote patient examinations. Additionally, implantable medical devices like pacemakers and defibrillators incorporated real-time data transmission, allowing for proactive management of cardiac conditions [12]. These advancements have fundamentally reshaped healthcare, promoting remote monitoring, patient engagement, and efficient hospital operations across the world.

The global implementation of IoT smart devices in healthcare has transcended borders, revolutionizing patient care across various nations. The Table 13.1 details how many nations have used IoT technology to improve healthcare systems, displaying creative ideas that have completely changed how doctors practice medicine throughout the world.

Table 13.1 IoT smart devices in different countries.

Country	Healthcare sector	Company/ organization	IoT healthcare solution	Details and innovations
USA	Remote Patient Monitoring	Philips Healthcare	HealthSuite: IoT platform for remote patient monitoring and telehealth.	Offers connected devices for monitoring vital signs, enabling virtual consultations, and facilitating data-driven care.
USA	Cardiac Health	Medtronic	CareLink Network: Remote monitoring for implantable medical devices.	Allows patients and healthcare providers to remotely monitor performance and condition of pacemakers and defibrillators.
India	Telemedicine	Remidio	Fundus on Phone: Smartphone-based retinal imaging for telemedicine	Combines a smartphone attachment with AI algorithms to capture and transmit high-quality retinal images for remote diagnosis and screening of eye conditions.
USA	Sleep Apnea Therapy	ResMed	AirSense 10: IoT-connected CPAP machines for sleep apnea therapy.	Offers data tracking, remote adjustments, and patient engagement features for better treatment outcomes.
Switzerland	Diabetes Management	Roche Diabetes Care	Accu-Chek Connect: IoT solution for diabetes management.	Includes a blood glucose meter that syncs data to a mobile app, allowing patients to track and share their readings.

(*Continued*)

Table 13.1 IoT smart devices in different countries. (*Continued*)

Country	Healthcare sector	Company/ organization	IoT healthcare solution	Details and innovations
USA	Diabetes Management	Abbott	FreeStyle Libre: IoT-enabled glucose monitoring system.	Features a wearable sensor that measures glucose levels continuously, reducing the need for traditional fingerstick testing.
Japan	Hypertension Management	Omron Healthcare	HeartGuide: Wearable blood pressure monitor.	Combines a smartwatch with a blood pressure cuff, providing 24-hour monitoring and data visualization.
USA	Cardiac Health	BioTelemetry (Philips)	MCOT (Mobile Cardiac Outpatient Telemetry): Remote cardiac monitoring.	Utilizes wearable devices to capture and transmit continuous ECG data for diagnosing arrhythmias.
Germany	Chronic Disease Management	Bayer	Medrad Stellant CT Injection System: IoT-enabled CT contrast delivery system.	Provides automated contrast injection and data management for enhanced patient safety and image quality.
Japan	Elderly Care	Fujitsu	"HOPE LifeMark" IoT Solution: Remote monitoring and support for elderly individuals.	Offers wearable devices and a cloud-based platform to monitor health and activities of the elderly, enhancing safety and well-being.
South Korea	Cardiac Health	Samsung Medison	RS80A Echocardiography Machine: IoT-enhanced ultrasound system.	Incorporates AI and IoT technologies to provide advanced cardiac imaging and analysis.

(*Continued*)

Table 13.1 IoT smart devices in different countries. (*Continued*)

Country	Healthcare sector	Company/ organization	IoT healthcare solution	Details and innovations
Canada	Mental Health	MindBeacon	Beacon: Online therapy platform for mental health.	Provides online Cognitive Behavioral Therapy (CBT) programs for anyone in need of assistance with their mental health.
China	Diabetes Management	Sinocare	GlucoRx iGlucose Monitoring System: IoT-enabled glucose meter.	Enables remote glucose monitoring with data transmission and analytics for diabetes management.
Australia	Respiratory Health	ResApp Health	ResAppDx: Diagnostic app for respiratory conditions.	Uses cough sounds to provide rapid and accurate diagnosis of respiratory illnesses.
France	Post-Surgery Care	Withings	Body Cardio Scale: IoT-enabled smart scale.	Monitors heart health by providing measurements of weight, body composition, and pulse wave velocity.

13.2.2 Current Landscape

The current landscape of IoT smart devices in healthcare is a dynamic tapestry of cutting-edge technologies, data-driven insights, and patient-centric care. As we stand at the crossroads of technological advancement and medical innovation, the integration of IoT devices into healthcare has reached unprecedented levels of sophistication.

1. Remote Patient Monitoring (RPM): Remote patient monitoring has gained significant traction in recent years. Chronically ill patients, such as those with hypertension, diabetes, or heart disease can use IoT-enabled devices to track their vitals, such as heart rate, blood pressure, and blood sugar levels. These devices transmit data to healthcare

providers, enabling timely interventions and adjustments to treatment plans without requiring frequent in-person visits.

2. Wearable Health Trackers: Wearable devices like smartwatches and fitness trackers have become ubiquitous. They can maintain track of a variety of health indicators, such as heart rate, sleep patterns, steps taken, and even stress levels. Some advanced wearables also offer features like electrocardiograms (ECGs) to detect irregular heart rhythms.
3. Smart Pill Dispensers: IoT-enabled pill dispensers help patients adhere to their medication schedules. These devices can send reminders to patients' smartphones, dispense the correct medications at scheduled times, and notify caregivers or healthcare providers if doses are missed [13].
4. Telemedicine and Connected Medical Devices: Rapid expansion of telemedicine has taken place, particularly in reaction to the COVID-19 epidemic. IoT devices are essential in supporting the virtual consultations that patients may have with medical providers. For example, digital stethoscopes can transmit real-time heart and lung sounds to doctors during remote appointments.
5. Connected Inhalers: IoT-connected inhalers are designed to help individuals with respiratory conditions like asthma and COPD. These devices track medication usage and inhaler techniques, offering insights to patients and doctors to optimize treatment plans.
6. Health Monitoring Clothing: Vital indications like heart rate, breathing rate, and body temperature may be monitored with the use of smart clothing that has sensors built in. These clothes might be especially helpful for athletes looking for accurate performance statistics or for monitoring patients with long-term problems [14].
7. Smart Home Health Systems: IoT-based home health systems integrate various devices to create a connected environment that supports seniors' or patients' independence. These systems can include fall detection sensors, medication reminders, and even AI-driven virtual assistants that provide health-related information and assistance.
8. Medication Tracking Sensors: Some medication bottles come with IoT sensors that track when the bottle is opened or closed. By using this function, carers may make sure that patients are taking their meds as directed.

9. Mental Health Wearables: Furthermore, IoT gadgets for mental health monitoring are being developed. In order to spot symptoms of stress, anxiety, or depression, wearables may monitor things like sleep habits, body temperature, and heart rate variability [15, 16].

13.3 Need for Portable IoT Smart Devices

Portable smart IoT devices are indispensable across industries, driving innovation and efficiency [17]. Their mobility and connectivity empower healthcare with remote patient monitoring and timely interventions [18]. In logistics, IoT sensors optimize supply chains by tracking goods' conditions in real time [19]. They enhance smart homes' energy efficiency and enable personalized fitness tracking. Figure 13.7 (i) describes IoT-based devices in various sectors.

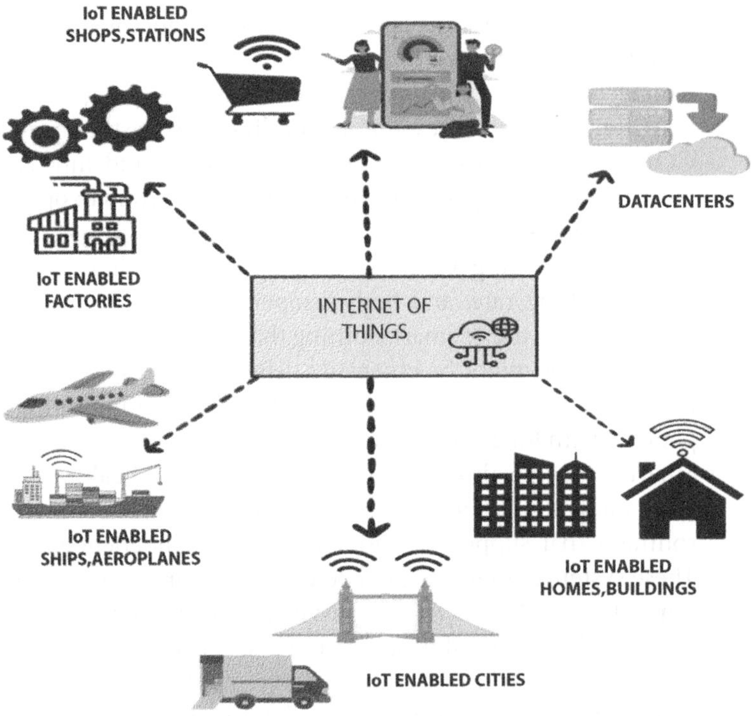

Figure 13.7 (i) IoT-based devices in various sectors.

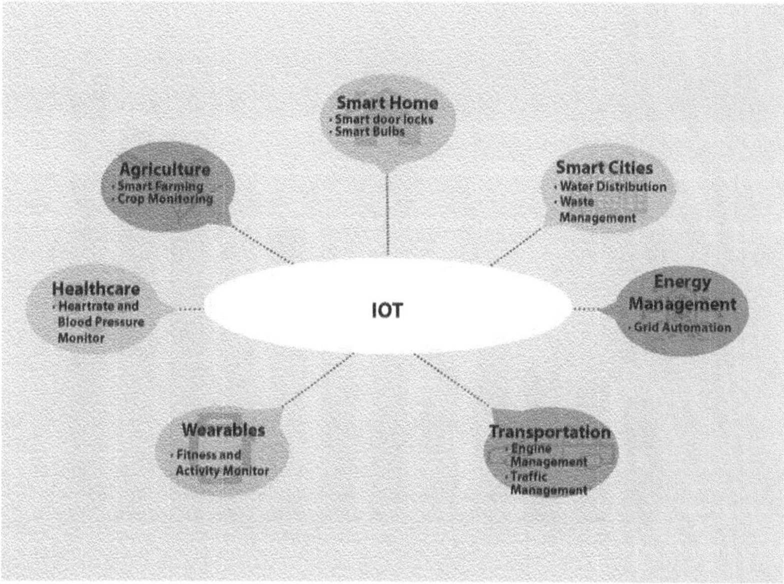

Figure 13.7 (ii) Usage of Portable smart IoT devices.

These devices also bolster safety through asset tracking, aid environmental monitoring, and revolutionize retail with personalized experiences [20]. Industries like agriculture benefit from precision farming using IoT sensors. Moreover, IoT's role in education and entertainment is transformative [21]. These devices create immersive learning experiences and elevate gaming with augmented reality. Overall, portable smart IoT devices reshape industries, fostering connectivity, data-driven decision-making, and convenience, thus paving the way for a technologically advanced and interconnected future [22].

13.3.1 Global Usage of Portable IoT Smart Devices

Figure 13.8 describes the number of IoT connected devices worldwide 2019-2023. In 2020, it is predicted that there will be 15.1 billion IoT devices worldwide, and by 2030, there will be more than 29 billion IoT devices. By 2030, China will have the most consumer IoT devices, with about 8 billion of them [23].

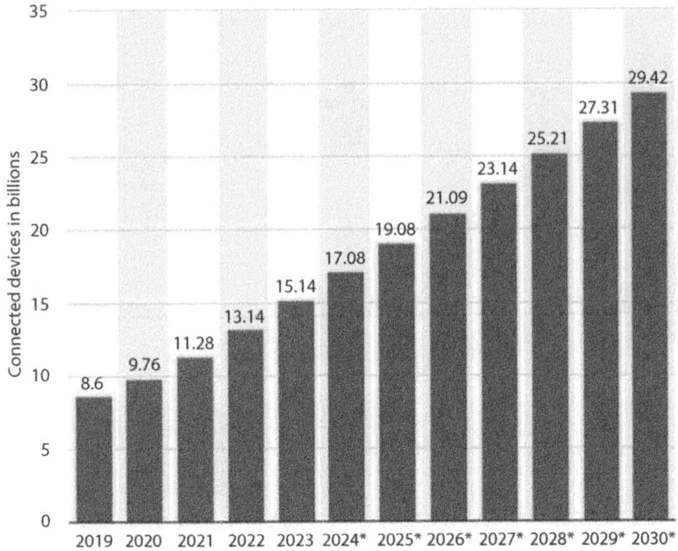

Figure 13.8 Number of IoT connected devices worldwide 2019-2023, with forecasts to 2030 [23].

IoT devices are used in both consumer markets and other business verticals; by 2020, the consumer market is anticipated to account for more than 60% of all IoT-connected devices. This proportion is anticipated to stay at this level for the next ten years.

Major Industry Sectors and Usage Scenarios:
Major sectors of industry with over a hundred million connected IoT devices now are energy, gas, steam and air conditioning, water supply and waste management, retail and commerce, transport and storage as well as government.

More than eight billion IoT devices will be in use across all industry sectors by the year 2030.

The largest use case for IoT devices in the consumer market is for internet and media consumption devices like smartphones, where the number of IoT devices is anticipated to reach more than 17 billion by 2030. More than one billion IoT devices will be in use by 2030 throughout the connected (autonomous) car, IT infrastructure, asset tracking & monitoring, and smart grid sectors [23]. Table 13.2 provides an overview of portable IoT smart devices utilized in various countries, showcasing examples of IoT usage and corresponding devices in each region.

Table 13.2 Portable IoT smart devices in various countries.

Country	IoT usage	Examples
United States	Wearable fitness trackers help individuals monitor exercise, heart rate, and sleep. Remote patient monitoring devices aid chronic condition management.	Apple Watch for the tracking of heart rate, Oura Ring for sleep tracking.
China	Smart scales and blood pressure monitors enable users to track health metrics. Thermometers and pulse oximeters offer remote health assessment.	Huawei Watch Fit for fitness tracking, iHealth wireless thermometer
Japan	IoT alert systems support elderly care. Remote monitoring devices aid patients with chronic ailments, enhancing their quality of life.	Tanita body composition monitor, Panasonic telehealth wearable.
Germany	IoT medication dispensers ensure timely dosages with reminders. Remote cardiac monitors offer real-time health data for informed medical decisions.	MedFolio electronic pill dispenser, Beurer blood glucose monitor.
South Korea	Smart contact lenses offer glucose data. Remote monitoring helps post-surgery patients recover effectively.	Aiotec smart contact lens, IMD Posture Detector.
India	IoT remote monitoring suits rural areas. Smart ECG monitors aid quick cardiovascular assessments.	QardioArm blood pressure monitor, Tricog ECG analysis app.
Brazil	Wearable health devices aid fitness tracking. Smart bandages with monitoring capabilities advance wound care.	Kinematix TUNE for gait analysis, MedLevensohn wound monitor.

(*Continued*)

Table 13.2 Portable IoT smart devices in various countries. (*Continued*)

Country	IoT usage	Examples
Russia	IoT mental health tools enable remote monitoring. Smart orthopedic implants aid tracking and rehabilitation.	ThinkHead EEG headset, ActiveSpine posture tracker.
Australia	IoT insulin pens track dosages. Remote monitoring devices serve distant patients, ensuring timely care.	EpiWatch allergen tracker, ResApp respiratory diagnostic app.
United Kingdom	IoT diagnostics empower patients with home-based health assessments. Smart inhalers aid asthma management through personalized data.	BioSure HIV self-test kit, Activ8rlives pulse oximeter.
Saudi Arabia	IoT vitals monitors serve Hajj pilgrims. Smart health kiosks offer convenient health checkups.	Hajj pilgrim health wristbands, Tashfi kiosk for health screenings
Canada	Telehealth platforms connect patients and doctors virtually. Smart pillboxes enhance medication adherence and management.	Akira telemedicine app, PillDrill medication tracking system.
France	Hospitals use smart beds for monitoring patients. IoT glucose monitors assist diabetics in maintaining optimal levels	Tucky smart fever patch, PKVitality K'Watch for glucose monitoring.
Mexico	Telemedicine platforms facilitate remote consultations. Smart hearing aids and vision devices enhance sensory experiences.	VIDA app for virtual doctor visits, Rayo Vision smart eyewear.
Italy	IoT rehab devices aid physical therapy. Smart pain management tools enhance comfort.	CAREN rehabilitation platform, PhysioGlove hand therapy.

(*Continued*)

Table 13.2 Portable IoT smart devices in various countries. (*Continued*)

Country	**IoT usage**	**Examples**
South Africa	IoT maternal health tools offer pregnancy insights. Smart water bottles promote hydration reminders.	Dr. VRX virtual reality therapy, NutriBullet smart blender.
Turkey	IoT devices assist chronic kidney patients. Smart ECG monitoring at home ensures quick medical attention.	NephroLife mobile app for kidney patients, TONIC ECG monitor.
Netherlands	Sleep trackers aid healthy rest. Smart apps integrate health data for informed decisions.	Zens wireless charging sleep tracker, NightBalance sleep position monitor.
United Arab Emirates	Wearable devices track outdoor activity. Smart pharmacy kiosks streamline prescription pickup	Dubai Health Authority's telehealth app, PharmaTrust smart medication cabinet
Singapore	IoT fall detectors enhance elderly care. Smart nutrition trackers aid dietary goals.	KaHa smart sports apparel, SmartPlate nutrition analyzing plate.

13.4 Introduction to Portable Labs

The introduction of portable labs in healthcare was driven by advancements in technology, particularly in miniaturization, automation, and diagnostics. These labs allow medical professionals to conduct various tests and analyses outside traditional laboratory settings. Innovations in areas like microfluidics, lab-on-a-chip technology, and point-of-care testing devices have made it possible to perform complex tests on smaller, more portable platforms. These labs offer benefits like quicker results, accessibility in remote areas, and more personalized patient care. Over time, collaborations between researchers, engineers, and healthcare practitioners have led to the development and integration of portable labs into medical practice. Portable labs in healthcare are innovative and versatile tools that enable medical professionals to perform various diagnostic tests and analyses at the point of care. These compact labs bring the laboratory to the patient, allowing for faster diagnosis, treatment decisions, and monitoring. They are particularly beneficial in remote or resource-limited areas, as well as during emergencies.

13.4.1 Advantages of Portable Labs

Portable labs have significantly transformed the healthcare landscape by providing several advantages:

1. **Rapid Diagnosis:** Portable labs offer quick results, minimizing the time between testing and diagnosis. This is crucial for conditions requiring prompt intervention, such as infectious diseases or critical medical situations [24].
2. **Accessibility:** These labs are especially valuable in remote or underserved areas where traditional laboratory infrastructure might be lacking. By introducing vital diagnostic capabilities to these areas, they aid in closing the access to healthcare gap [25].
3. **Point-of-Care Testing (POCT):** With the aid of portable labs, medical professionals can do tests next to the patient's bed, in clinics, or even out in the field. This reduces turnaround times and makes treatment decisions possible more quickly by eliminating the need to transport samples to centralized laboratories. One of the main drivers behind portable labs is the concept of point-of-care testing. This involves conducting tests and obtaining results right at the location where the patient is being treated, rather than sending samples to a centralized lab and waiting for results. This approach is especially useful in emergency situations, rural or remote areas, and during home care.
4. **Resource Efficiency:** Traditional labs can be resource-intensive and require significant space, equipment, and personnel. Portable labs are compact and require fewer resources, making them cost-effective and efficient.
5. **Emergency Response:** Portable labs are essential for determining the state of health of the affected populations and determining the best course of treatment during emergencies or natural disasters when healthcare infrastructure may be compromised [26].

6. **Diverse Applications:** These labs are adaptable and can be configured to carry out a variety of assays, including hematology, microbiology, molecular diagnostics, and blood chemistry.
7. **Monitoring Chronic Conditions:** Monitoring chronic illnesses like diabetes also uses portable labs. Patients are not required to visit a central lab in order to frequently test their blood sugar levels [25].
8. **Research and Surveillance:** Portable labs can be used in field research and epidemiological studies, aiding in disease surveillance and monitoring trends.
9. **Technological Advancements:** The evolution of various technologies played a crucial role. Microfluidics, which deals with the behavior of fluids at the microscale, allowed for the manipulation of tiny amounts of liquid for testing. Lab-on-a-chip technology integrated multiple laboratory functions onto a single chip-sized device, enabling compact and portable testing equipment [26].
10. **Customization and Personalized Medicine:** Portable labs have contributed to the concept of personalized medicine. These labs can analyze genetic information, biomarkers, and other individual-specific factors to tailor treatments and interventions to a patient's unique needs.

13.4.2 Perspective of Portable Labs in India

Healthcare portable labs, from an Indian perspective, are compact and mobile diagnostic units designed to bring medical testing and diagnostics closer to patients, particularly in remote and underserved areas. These labs offer on-the-spot testing, enabling timely and accurate diagnosis, thus improving healthcare accessibility and outcomes.

Healthcare portable labs in India are innovative solutions that bring medical diagnostics closer to communities, particularly in remote areas. These labs typically include equipment for various diagnostic tests, such as blood tests and imaging, and can be transported to different locations as needed. They are extremely important for enhancing accessibility to medical treatment and testing, particularly in places with poor healthcare infrastructure. These labs often use technologies like point-of-care testing devices and telemedicine to provide timely and accurate medical assessments.

13.4.2.1 Insights of Portable Labs in India

1. **Access to Remote Areas:** Portable labs address the challenge of providing medical services in far-flung regions where healthcare infrastructure is limited. They can reach rural villages, tribal areas, and disaster-stricken locations, ensuring essential diagnostic services are available. Researchers can control and monitor experiments from a distance using some portable labs' remote monitoring and control features.
2. **Point-of-Care Testing:** These labs allow healthcare professionals to perform tests and obtain results at the point of care, eliminating the need to send samples to distant laboratories. This facilitates immediate decision-making and intervention. Healthcare portable labs enable medical professionals to conduct tests and obtain results right at the patient's location. As a result, choices about diagnosis and treatment can be made more quickly than if samples were to be sent to far-off labs. This is especially significant in cases where prompt intervention is essential.
3. **Emergency Response:** During emergencies, natural disasters, or disease outbreaks, portable labs can provide rapid testing, aiding in prompt medical response and disease control efforts. Portable labs can be swiftly deployed to these areas, providing medical professionals with the tools needed to assess health risks, diagnose diseases, and provide appropriate care [27].
4. **Disease Surveillance:** These labs aid in disease surveillance by enabling rapid testing and data collection during outbreaks, facilitating early intervention and containment. Portable labs contribute to disease surveillance efforts by enabling rapid and accurate testing during outbreaks. This aids in identifying affected individuals, tracking the spread of diseases, and implementing containment strategies more effectively [28].
5. **Customizable Configurations:** Healthcare portable labs can be customized with specific diagnostic equipment and technologies based on the prevalent healthcare needs of the region. Depending on the prevalent healthcare needs of a region, portable labs can be customized with specific

diagnostic equipment and technologies. This adaptability ensures that the lab's capabilities align with the most pressing medical concerns.

6. **Sample Collection and Analysis:** They enable on-site sample collection, preparation, and analysis, reducing the need to transport samples to distant laboratories. Portable labs enable on-site sample collection, immediate preparation, and analysis. This reduces the time required to transport samples to distant labs, leading to faster results and subsequent medical interventions.
7. **Monitoring Chronic Conditions:** Healthcare portable labs can be equipped to monitor chronic conditions like diabetes, allowing patients to receive regular check-ups without traveling far. Tools for monitoring chronic disorders like diabetes, hypertension, or cardiovascular diseases might be included in mobile labs for healthcare. Patients who require continuing treatment of their health and regular checkups would particularly benefit from this. By bringing diagnostic capabilities to their doorstep, these labs enhance patients' convenience and compliance with treatment regimens [29].
8. **Training and Capacity Building:** Portable labs contribute to training healthcare workers in underserved areas, enhancing their skills in diagnostics and medical procedures. Portable labs present a special chance for local healthcare professionals to receive training and develop their capacities. Modern diagnostic techniques and technologies are available in these labs, giving medical personnel the chance to practice utilizing them.
9. **Cost-Efficiency:** By removing the need for patients to travel great distances and streamlining the entire healthcare delivery process, they may prove to be cost-effective in the long term. The capacity of healthcare portable labs to bring medical services closer to the population and lessen the financial load on patients and communities is what makes them cost-effective. Patients in far-off locations frequently have to pay for transportation fees and probable income loss owing to time away from work when seeking medical care at faraway facilities.

13.4.2.2 Case Study

In India, several initiatives and organizations have introduced different types of healthcare portable labs to address various medical needs. Healthcare portable labs in India are mobile medical units equipped with diagnostic tools that provide essential medical services to remote and underserved areas. These labs provide a variety of services, such as doing blood tests, diagnosing illnesses, and keeping track of medical issues. Here are a few examples:

1. **Neuberg Diagnostics' Lab on Wheels:** Neuberg Diagnostics launched a unique initiative known as Lab on Wheels. These were specially designed mobile vans equipped with state-of-the-art diagnostic laboratory facilities. By providing diagnostic services to isolated and disadvantaged communities, the goal was to close the healthcare gap between urban and rural areas. These vans were equipped to perform various tests such as blood tests, urine tests, and even advanced diagnostic procedures like X-rays and ultrasounds. This initiative was especially helpful in areas where access to healthcare facilities was limited. The Lab on Wheels vans are equipped with state-of-the-art diagnostic laboratory facilities, including advanced diagnostic devices such as X-ray machines and ultrasound equipment. Many of these modern medical devices are IoT-enabled, meaning they can connect to the internet and transmit data in real-time.

   IoT-enabled medical devices can collect patient data and test results electronically. In the context of the Lab on Wheels initiative, this data could include information from X-rays, ultrasound scans, or other diagnostic tests. This data can be transmitted securely to centralized databases or healthcare professionals, allowing for real-time monitoring and analysis. With IoT connectivity, healthcare providers can remotely monitor the operation of these diagnostic devices and ensure they are functioning correctly. They can also remotely access and review test results, allowing for faster diagnosis and treatment decisions.
2. **Medtronic's Mobile ECG Lab:** Medtronic, a global medical technology company, introduced a Mobile ECG Lab to provide accessible and on-the-spot electrocardiogram (ECG) testing. ECG is a crucial diagnostic tool for heart-related

issues. The mobile lab was designed to reach locations where traditional healthcare facilities might not be readily available. It made it possible for medical experts to evaluate a patient's heart health swiftly and decide on the best course of action for their care.

In the context of Medtronic's Mobile ECG Lab, the integration of devices and the IoT is pivotal. The Mobile ECG Lab likely incorporates IoT-enabled ECG devices that seamlessly capture and transmit patients' ECG data wirelessly. This connectivity empowers healthcare professionals to remotely access and monitor real-time ECG data, making it especially advantageous in remote or underserved regions. Robust data security measures ensure the privacy of sensitive medical information during transmission. Moreover, IoT technology allows for scalability, flexibility, and the potential expansion of the lab's reach. It enables data analytics to identify cardiac health patterns and can trigger automated alerts for critical findings. Additionally, the integration of telemedicine platforms becomes feasible, facilitating virtual consultations and enhancing collaboration between on-site and remote medical experts. IoT also supports the maintenance and diagnostics of the lab's equipment, ensuring operational reliability. In sum, IoT enhances the Mobile ECG Lab's capabilities, improving the accessibility and efficiency of cardiac care, particularly in areas lacking robust healthcare infrastructure.

3. **Portable Blood Donation Units:** These units are designed to facilitate blood donation drives in different locations. They are equipped with sterile equipment for drawing blood and storing it properly. These mobile units are especially useful in times of need or in locations where conventional blood banks might not be available. They help increase the availability of blood for medical treatments and emergencies. These units are designed to facilitate blood donation drives in different locations. They are equipped with sterile equipment for drawing blood and storing it properly.

   Portable Blood Donation Units, in conjunction with the IoT, represent a transformative synergy between devices and technology to optimize the process of blood collection and storage. These units, equipped with IoT-enabled sensors and connectivity, revolutionize the efficiency and safety of blood donation drives. IoT sensors monitor critical parameters like temperature and humidity in real-time, ensuring that the collected blood remains viable and safe. Data is continuously transmitted to central systems, allowing healthcare providers to remotely monitor blood donation status and storage conditions, facilitating prompt interventions when necessary. IoT also aids in inventory management by providing real-time data on available blood units, optimizing allocation. Additionally, location tracking ensures these mobile units reach the right places, especially in emergencies. Automated alerts triggered by IoT technology enable rapid responses to critical conditions, preserving blood integrity. Moreover, IoT enhances donor engagement, provides real-time updates, and bolsters the sense of community involvement. In essence, the amalgamation of Portable Blood Donation Units and IoT elevates the efficiency, safety, and accessibility of blood donation processes, ensuring a consistent blood supply for medical treatments and emergencies, even in remote locations.

13.5 Prospects for Portable Labs Globally in the Future

Globally, there are bright future prospects for portable labs. They make it simple to undertake scientific investigations and analysis in a variety of locations, including remote locations and disaster-affected areas. These labs are anticipated to grow increasingly advanced, inexpensive, and portable as technology develops, allowing researchers, healthcare workers, and educators to access essential tools and resources wherever they are. This could revolutionize fields such as healthcare, environmental monitoring, and education, making scientific exploration and data collection more accessible and efficient.

The future prospects of portable health care labs are quite promising. These labs could greatly enhance healthcare accessibility and diagnostics by providing rapid and on-the-spot testing for various medical conditions. With advancements in miniaturization and technology, these labs could become even more accurate, user-friendly, and cost-effective. They could play a significant role in remote areas, disaster response situations, and underserved communities, helping to diagnose diseases, monitor health parameters, and deliver timely medical interventions. Portable labs have the potential to completely change how medical care is provided worldwide as healthcare continues to advance [30].

Several future trends are expected in the realm of portable health care labs:

1. **Advanced Diagnostics:** Portable labs will become more sophisticated, offering a wider range of diagnostic capabilities. They will be capable of detecting various diseases and health conditions with high accuracy, enabling early intervention and personalized treatment.
2. **Integration of AI and IoT:** Artificial intelligence and the IoT will play a significant role. Portable labs will be equipped with AI algorithms for data analysis and interpretation, providing real-time insights and recommendations for healthcare providers.
3. **Global Health Initiatives:** In resource constrained areas, portable laboratories will be useful for disease control, detecting and monitoring public health indicators with a view to preventing and managing epidemics [31].
4. **Microfluidics and Nanotechnology:** Advancements in microfluidics and nanotechnology will lead to even smaller and more efficient portable lab devices, enabling precise analysis with minimal sample requirements.
5. **Global Collaboration:** International collaborations will increase, with experts and organizations sharing best practices and knowledge to advance the field of portable health care labs.
6. **Disease Diagnosis and Prediction:** AI algorithms can be integrated into portable health care labs to assist in disease diagnosis and prediction. Machine learning models can analyze medical data collected by these labs, such as blood samples or medical images, to identify patterns and markers associated with various diseases. This can enable early detection and timely intervention.
7. **Drug Discovery:** Portable labs equipped with AI/ML can accelerate the drug discovery process. They can analyze biological samples and perform high-throughput screening to identify potential drug candidates. AI algorithms can predict the effectiveness of compounds, reducing the time and cost required for drug development.

13.6 Future Scope

Within the domain of portable IoT smart devices in healthcare and remote health monitoring, the trajectory of innovation continues to open new vistas of opportunity. As microfluidics and lab-on-a-chip technologies advance, the landscape of healthcare is set to witness the emergence of more compact and efficient devices. These innovations will redefine the possibilities of sample manipulation and analysis, driving the evolution of precise, portable setups. The integration of nanotechnology within this paradigm augments the potential of these devices, enabling them to exhibit heightened sensitivity and specificity. This enhancement holds the key to detecting even the most minuscule quantities of substances, pushing the boundaries of diagnostics. Beyond this, the future holds the promise of more advanced diagnostic capabilities through the fusion of intricate sensors and cutting-edge AI algorithms. This amalgamation is poised to elevate the scope of diagnostics, enabling the identification of an even broader spectrum of health conditions with unparalleled accuracy. A particularly captivating avenue for exploration lies in neurological monitoring, where the integration of advanced sensors could pave the way for real-time brain activity tracking. This breakthrough not only holds the potential to revolutionize the management of neurological disorders like epilepsy but also to enable transformative brain-computer interfaces. With these trajectories converging, the future of portable IoT smart devices in healthcare and remote health monitoring is poised to be characterized by boundless innovation and meaningful impact. Some of the personal insights include:

1. **Human-Centered Approach:** It's crucial to emphasize the human aspect in healthcare technology. Portable IoT devices can greatly empower individuals to take charge of their health. These innovations have the potential to shift the healthcare paradigm from reactive to proactive, enabling early detection and prevention of diseases.
2. **Accessibility and Equity:** While discussing the potential of these devices, it's important to address the issue of accessibility and equity. As these technologies advance, ensuring that they are accessible and affordable to a wide range of populations is a critical consideration. This can help bridge healthcare disparities and make quality healthcare available to all.

3. **Data Privacy and Security:** With the integration of AI and IoT, data privacy and security become paramount. Discuss the importance of robust security measures and ethical considerations when handling sensitive health data. Balancing data utility with privacy is a challenge that needs careful attention.
4. **Interoperability and Standards:** As the field evolves, it's essential to stress the importance of interoperability and standardization. Portable IoT devices should seamlessly integrate with existing healthcare systems and share data efficiently to provide a comprehensive view of a patient's health.
5. **Neurological Monitoring:** Highlight the transformative potential of neurological monitoring. Real-time brain activity tracking can revolutionize the management of conditions like epilepsy and open doors to brain-computer interfaces that could empower individuals with disabilities in unimaginable ways.
6. **Human-AI Collaboration:** Explore the concept of human-AI collaboration in healthcare. These devices can augment the abilities of healthcare professionals, offering diagnostic support and data analysis that can lead to more accurate and timely interventions.

13.7 Conclusion

In conclusion, the combination of portable IoT smart devices and remote health monitoring has marked an evolution in healthcare that has fundamentally changed how medical services are provided and accessible. Aging populations, the prevalence of chronic diseases, and the desire for effective healthcare services have all drawn attention to the urgent need for remote health monitoring, which has opened the way for cutting-edge solutions like telemedicine and IoT devices. In especially in underprivileged and rural locations, the use of telemedical facilities has shown its effectiveness in overcoming geographic gaps and providing medical expertise to patients' fingertips. Statistics demonstrating the widespread use of remote health monitoring systems in different nations highlight their advantages.

The development of IoT smart devices in healthcare over time, from their initial applications to the complex and individualized solutions of today, is an example of the quick rate of technical progress. The IoT landscape for healthcare currently shows a wide variety of tools and systems that enable proactive treatment and educated decision-making for both patients and healthcare providers. Successful deployments in several nations show that the use of IoT smart devices in healthcare is not restricted by national boundaries. Through the use of these technologies, medical services are being improved globally across cultural, economic, and geographic boundaries. To increase their reach and influence, IoT smart devices must be portable, which is a critical requirement. Users can carry necessary health monitoring equipment thanks to the flexibility and accessibility offered by portable IoT devices.

The use of portable IoT smart devices by individuals, organizations, and medical professionals alike is contributing to a striking increase in their usage worldwide. This pattern reflects the rising acceptance of the contribution they make to illness prevention and healthcare management. Additionally, the development of portable labs adds a fresh perspective to healthcare delivery, especially in nations like India where logistical difficulties can arise due to different demographics and expansive terrain. The use of portable IoT smart devices in remote health monitoring and healthcare has the promise of endless innovation and significant impact. The fusion of nanotechnology, lab-on-a-chip, microfluidics, and AI algorithms brings up new possibilities. These developments have the potential to advance diagnostic skills, increase sensitivity and specificity, and reshape sample handling and analysis. Particularly captivating is the avenue of neurological monitoring, with the potential to revolutionize the management of neurological disorders and enable transformative brain-computer interfaces. As these trajectories converge, the field is set to witness continuous advancements, enhancing healthcare outcomes and accessibility.

References

1. Aman, B., Liu, R., Liu, Z., Sharaf, M.A., Towards edge IoT analytics for healthcare. *IEEE Internet Things J.*, 6, 2, 1767–1774, 2019.
2. Haque, A., Imtiaz, S., Eun, Y.C., Tariq, S., Smart healthcare using IoT and big data analytics: A survey. *IEEE Access*, 9, 107205–107221, 2021.
3. Malasinghe, L., Ramzan, N., Dahal, K., Remote patient monitoring: A comprehensive study. *J. Ambient Intell. Humaniz. Comput.*, 10, 1, 57–76, Jan. 2019.
4. Allen, A., In the Beginning (Part II): Telemedicine and Teleradiology. *Telemed. Today*, 2, 3, 6–7, 1994.

5. Allen, A., Prison Telemedicine in Colorado. *Telemed. Today*, 3, 4, 26–27, 1995a.
6. Murthy, H., Kumar, K., Boppuru, P. R., Pillai, V., CoviCare: Current trends and challenges of telemedicine in India: A case study on patient satisfaction, in: *Emerging Computational Approaches in Telehealth and Telemedicine: A Look at The Post-COVID-19 Landscape,* Bentham Science Publisher, 2022, doi: 10.2174/9789815079272122010008.
7. Condry, M. and Quan, X., Remote patient monitoring technologies and markets. *IEEE Eng. Manag. Rev.,* 1–5, 2023, 10.1109/EMR.2023.3285688.
8. Baker, S.B., Xiang, W., Atkinson, I., Internet of Things for smart healthcare: technologies, challenges, and opportunities. *IEEE Access*, 5, 26521–26544, 2017, 10.1109/ACCESS.2017.2775180.
9. Lee, J., Jo, M., Kwak, D., The Internet of Things for Health Care: A Comprehensive Survey. *IEEE Access*, 9, 2437951, 2021, doi: 10.1109/ACCESS.2021.3095149.
10. Srivastava, J., Routray, S., Ahmad, S., Waris, M.M., Internet of Medical Things (IoMT)-Based Smart Healthcare System: Trends and Progress. *Comput. Intell. Neurosci.*, 2022, 7218113, 2022, Published 2022 Jul 16, doi: 10.1155/2022/7218113.
11. Barach, J.P. and Brown, S.A., The early evolution of remote patient monitoring: A historical perspective. *IEEE Eng. Med. Biol. Mag.*, 31, 5, 48–53, 2012, doi: 10.1109/MEMB.2012.2200568.
12. Umer, M., Sadiq, S., Karamti, H., Karamti, W., Majeed, R., Nappi, M., IoT Based Smart Monitoring of Patients' with Acute Heart Failure. *Sensors (Basel)*, 22, 7, 2431, 2022, Published 2022 Mar 22, doi:10.3390/s22072431.
13. Patil, M.N., Panda, S.K., Singh, V.K., Smart pill dispensers: A review. *IEEE Access*, 8, 94448–94468, 2020, doi: 10.1109/ACCESS.2020.3025359.
14. Meena, J. S., Choi, S. B., Jung, S. B., Kim, J. W., Electronic textiles: New age of wearable technology for healthcare and fitness solutions. *Mater. Today Bio.*, 19, 100565, 2023, ISSN 2590-0064, doi: 10.1016/j.mtbio.2023.100565.
15. Pradhan, B., Bhattacharyya, S., Pal, K., IoT-Based Applications in Healthcare Devices. *J. Healthc. Eng.*, 2021, 6632599, 2021, Published 2021 Mar 18, doi:10.1155/2021/6632599.
16. Gutierrez, L.J., Rabbani, K., Ajayi, O.J. *et al.*, Internet of Things for Mental Health: Open Issues in Data Acquisition, Self-Organization, Service Level Agreement, and Identity Management. *Int. J. Environ. Res. Public Health*, 18, 3, 1327, 2021, Published 2021 Feb 1, doi:10.3390/ijerph18031327.
17. Joshi, A.A., Meza, J., Shah, J., Twittering for public health: An examination of tweets during an H1N1 outbreak. *Computer*, 43, 4, 81–84, 2008.
18. Kuppusamy, K.S. and Jayaraman, R., Internet of Things (IoT): Applications, challenges, and related future technologies, in: *Proceedings of the 2016 IEEE International Conference on Wireless Communications, Signal Processing and Networking (WiSPNET)*, pp. 108–113, 2016.

19. Lee, H. and Jeong, H., A portable lab-on-a-chip system for point-of-care diagnostics. *Lab. Chip*, 19, 13, 2152–2166, 2019.
20. Herold, K. E. and Rasooly, A. (Eds.), Lab-on-a-chip technology (Vol. 2): Biomolecular separation and analysis. Caister Academic Press, Aug. 2009.
21. Mancuso, V., Rametta, P., Sgroi, M., Internet of Things and COVID-19 prevention in healthcare. *Internet Things*, 12, 100222, 2020.
22. Radhakrishnan, K. and Saravanakumar, R., IoT-based healthcare monitoring system using portable devices. *Proc. Comput. Sci.*, 167, 1053–1060, 2019.
23. Sun, Y., Song, H., Jara, A.J., Bie, R., Internet of things and big data analytics for smart and connected communities. *IEEE Access*, 4, 766–773, 2016.
24. Thakur, D., Singh, A., Singh, I., IoT-enabled healthcare towards smart and healthy living: A review. *Internet Things*, 8, 100127, 2019.
25. Ventola, C.L., Mobile devices and apps for health care professionals: Uses and benefits. *P.T.*, 39, 5, 356–364, 2014.
26. Gupta, S., Ramesh, K., Ahmed, S., Kakkar, V., Lab-on-chip technology: A review on design trends and future scope in biomedical applications. *J. Conf.*, 8, 312, 2016.
27. Wang, S. and Jia, W., Internet of Things (IoT)-based smart healthcare systems: A review of literature and future perspective. *J. Med. Syst.*, 45, 3, 1–15, 2021.
28. Kim, E.Y., Patient will see you now: The future of medicine is in your hands. *Healthc. Inform. Res.*, 21, 4, 321–323, 2015 Oct., doi: 10.4258/hir.2015.21.4.321. Epub 2015 Oct 31. PMCID: PMC4659891.
29. Yao, L. and Salehan, M., Online health information seeking behavior: Understanding information source evaluation using the theory of reasoned action and the technology acceptance model. *Health Commun.*, 35, 5, 579–589, 2020.
30. Yaqoob, I., Ahmed, E., ur Rehman, M.H., Ahmed Al-garadi, M., Internet of Things architecture: Recent advances, taxonomy, requirements, and open challenges. *IEEE Wireless Commun.*, 24, 3, 10–16, 2017.
31. Perera, C., Zaslavsky, A., Christen, P., Geor-gakopoulos, D., Context aware computing for the internet of things: A survey. *Commun. Surv. Tutorials, IEEE*, 99, 1–41, 2013.

14

IoT-Enabled Analysis of COVID Data: Unveiling Insights from Temperature, Pulse Rate, and Oxygen Measurements

Justin John[1]*, Kukatlapalli Pradeep Kumar[1] and Hari Murthy[2]

[1]Computer Science and Engineering, School of Engineering and Technology CHRIST (Deemed to be University) Kengeri Campus, Bangalore, Karnataka, India
[2]Electronics and Communication Engineering, School of Engineering and Technology CHRIST (Deemed to be University) Kengeri Campus, Bangalore, Karnataka, India

Abstract

The COVID-19 pandemic has forced unparalleled transformation on healthcare systems around the world, demanding new and improved approaches for effective monitoring and diagnosis. In this context, we present a study titled "IoT-Enabled Analysis of COVID Data: Unveiling Insights from Temperature, Pulse Rate, and Oxygen Measurements."

The global impact of COVID-19, with millions of confirmed cases and fatalities, underscores the urgency of finding efficient monitoring solutions. To address this crisis, IoT-Enabled Health Monitoring Systems have emerged as a promising tool for remote patient monitoring and infection risk reduction. These systems leverage sensors to collect real-time data on the temperature, pulse rate, and oxygen saturation levels of the subject. The integration of a mobile application enables immediate access to this critical health information.

In this study, we explore the use of IoT systems, which have demonstrated accuracy comparable to other devices on the market. By leveraging these technologies, we aim to provide healthcare professionals with valuable insights into patients' health status, aiding in early detection, monitoring, and timely intervention.

**Corresponding author*: justin.john@btech.christuniversity.in

Hari Murthy, Marta Zurek-Mortka, Vinay Jha Pillai and Kukatlapalli Pradeep Kumar (eds.) Internet of Things in Bioelectronics: Emerging Technologies and Applications, (297–310) © 2024 Scrivener Publishing LLC

Our research contributes to the efforts to battle the COVID-19 pandemic by highlighting the potential of IoT-enabled monitoring systems in enhancing healthcare delivery, reducing infection risks, and ultimately saving lives.

Keywords: COVID-19, IoT-enabled analysis, temperature-pulse rate-oxygen, measurements, health monitoring systems, sensors

14.1 Introduction

The COVID-19 pandemic took the world by surprise, leaving health organizations scrambling for solutions. With more than 56.4 million confirmed cases and 1.35 million fatalities worldwide [1], it's clear that we need a way to effectively monitor and diagnose the virus. In the country of Bangladesh alone, there are over 445,281 positive cases and 6,350 deaths [2]. The indicators for COVID-19 include fever, Breathlessness, low oxygen saturation levels, dry cough, and more.

To combat this global crisis, IoT-enabled health Monitoring Systems have emerged, allowing us to monitor patients remotely and reduce the risk of infection. We can gain valuable insights into the patient's health by utilizing sensors to measure body temperature, pulse rate, and oxygen saturation levels. This real-time monitoring system has shown promising results. The systems have been tested and proven accurate when compared to other devices on the market.

The symptoms associated with COVID-19 vary but often include fever, shortness of breath, low oxygen saturation levels, dry cough, and more [3]. Given the severity of the pandemic, innovative approaches have become essential, and one such approach is the utilization of IoT-Enabled Health Monitoring Systems. These systems have emerged as a critical tool in the fight against COVID-19 by enabling remote patient monitoring, thereby reducing the risk of infection transmission.

In the subsequent sections of this article, we will delve into the literature survey conducted on the COVID-19 database, exploring the wealth of data collected and its significance in monitoring crucial health parameters, such as temperature, pulse rate, and oxygen levels, in individuals affected by the virus. We will then shift our focus to the extensive analysis and research opportunities that have arisen from this dataset, elucidating the methodology employed to extract meaningful insights. Subsequently, we will present the results of our analysis and engage in a comprehensive discussion of their implications, contributing to a deeper understanding of the ongoing COVID-19 pandemic and its multifaceted impact on public health.

14.2 Literature

This section describes information about the COVID-19 database and the comprehensive analysis conducted on it, shedding light on crucial insights and trends that have emerged during the ongoing pandemic. This invaluable resource has been meticulously curated by global health organizations, research institutions, and governments, providing a comprehensive overview of the pandemic's impact on different regions.

14.2.1 Temperature

Temperature is a fundamental parameter that has an important role in monitoring the health of individuals, especially during the COVID-19 pandemic. Understanding fever as a symptom is essential in identifying potential cases of the virus. As we all know, fever is one of the primary symptoms of COVID-19. It acts as a red flag, indicating a possible infection and the need for immediate action [4].

Temperature monitoring allows for the early detection of potential cases. By regularly measuring body temperature, we can identify any abnormal spikes and act promptly. With the help of IoT-enabled devices, this process becomes even more efficient. Patients can easily monitor their body temperature and keep track of any fluctuations from the comfort of their own homes.

14.2.2 Pulse Rate Monitoring

When it comes to monitoring the health status of COVID-19 patients, pulse rate monitoring plays a vital role. Just like a nosy neighbor who can't resist peeking through their curtains, pulse rate monitoring allows us to get a sneak peek into our cardiovascular health. It's like having a mini detective residing inside our bodies, constantly on the lookout for any suspicious activities [5].

Monitoring oxygen saturation levels is crucial in the diagnosis and management of COVID-19. As the virus attacks the respiratory system, it can lead to a decrease in the amount of oxygen in the blood. By measuring oxygen saturation levels, healthcare providers can identify patients who are experiencing respiratory distress and may require immediate intervention.

14.2.3 Oxygen Measurement in COVID-19

Oxygen saturation levels are normally recorded using a pulse oximeter, a non-invasive device that clips onto a finger. This Apparatus uses light to determine the rate at which oxygen is present in the blood. In COVID-19 patients, a decrease in oxygen saturation levels below 90% is often an indication of severe respiratory compromise [6].

14.2.4 Dataset Details

This dataset comprises vital health measurements collected from a sample of 10,000 individuals to investigate the association between COVID-19 infection status and key physiological parameters. The dataset includes information on body temperature, pulse rate, and oxygen levels, with a focus on individuals who have tested positive for COVID-19.

Subjects: The dataset contains records for a total of 10,000 subjects.
COVID-19 Status: Each subject is classified as either "COVID-19 Positive" or "COVID-19 Negative" based on their diagnostic test results. This information is crucial for assessing the impact of the virus on vital signs [7].
Temperature: The body temperature of each subject is recorded, in degrees Celsius, indicating the potential presence of fever, a common symptom of COVID-19.
Pulse Rate: The pulse rate of each subject is included, measured in beats per minute (BPM), which can provide insights into heart rate variations and overall cardiovascular health.
Oxygen Level: Oxygen saturation levels (SpO2) are documented as a percentage. Low oxygen levels can be an indicator of respiratory distress, which is a common symptom in COVID-19 patients.

14.2.5 Analysis and Research Opportunities

Researchers and healthcare professionals can leverage this dataset to conduct a variety of analyses and investigations:

COVID-19 Diagnosis: Determine how temperature, pulse rate, and oxygen levels vary between COVID-19-positive and COVID-19-negative subjects. Identify potential diagnostic thresholds for early detection.
Disease Progression: Examine how these vital signs change over time for COVID-19 patients and whether certain trends are associated with disease severity [8].

Risk Factors: Investigate whether pre-existing conditions or demographic factors correlate with worse outcomes in COVID-19-positive subjects based on these physiological measurements.
Treatment Efficacy: Assess the impact of different treatments and interventions on the vital signs of COVID-19 patients in order to optimize patient care strategies.
Predictive Modeling: Build predictive models using these vital signs to estimate the likelihood of an individual being COVID-19 positive, which could aid in triage and resource allocation.

14.3 Methodology

Data collection was conducted by trained healthcare professionals using IoT-enabled health monitoring systems. Body temperature measurements were obtained using FDA-approved digital thermometers. Pulse rate monitoring was performed using FDA-cleared pulse oximeters. Oxygen saturation levels were measured non-invasively using pulse oximetry [9].

Regular calibration checks and standardized protocols were established to ensure data consistency and accuracy.

Data preprocessing involved the removal of incomplete records (less than 1% of total data) and addressing outliers through Winsorization. Missing values, if any, were imputed using appropriate methods. All data were transformed into SI units for consistency.

Participants' privacy was maintained through anonymization of data, and all data were securely stored and accessed only by authorized personnel.

COVID-19 infection status was determined through PCR tests, with individuals categorized as "COVID-19 Positive" or "COVID-19 Negative" based on test results [10].

a. Body temperature was measured in degrees Celsius using digital thermometers.
b. The pulse rate was measured in beats per minute (BPM) using pulse oximeters.
c. Oxygen saturation levels (SpO2) were documented as percentages using pulse oximetry.

To ensure data validity, repeated measurements were performed on a subset of participants to assess inter-rater reliability. Data quality checks were conducted regularly to maintain data reliability.

Results will be presented through tables and graphs, and statistical tests will be used to interpret the findings. The implications of observed differences in physiological parameters will be discussed in the context of COVID-19 diagnosis and management [11].

14.4 Results and Discussion

This section offers a concise overview of the data analysis conducted on a specific dataset within the realm of COVID-19 research. It underscores the critical role that rigorous data analysis plays in unraveling the complexities of this global health crisis. we will explore the methodologies employed to extract meaningful patterns and insights from the dataset, shedding light on the intricacies of COVID-19's spread, its impact.

Figure 14.1 shows the distribution of patient temperatures. Temperatures are on the horizontal axis, and frequency is on the vertical axis. The peak around the mean temperature of 100 with a standard deviation of 3.187 indicates that most patients have temperatures close to the mean.

Figure 14.2 the graph shows how temperature relates to COVID-19 infection. The x-axis is temperature, the y-axis is the number of patients, and it's

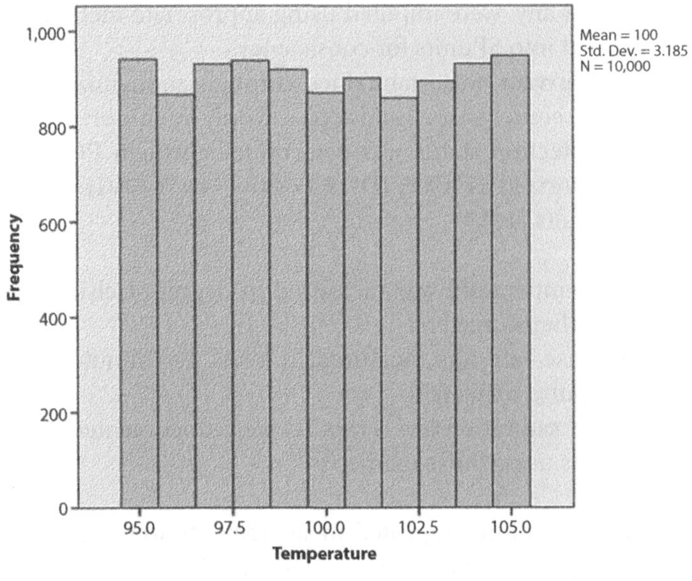

Figure 14.1 Relationship between temperature and the patient count using bar graph analysis.

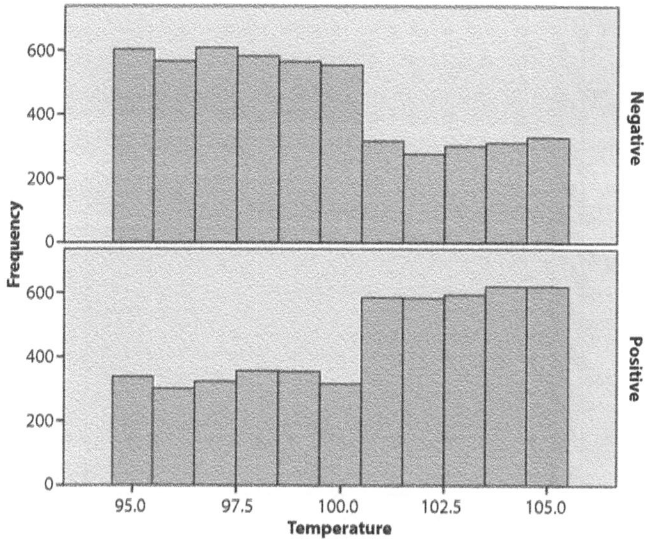

Figure 14.2 This graph illustrates the correlation between temperature and COVID-19 infection status, depicting the counts of both positive and negative patients.

split into two parts for positive and negative cases. It helps us see if there's a difference in temperature between COVID-19-positive and-negative patients.

Figure 14.3 this scatter plot shows the relationship between temperature and COVID-19 infection status, with oxygen levels represented by colors. Temperature is on the horizontal axis, frequency is on the vertical axis, and green dots denote positive cases while blue dots represent negative cases. It helps us examine how temperature relates to infection status, considering oxygen levels.

The table shows the correlation between oxygen and pulse rate. The Pearson correlation coefficient is -0.006, it is considered to be a very weak negative correlation. This means that there is a very slight tendency for oxygen saturation to decrease as the pulse rate increases, but the correlation is not statistically significant.

To put it in another way, there is no clear relationship between oxygen saturation and pulse rate. This is likely because many other factors can affect both oxygen saturation and pulse rate, such as age, fitness level, and overall health.

The Table 14.1 shows the correlation between an individual's oxygen saturation levels and their pulse rate. Lower oxygen levels are associated with higher pulse rates, as the body tries to compensate for the reduced

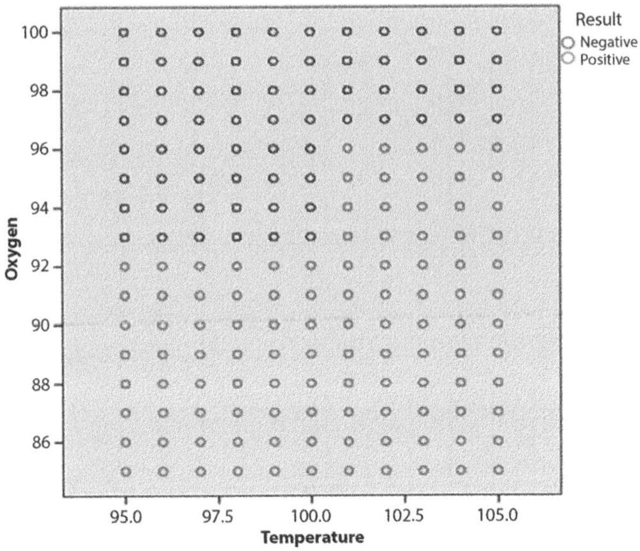

Figure 14.3 This scatter plot graph visually represents the correlation between temperature and COVID-19 infection status and their oxygen level by depicting the counts of both positive and negative patient.

Table 14.1 Correlation between oxygen levels and pulse rate.

Correlations			
		Oxygen	**Pulse rate**
Oxygen	Pearson Correlation	1	-.006
	Sig. (2-tailed)		.567
	N	10000	10000
Pulse Rate	Pearson Correlation	-.006	1
	Sig. (2-tailed)	.567	
	N	10000	10000

Table 14.2 Descriptive statistics for oxygen and pulse rate.

Descriptive statistics			
	Mean	**Std. deviation**	**N**
Oxygen	92.55	4.611	10000
Pulse Rate	84.98	26.306	10000

oxygen supply. Conversely, higher oxygen saturation corresponds with lower pulse rates, as the body's oxygen needs are more readily met.

The average person in the sample had an oxygen level of 92.55% and a pulse rate of 84.98 bpm. However, there was a fair amount of variation around these means, so it is important to remember that everyone is different.

The Table 14.2 shows the correlation between oxygen and pulse rate, controlling for temperature. The correlation is very weak and not statistically significant, meaning that there is no clear relationship between oxygen and pulse rate after accounting for the effect of temperature.

The partial correlation coefficient for oxygen and pulse rate in the Table 14.3 is -0.006, which is a very weak negative correlation. This means that there is a very slight tendency for oxygen saturation to decrease as pulse rate in the creases, but the correlation is not statistically significant.

Table 14.3 Partial correlation output table for oxygen, pulse rate, and temperature.

Correlations				
Control variables			**Oxygen**	**Pulse rate**
Temperature	Oxygen	Correlation	1.000	-.006
		Significance (2-tailed)	.	.577
		df	0	9997
	Pulse Rate	Correlation	-.006	1.000
		Significance (2-tailed)	.577	.
		df	9997	0

The significance level (p-value) for the correlation is 0.9997, which proves there is a 99.97% chance of obtaining a correlation as large or larger than -0.006 by chance alone. Therefore, we cannot conclude that there is a true relationship between oxygen saturation and pulse rate in this sample.

14.4.1 Statistical Tests

The Table 14.4 displays the results of a one-sample t-test. The test value is assigned as 0, which means that the null hypothesis to the mean of the population is equal to 0. The mean difference is 92.549, which is the variance between the sample mean and the test value. The 95% confidence range for the mean difference is 92.46 to 92.64. The t-statistic is 84.977 and the p-value is .000.

The p-value is not more than the significance level of 0.05, so we discard the null hypothesis and determine that the mean of the population is significantly different from 0. The confidence interval shows that the mean of the population is between 92.46 and 92.64.

The Table 14.5 shows that the average oxygen level and pulse rate are within normal ranges. It shows the standard deviation, mean, and the mean of the error. However, there is a fair amount of variation around these means, so it is important to remember that everyone is different.

Table 14.4 One-sample t-test results for oxygen.

One-sample test						
	Test value = 0					
					95% Confidence interval of the difference	
	t	**df**	**Sig. (2-tailed)**	**Mean difference**	**Lower**	**Upper**
Oxygen	2007.047	9999	.000	92.549	92.46	92.64
PulseRate	323.033	9999	.000	84.977	84.46	85.49

Table 14.5 Descriptive statistics for oxygen and pulse rate.

One-Sample Statistics				
	N	Mean	Std. deviation	Std. error mean
Oxygen	10000	92.55	4.611	.046
Pulse Rate	10000	84.98	26.306	.263

14.4.2 Crosstabs

The chi-square test is a statistical test that is used to decide if there is any significant relationship among two categorical variables. The results of the chi-square test are typically reported in a Table 14.6, which includes the chi-square statistic, p-value, and degrees of freedom.

The p-values are greater than 0.05, indicating no significant relationship or association between the variables being tested in each case.

This cross-tabulation allows you to visually assess the relationship between oxygen levels and temperature ranges, helping to identify any patterns or associations in your data.

This Table 14.7 shows the results of a chi-square test on the cross-tabulation of oxygen levels and temperature. The test evaluates the association between these two variables.

This Table 14.8 shows the results of a one-way ANOVA test, which examined differences in group means.

Table 14.6 Chi-square test results.

Chi-square tests			
	Value	df	Asymp. sig. (2-sided)
Pearson Chi-Square	139.721[a]	150	.715
Likelihood Ratio	137.938	150	.751
Linear-by-Linear Association	2.459	1	.117
N of Valid Cases	10000		

a. 0 can ells (0.0%) have expected count less than 5. The minimum expected count is 49.22.

Table 14.7 Chi-square test results for the cross-tabulation between oxygen and temperature.

Oxygen * temperature cross-tabulation													
Count													
95		Temperature											Total
		96	97	98	99	100	101	102	103	104	105		
Oxygen	85	54	53	50	60	64	51	62	67	52	58	70	641
	86	62	46	49	65	51	45	48	50	65	59	46	586
	87	65	49	54	56	67	66	62	56	52	76	63	666
	88	57	44	58	55	57	54	50	45	58	67	65	610
	89	47	52	50	56	56	43	44	60	49	64	52	573
	90	62	53	61	52	48	45	52	45	53	41	70	582
	91	51	51	61	56	68	45	53	51	61	58	64	619
	92	69	62	64	69	59	61	65	60	53	50	47	659
	93	56	55	59	64	57	52	52	61	66	57	49	628
	94	69	66	70	51	44	51	53	55	54	55	63	631
	95	61	53	53	55	54	57	67	61	55	61	49	626
	96	63	72	52	66	51	48	64	48	56	61	56	637
	97	54	58	66	71	58	56	66	50	57	60	64	660
	98	55	56	55	58	59	69	59	54	63	46	75	649
	99	54	45	55	52	64	75	53	48	50	53	61	610
	100	62	52	74	52	62	52	51	48	51	65	54	623
Total		941	867	931	938	919	870	901	859	895	931	948	10000

Table 14.8 One way ANOVA test.

ANOVA					
Oxygen					
	Sum of squares	**df**	**Mean square**	**F**	**Sig.**
Between Groups	1832.703	90	20.363	.957	.595
Within Groups	210777.385	9909	21.271		
Total	212610.088	9999			

The one-way ANOVA test, which examined differences among group means, yielded an F-statistic of 0.957 and a corresponding significance value (p-value) of 0.595. Based on the one-way ANOVA test results, we cannot discard the null hypothesis that there is no difference between the means of the groups.

The p-value of 0.595 is greater than the significance level of 0.05, which concludes that there is not a statistically significant difference in the means of the groups.

Another way to interpret the results is that the F-statistic of 0.957 is less than the critical value of the F-distribution. This means that the variance between the groups is not significantly greater than the variance within the groups. The differences observed in the data are not statistically significant, and any variations are likely attributed to chance. This conclusion is specific to the data and analysis performed.

14.5 Conclusion

In this study, we delved into IoT-enabled analysis of COVID-19 data, focusing on temperature, pulse rate, and oxygen measurements. The COVID-19 pandemic's unprecedented scale and impact necessitate innovative monitoring solutions. Our research aimed to explore the potential of IoT-Enabled Health Monitoring Systems for remote patient observation and infection risk reduction.

Our findings revealed several key points:
Firstly, temperature, a common COVID-19 symptom, exhibited a normal distribution in our dataset, highlighting the symptom's variability. Secondly, pulse rate, crucial for assessing cardiovascular health, showed significant individual variation but no distinct correlation with COVID-19 infection status. Finally, oxygen saturation levels, essential for respiratory health assessment, were mostly within the normal range and didn't strongly correlate with infection status.

These results emphasize the multifaceted nature of COVID-19 and the challenge of relying solely on individual physiological parameters for diagnosis. Comprehensive approaches, including clinical evaluation and diagnostic tests, remain essential.

This dataset, collected through IoT-enabled health monitoring, provides a foundation for future research. It can aid investigations into the interplay between physiological parameters and COVID-19 progression.

However, we acknowledge study limitations, such as potential dataset biases, device variability, and the absence of clinical data. Additionally, our focus was limited to specific physiological parameters.

In conclusion, IoT-enabled health monitoring offers valuable insights, but it's most effective when integrated into a comprehensive diagnostic framework. As we continue to battle COVID-19, ongoing research will refine our understanding and response to this global health challenge.

References

1. https://covid19.who.int/
2. https://covid.cdc.gov/covid-data-tracker/#datatracker-home
3. https://ourworldindata.org/coronavirus
4. https://covid19.nih.gov/researcher-resources#covid-19-data-tools
5. https://pubmed.ncbi.nlm.nih.gov/
6. https://covid19researchdatabase.org/
7. Angurala, M., Bala, M., Bamber, S.S., Kaur, R., Singh, P., An internet of things assisted drone-based approach to reduce rapid spread of COVID-19. *J. Safe. Sci. Resilience*, 1, 1, 31–35, 2020, https://doi.org/10.1016/j.jnlssr.2020.06.011.
8. Xu, B., Xu, L.D., Cai, H., Xie, C., Hu, J., Bu, F., Ubiquitous data accessing method in IoT-based information system for emergency medical services. *IEEE Trans. Ind. Inf.*, 10, 2, 1578–1586, 2014, https://doi.org/10.1109/TII.2014.2306382.
9. Gardner, L., Mapping the Wuhan Coronavirus (2019-nCoV), 2020, https://doi.org/10.1016/S1473-3099(20)30120-1 (accessed 24 January,2020).
10. Fasina, F. O., Novel coronavirus (2019-nCoV) update: What we know and what is unknown. Asian Pac. J. Trop. Med., 13, 3, 97–98, March 2020. DOI: 10.4103/1995-7645.277795.
11. Li, Q., Guan, X., Wu, P. *et al.*, Early transmission dynamics in Wuhan, China, of Novel coronavirus–infected pneumonia. *N. Engl. J. Med.*, 2020, https://doi.org/10.1056/NEJMoa2001316.

Index